PERSONAL THERAPY
for SCHIZOPHRENIA
and RELATED DISORDERS

PERSONAL THERAPY
FOR
SCHIZOPHRENIA
AND
RELATED DISORDERS

A Guide to Individualized Treatment

Gerard E. Hogarty

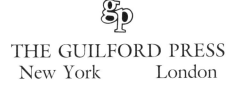

THE GUILFORD PRESS
New York   London

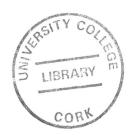

© 2002 The Guilford Press
A Division of Guilford Publications, Inc.
72 Spring Street, New York, NY 10012
www.guilford.com

Printed in the United States of America

This book is printed on acid-free paper.

Last digit is print number: 9 8 7 6 5 4 3 2 1

Library of Congress Cataloging-in-Publication Data

Hogarty, Gerard E.
    Personal therapy for schizophrenia and related disorders : a guide to individualized treatment / Gerard E. Hogarty.
        p. cm.
    Includes bibliographical references and index.
    ISBN 1-57230-782-X (alk. paper)
    1. Schizophrenia.   I. Title.
RC514 .H584 2002
616.89′8206—dc21

                                                                        2002006579

To my wife, Susan, whose support and gentle insistence about the value of personal therapy resulted in this offering to those who live and work with schizophrenia

About the Author

Gerard E. Hogarty, MSW, is Professor of Psychiatry in the Western Psychiatric Institute and Clinic at the University of Pittsburgh Medical Center. He received both his undergraduate and graduate degrees from the Catholic University of America in Washington, D.C. Early in his career, he served as clinician and research social worker on the initial National Institute of Mental Health (NIMH) Collaborative Study of antipsychotic drugs.

Following an appointment at NIMH, Professor Hogarty became Chief of Social Science Research at the Friends Medical Science Research Center in Baltimore, where he conducted the first posthospital, controlled maintenance studies of drug and psychosocial interventions with schizophrenia patients. Since coming to Pittsburgh, he and his colleagues have continued to develop and test integrated medication and psychosocial approaches. Among these have been tests of the minimum effective antipsychotic dose appropriate to acute and maintenance treatment, studies addressing the nature and pharmacological treatment of impaired affect in recovering schizophrenia, as well as the development and testing of the now popular family psychoeducation approach. His current research program centers on the study of disorder-relevant, individual psychosocial treatments for schizophrenia, including a novel cognitive rehabilitation approach. These initiatives have received over 30 years of NIMH support.

Professor Hogarty has authored numerous articles, book chapters, and books, and has lectured extensively throughout the United States,

Canada, and Europe. He is an elected member of the American College of Neuropsychopharmacology, a fellow of the Association for Clinical Psychosocial Research, and has served as advisor or consultant to numerous agencies. He was the recipient of the Stanley R. Dean Award from the American College of Psychiatrists, as well as an NIMH MERIT award. He was also designated the Hall–Mercer Scholar by the Pennsylvania Hospital, and received the Armin Loeb Research Award from the International Association of Psychosocial Rehabilitation Services, the Arthur P. Noyes Award from the State of Pennsylvania and its Departments of Psychiatry, as well as an Outstanding Research Award for the study of personal therapy from the Society for Social Work and Research. Most recently, he received the Paul Hoch Award for lifetime achievements from the American Psychopathological Association.

Preface

Throughout history, including the modern era of clinical psychopharma-cology, the mainstay of treatment for schizophrenia disorders has relied on talking with patients—to offer them psychological and material sup-port and to facilitate greater awareness, adaptive skills, and, above all, hope. However, with the exception of time-limited, problem-focused skills training, cognitive-behavioral interventions, and family psychoedu-cational approaches, attempts to document the efficacy of a *formal* psycho-therapy for treating schizophrenia have been largely unsuccessful, as the brief review offered elsewhere in this volume will illustrate. This is true whether the psychotherapy in question is supportive, insight-oriented, or interpersonal in nature. Despite the absence of clear efficacy, psychothera-py has, however, remained the primary form of nonsomatic treatment for schizophrenia throughout much of the past century (Fenton, 2000). For-tunately, the Personal Therapy (PT) approach—a well-tested, disorder-relevant psychotherapy that integrates many of the most efficacious practice principles available—has now been developed. This volume was written as an introduction to the rationale, process, and content of PT for those who seek a more cost-effective treatment approach for patients with schizophrenia. I mention cost because *avoidable* hospitalizations represent the principal financial expenditure for schizophrenia and related disorders, more so when coupled with the price of what is often an unnecessary so-cial and vocational incapacity.

PT was developed as a graduated program of biopsychosocial practice principles that were designed to facilitate the typically slow process of clinical stabilization and community reintegration that follows an episode of psychosis. Those who live and work with schizophrenia know that recovery is most often measured in years, rather than weeks or months. There is no "quick fix" for schizophrenia. Multidimensional impairments, disabilities, and social handicaps that evolved over many years in a patient's life require a longitudinal, multidimensional response. PT selects the better established psychotherapeutic components and uniquely incorporates them in a way that accommodates both the phase of illness and the needs of the individual outpatient. This approach has stood both the test of rigorous scientific scrutiny among challenging samples of patients, as well as the critical review of experts. The effects of PT and medication on the adjustment of patients with schizophrenia, for example, far exceed the effects of what could be considered state-of-the-art routine care. These encouraging results apply to younger patients who continue to reside with their families as well as older, more persistently ill patients who go it alone.

While I intended this book to serve the dual purposes of textbook and treatment manual, I have approached the writing as if I were having a personal conversation with you, the reader. The results of several decades of systematic research, including the process and content of PT, are shared and interspersed with my personal value system and clinical opinions. If at times I tend to emphasize research considerations (including an Appendix that describes the statistical procedures commonly used in clinical trials), it is because I remain strongly committed to the belief that the more completely informed clinician is the best resource that a patient can have.

PT principles are offered as practical suggestions for a wide range of problems that conspire against stabilization, relapse prevention, and social recovery. Whether it be patient education or the application of specific coping strategies, the techniques of PT should foster a greater understanding, control, and mastery of the devastating effects of schizophrenia. While a cure is clearly unrealistic in the absence of the known causes of this severe mental illness, opportunities for a less symptomatic and more satisfying life have been shown to be within reach for most PT recipients. Obviously, no clinical practice guide can presume to address the unique needs of each patient. Research findings apply to groups of patients and cannot always be validly attributed to a specific individual. If the practice principles described in this volume appear contraindicated for an individual patient or extend beyond the training, experience, and personal comfort of the clinician, clearly one's clinical judgment should be used, and the counsel of a more knowledgeable professional, or a more appropriate referral, should be sought. This said, however, a majority of patients truly value the individual psychotherapy they receive, and PT is a way to assure that their psychotherapy remains goal directed, meaningful, and as effective as possible.

In an era of managed care, cost containment, and staff demoralization, I sincerely hope that this book will become a source of confidence, assistance, satisfaction, and renewal for patients with schizophrenia and those who serve them.

GERARD E. HOGARTY

Acknowledgments

Personal therapy (PT) was developed and tested by the *Environmental–Personal Indicators in the Course of Schizophrenia* (EPICS) Research Group. The work was generously supported by a MERIT extension of Grant No. MH-30750 from the National Institute of Mental Health to the author. Clinician orientation to PT was guided initially by a preliminary manual that represented the contributions of many individuals, principally Douglas J. Reiss, PhD, Deborah P. Greenwald, PhD, Sander J. Kornblith, PhD, and the author. Once PT was implemented, the content evolved in the manner described in this text.

I thank the following individuals for their various contributions to this volume:

Sander J. Kornblith, PhD, provided advice and commentary on the components of each PT phase described in Chapters 4, 5, and 6, particularly the discussions of internal coping in these three chapters as well as the descriptions of conflict resolution and criticism management (Chapter 6).

Samuel Flesher, PhD, offered extensive commentary and guidance related to Social Security benefits (Chapter 3), adjustment to disability (Chapter 5), and social and vocational issues (Chapter 6).

Deborah P. Greenwald, PhD, contributed advice and commentary on basic social skills training (Chapter 4), intermediate skills training and deep breathing (Chapter 5), and progressive relaxation (Chapter 6).

Richard F. Ulrich, MS, provided data analyses for Chapter 2 and commentary on the statistical procedures that are described in Appendix A.

Hari Parepally, MD, offered critical commentary and suggestions regarding medication management that are elaborated in Chapters 3, 4, and 5.

Susan Cooley, MNEd, contributed reference materials related to the format of psychoeducation (Chapters 4 and 5), the relaxation response (Chapter 5), and guided imagery (Chapter 6).

Ann Louise DiBarry, MSN, provided critical commentary on the content and process of PT, and Mary Carter, PhD, assisted in accessing the extensive bibliography used to support PT and its rationale.

Finally, the extraordinary typing and retyping of the manuscript, the format of the chapters and appendices, table construction, and graphics represent the dedicated and generous effort of Michele Bauer. I also thank former members of the research team: George Alexander, MD, Patricia Bartone, MSN, Ann Garrett, PhD, Kathleen Hammil, MSN, Harry Levin, MD (deceased), Douglas Reiss, PhD, and Elizabeth Venditti, PhD, for their assistance and skill in conducting the studies of PT. I am especially grateful for the sustaining support of David Kupfer, MD, Chair of the Department of Psychiatry at the University of Pittsburgh Medical Center.

In gratitude, I will donate a portion of the proceeds from this book to support the patient activities of the Western Psychiatric Institute and Clinic's schizophrenia outpatient program.

Contents

CHAPTER ONE

Introduction, Background, and Rationale

INTRODUCTION

The status of psychotherapy among contemporary treatments for schizo-phrenia has been succinctly captured by McGlashan (1994, p. 147): "What has become of the psychotherapy of schizophrenia can be sum-marized briefly in two sentences. The bad news is that it is currently en-dangered, at least in America, by stigma and acute fiscal concerns. The good news is that psychotherapy has been evolving and continues to evolve in a healthy manner as we understand schizophrenia better." Per-sonal therapy (PT) is the most recent product of this evolution. It is an empirically tested approach that has been found to be effective for the clinical stabilization and psychosocial recovery of persons who suffer schizophrenia and schizoaffective disorders. The evidence regarding the efficacy of PT extends to the broadest areas of interpersonal relationships and instrumental role performance (Hogarty, Greenwald, et al., 1997). PT was designed as an *integrated* composite of various techniques that could be strategically tailored to individual patient needs and preferences according to clinical state, strengths and deficits. While conceptualized in light of the cognitive and affective features of schizophrenia, there are no principles of PT practice, to the present author's knowledge, that would intrinsically appear to be contraindicated in the management and care of

1

other functional psychotic conditions, although requisite evaluations among nonschizophrenia samples have not been made to date.

The primary objective of PT is to achieve and maintain clinical stability. It does so using appropriate pharmacotherapy and the acquisition of adaptive strategies sufficient for the management of stressful relationships and life events that might provoke the prodromes of psychosis. Through the provision of individually tailored coping skills, the secondary goals of interpersonal, social, and vocational adjustment are sought. PT is intended for the clear majority of schizophrenia patients who, by history or clinical state, appear to be at continuing risk for psychotic decompensation and/or continuing poor adjustment, including first-episode patients. PT was designed to be applied in three distinct phases that accommodate the stages of clinical recovery and reintegration that follow a psychotic episode, a concession made to the well-known vulnerability of schizophrenia patients to environmental overload, whether therapeutic or otherwise. When "investigative" psychotherapeutic tasks are reserved to the relatively few eligible patients, PT is congruent with contemporary recommendations for a phase-relevant, "flexible individual psychotherapy" of schizophrenia (Fenton, 2000). PT is a treatment that acknowledges the *biology* of a brain disorder, the *psychology* of the person so affected, and the *sociology* of the environment that influences the course of the disorder, whether positively or negatively.

This volume is offered as a working manual for the provision of PT. As shall be emphasized throughout, it is not intended to be a "cookbook" of rigid practice strategies that are narrowly focused on a specific problem. Rather, the manual attempts to provide a variety of clinical approaches to the multiple problems that characterize the individual patient as he or she struggles to achieve and maintain postepisode stabilization. When a patient appears not to profit from a specific technique, rather than continuing to provide the same ineffective approach, PT offers a range of options within and across the treatment phases that can counter this all-too-common therapeutic stalemate. While services for the severely mentally ill are increasingly provided in team approaches, even within these systems most patients are motivated to seek an alliance with an individual clinician. PT provides a way to use this crucial collaboration in a goal-directed and efficacious manner.

Following the formation of a treatment contract and the establishment of a working therapeutic alliance, PT unfolds as a graduated series of strategies designed to achieve and maintain clinical stabilization and functioning. These principles of practice are prescribed in distinct phases that broadly reflect the patient's current level of clinical stability. Most often, candidates for PT will find themselves recovering from a recent episode of schizophrenia for which basic-phase techniques are most appropriate. Later, as symptoms remit and the need to maintain stability achieves paramount importance, the PT techniques of the intermediate phase rise to prominence. Later, as the energy for resuming a fuller social and vocational life returns, advanced-phase strategies should help ensure a safe and rewarding reintegration into the community. By design, there is an intentional redundancy to the PT techniques across the three treatment phases, with only the depth, scope, and skill level of a specific strategy changing as the patient achieves greater symptom stabilization.

These recurrent themes first include *psychoeducation* that increases in content from contemporary information about schizophrenia and its treatment in the basic phase to an intermediate-phase understanding of personal vulnerability, including problems in adjustment to residual disability, and its effect on the ebb and flow of symptoms. Later, an individualized tailoring of this knowledge to the demands of community reentry occurs in the advanced phase. A similar progression characterizes the *assumption of responsibilities* across phases, from self-care to the resumption of personally valued social and vocational roles. *Internal coping* is the centerpiece of PT that begins in the basic phase with a personal definition of stress and its relationship to major prodromal signs of relapse. The concurrent application of individually generated "autoprotective" or survival strategies and the tried-and-true skills-training techniques of role restructuring, conflict avoidance, and positive assertion are introduced as strategies to counteract stress. In the intermediate phase, internal coping proceeds to a better appreciation of the "march of symptoms" that begins with the earliest cues of subject distress and might end with the manifestation of minor or major symptoms. Coping strategies designed to abort this process increase in sophistication and include deep breathing, simple relaxation, and the interpersonal skills embodied in social perception training (learning to take the emotional temperature of other key persons in the patient's life). In the advanced phase, internal coping reaches the apex of skills development through a highly individualized selection of perceived cues of distress and their associated adaptive strategies. In addition to the techniques of progressive relaxation and guided imagery, adaptation addresses the reality of behavioral reciprocity, a "reflective consideration" of how one's newly acquired coping skills might impact, both positively and negatively, on the behavior of others. Conflict resolution and criticism management become key coping techniques designed to facilitate the resumption of social and vocational roles. An *in vivo* consideration of historical sources of interpersonal and vocational stress, past coping successes and failures, and the integration of newly acquired knowledge and skills complete the sequence of PT practice principles. This manual attempts to illustrate how these recurrent themes can be blended *within* and *across* phases in a seamless set of exercises. The incremental development of an individual repertoire of interpersonal and role performance skills will hopefully serve to keep the patient free of disabling symptoms and able to enjoy a satisfying quality of life.

The preceding remarks aside, it is necessary to say that PT is not a panacea. A minority of study patients managed to achieve outcomes with PT that were as likely to be attained with medication and a less intensive supportive therapy. (I attempt to identify these patients in Chapter 2.) Further, a number of PT recipients who lived independent of family fared less well than control subjects regarding the prevention of psychotic relapse in the first year following hospital discharge, although we are now able to make recommendations that should dramatically decrease early relapse for these highly vulnerable patients. (However, the *adjustment* of these patients did improve significantly with PT.) Also, many patients found progress through all three phases of PT difficult to achieve in a reasonable period of time. For example, only 54% of patients in our studies achieved the advanced phase of PT skills acquisition during the 3-year treatment trials. On the other hand, nearly all patients successfully mastered the basic-phase skills that might characterize the practice of better ambulatory programs, and 93% were able to progress through the intermediate level of skills and adaptive strategy training that is rarely made available to schizophrenia patients. PT continues a century-old process of "aftercare" following a psychotic episode and/or hospitalization and is best viewed as a recent step in the evolution of interventions that have been addressed to achieving stabilization, forestalling relapse and restoring functional capacity in the areas of personal and social adjustment. When compared to patients who received a comprehensive supportive therapy and/or a family psychoeducation management approach, life was distinctly better for the group of PT recipients. But the course of schizophrenia had neither been reversed nor entirely addressed regarding the factors that limit *optimal* remission and recovery. While some might argue that the glass is mostly empty, 26% of PT recipients were able to *exceed* their best premorbid levels of major role adjustment, a goal that to date has typically eluded most treatment efforts made in behalf of schizophrenia patients.

Reasons for Developing PT

Given these caveats, why would a group of experienced and dedicated research clinicians have each spent 9 years of their collective lives, let alone institutional resources and a considerable quantity of taxpayer dollars, developing and testing a form of care that held expectations for only modestly advancing outcomes beyond those possible with existing interventions? The reasons were many and included the incomplete testing of formal psychotherapies in past studies, an issue that called for a redress since many otherwise skillful clinicians had persisted in a belief in various forms of psychotherapy in spite of negative findings. Individual psychotherapy had been and continues to be the most common nonsomatic treatment for schizophrenia despite the absence of supporting evidence. Fenton (2000), in an overview of the field through the mid-1990s, surmised, "With virtually no data to support its efficacy, individual psychotherapy had been the cornerstone of treatment for schizophrenia for decades" (p. 47). Compared to the countless pharmacotherapy studies, the dearth of well-controlled psychotherapeutic trials in schizophrenia has been something of a tragedy.

Other reasons extended to an apparent decay of psychosocial treatment effects over time, primarily when treatment was terminated, as well as the relative absence of evidence that the addition of a psychosocial treatment to medication did anything for patient *adjustment* beyond the gains achieved by forestalling relapse (see Hogarty, Greenwald, et al., 1997, for a review). Important effects were indeed associated with existing psychosocial approaches, but the benefits were clearly circumscribed (Lehman, Carpenter, Goldman, & Steinwachs, 1995). Insurers were also increasingly reluctant to underwrite the costs of psychotherapy, alleging there was no evidence that it influenced the core neurobiological processes of schizophrenia—or that it even "worked." Otherwise, psychosocial treatments had not exceeded 2 years of controlled study, thereby limiting inferences of efficacy to the intermittent crises that often characterized the early stages of recovery from an episode. "Time-limited" programs might provide for some greater stabilization of symptoms or the acquisition of a coping strategy or two, but the cognitive mastery needed to understand and manage one's illness was clearly beyond the scope of brief treatment approaches, as we hope to demonstrate in this volume.

More than anything, comprehensive service systems were bending under the yoke of cost containment, as well as the managed behavioral health care constraints on the quality and number of therapeutic contacts.

In fact, the cost of maintaining seriously ill Medicare beneficiaries has led many for-profit health maintenance organizations (HMOs) to abandon this patient population as government programs reduced their reimbursements for care. While it was hoped that a reduction in state hospital reimbursements and lengths of stay would translate into more dollars for ambulatory care, unfortunately outpatient reimbursements have appeared to decline as well (Leslie & Rosenheck, 1999; Huskamp, 1998). Clinicians in turn have been pressured to achieve better outcomes for more patients with fewer therapeutic and material resources. Thus, an easily acquired yet effective intervention that would be less dependent on external resources seemed to be a goal worthy of pursuit. The "downsizing" of staff and resources also appeared to coincide with the increasing rationalization that optimal functioning would be within the easy reach of one or another of the new antipsychotic medications that might be sufficient for recovery when prescribed with support and encouragement, that is, the "warm medication" approach. The seductive promise of eminent discovery that would reveal the defective gene(s), the covert lesion, the disrupted neural circuit, or the offending toxin(s) might also have served to encourage a fiscally conservative, minimally responsive and micromanaged behavioral health delivery system to adopt the false assurance that the limited but "cost-effective" services being provided for schizophrenia patients were sufficient. The remediation of residual dysfunctioning might simply be another discovery away (see Gabbard, 1992, for a discussion of psychotherapy in the era of modern neurobiology). Unfortunately, as patients, families and their providers well know, this promise has remained an exercise in wishful thinking.

In recent decades, an ominous reorganization of services also began to emerge. With diminishing resources, the closing of public psychiatric inpatient units and increasingly large outpatient caseloads, the ultimate management of the patient with schizophrenia has been devolving to a very brief "one-*on*-one" therapeutic encounter, or worse yet to assembly hall therapeutics where patients would "one *by* one" petition the dais for their minute or two of counsel and prescription (Young, Sullivan, Burnam, & Brock, 1998). The first surveys designed to assess concordance with empirically established treatment recommendations have revealed chasmic differences between what is possible and the reality of schizophrenia undertreatment (see Lehman & Steinwachs, 1998; Dixon et al., 1999; Young et al., 1998). To complicate matters even more, psychosocial treatment responsibilities seem to have been increasingly placed on the already burdened shoulders of case managers or mental health "technicians," many of whom appeared to have little knowledge, let alone formal training, regarding the nature and treatment of severe mental disorders. As a thinly disguised attempt at cost reduction, patients and families themselves have been actively recruited to the "self-help" enterprise. Meanwhile, those with better credentials and experience have continued their practice of psychotherapy following the tenets of one or more of the hundreds of "therapies" available, few of which have been empirically tested, and even fewer have been designed with the schizophrenia patient in mind. As public reimbursement systems increasingly tend toward the severely mentally ill, many private practitioners have felt the need to incorporate a disorder-relevant and well-tested intervention into their practice.

Thus, it seemed that while the world awaited the new technologies of rehabilitation (that are in development) or the latest neuroimage or compound from the laboratory, it might well have been a service to those who continued to struggle with schizophrenia in the face of diminishing resources for us to select, integrate, develop, and test practice principles that had either shown efficacy in prior research, claimed the strong allegiance of experienced clinicians, or seemed theoretically compelling. It was in this scientific and political environment that PT was conceived in 1985 and brought to its development, testing, and ultimate publication by late 1997. As long as a provider had some time to spend with a schizophrenia patient, why not use it in a more empirically supported, efficacious, disorder-relevant, and humane way? Seemingly less costly psychosocial alternatives (e.g., support or activities therapy) could be far more expensive in the long run if shown to be ineffective or minimally effective compared to an individual psychosocial treatment that had demonstrated clear efficacy in a scientifically valid study (see Liberman et al., 1998, for a relevant example). Money and resources are not always the problem in managed care; rather, an administrative incentive for clinicians to provide treatments of demonstrated efficacy could contribute to achieving optimal outcomes in a cost-managed system.

Finally, it seemed worthwhile to provide a volume that could serve both as a basis for therapeutic optimism as well as a rejoinder to the explicit (or more often covert) *therapeutic nihilism* that often influences the judgment of mental health providers, insurers, health policy planners, politicians, and even some scientists when it comes to supporting treatment initiatives for schizophrenia patients.

The Knowledge Base of PT

Having defined a need was one thing; finding the rationale and strategies for implementing an appropriate therapeutic response proved to be something else. Where does one turn in the search for valid and promising psychosocial techniques that might nip a pending psychotic episode in the bud or independently enhance functioning? The choices seemed narrowly drawn to four sources of potential insight: the clinical experience at our program, the experiences of patients themselves, the "practice wisdom" of other clinicians, and the empirically tested principles derived from controlled clinical trials. We feel that it is important for the reader to know the value system that influenced our search for a credible knowledge base to PT, prior to a discussion of its rationale, content, and process. While each source of potential insight had its own inherent benefits and constraints, our decision to rely more heavily (but not exclusively) on empiricism will come as no surprise to those who have followed the work of our research group. Our theoretical emphasis and clinical content have not only reflected personal values but have extended to a concern that the very survival of psychosocial forms of healing in a cost-managed environment will likely depend on empiricism. In recent years, the leadership of many professional groups has gratefully begun to appreciate that the future of their organizations will likely turn on the adoption of evidenced-based practice.

We do acknowledge that the insight born of patient experience represented something of a paradox, since PT's response to the affect dysregulation that appeared to precede schizophrenia relapse was a primary strategy. A considerable literature had addressed the personal or "subjective" experiences of schizophrenia patients, one that appeared particularly relevant to our basic objectives and one that we have tried to responsibly accommodate. Included in this legacy were the historical accounts provided by individual patients, theoretical speculation on the origin and meaning of symptoms and experience as well as associated adaptive techniques, and recommended clinical procedures that followed upon these observations. In many ways, however, this excess of clinical wisdom also represented a deterrent to systematic treatment development. Whose insights, for example, were to be preferred? Those that made the most clinical sense? Those whose proponents enjoyed a greater reputation among peers? Or those that most closely reflected the experience and training associated with our own respective disciplines? The task was made greater when one considered potential insights from such diverse fields as cultural anthropology, sociology, philosophy, theology, and developmental psychology. We concluded that whatever the limitations of empiricism might be, not to be ignored was the protection from "information overload" that was offered by well-reasoned, appropriately designed, and carefully executed studies. In spite of strong feelings that are often held by individual clinicians, empiricism need not be devoid of humanism. "Guided" principles of practice that result from empirical scrutiny do not ignore the individual; rather, they respond to important needs that are often common to the *majority* of individuals that suffer the disorder. Explicit practice principles can inevitably be adapted to the special or multiple needs of the individual patient, as this volume attempts to show. Whether developmental, behavioral, interpersonal, or educational in nature, each of our own and most other empirically established psychosocial interventions have had their theoretical roots well grounded in the clinical observation and accounts of individual patients.

Where we take exception to the contemporary emphasis on "subjective experience" as the centerpiece for the individual psychotherapy of schizophrenia patients is when phenomenology becomes the explanatory model for the disorder itself. Other models that are supported by extensive and scientifically valid studies of an underlying neurobiological basis seem far more compelling, in our opinion (e.g., see Keshavan & Murray, 1997, or Keshavan & Hogarty, 1999, for relevant reviews). Public and personal commentary regarding our prior efforts have sometimes implied that an acknowledgment of a pervasive pathophysiology in schizophrenia constituted an implicit endorsement of "biological reductionism," ignoring for the most part that the "psycho" and "social" contributions to onset, treatment response, course, and outcome had been given equal weight in the equations of theory building. Close examination of the theoretical premises that have supported our efforts, including PT, would reveal that they are neither deterministic, linear, nor reductionistic in nature. For example, we have tried to avoid the implication of an "inside-out" cascade of effects that begins with impairments in neuroanatomy, extends to those that are neurochemical and neuropsychological in nature, and subsequently results in cognitive deficits, symptom presentation, and dysfunctional behavior. This frequently assumed connection between "neuroscience and phenomenology" seems decidedly incomplete at the moment (Mortimer & McKenna, 1994). Rather, our postulates have attempted to recognize the inevitable synergy and hence interaction between neurocognitive impairment, the individual affective and behavioral adaptations to such, and the *reciprocal* influence of experience, including psychosocial treatment. One's own social-ecological "niche" clearly shapes cognition, affect, and hence individual differences in abilities and behavior (Eisenberg, 1995), but we are ever mindful that problems in neural structure and connectivity, as well as the associated difficulties in hormonal or neurochemical activation and inhibition, often disrupt the lawful processes of stimuli identification, incorporation, synthesis, and expression among schizophrenia patients (Keshavan & Hogarty, 1999). The reader will, we hope, shortly come to appreciate that we have nevertheless relied heavily on the subjective experience of schizophrenia as a point of therapeutic entry not only as the medium for developing a deeper understanding of personal suffering (including the constraints on adjustment, coping strategies, hopes, and aspirations) but also as the linchpin for establishing correct empathy and a positive transference that facilitates the therapeutic alliance. The proper integration of subjective experience and objective assessment of psychotic behavior is both necessary and possible, as clearly described elsewhere (Davidson, Stayner, & Haglund 1998).

We have deliberately sought to avoid the *interpretation* of psychotic content by not endowing such with special meaning; that is, we see no particular value in the symbolic representation of psychotic material as the foundation for therapeutic intervention. We believe that there is an important difference between romanticizing representations of psychotic material (other than accepting the existence of psychosis) and the clinical obligation to serve as a "beacon of reality" for our thought-disordered patients. For those that do see the content of a bizarre delusion or hallucination as holding imperative "clinical meaning," we feel that there is a professional, if not moral, obligation to conduct an experiment on the healing methods that would follow upon this belief. The sensorimotor, perceptual, and cognitive experiences of patients who are often poorly differentiated from the world, poorly organized in terms of self-identity, and poorly integrated into an affective and cognitive life that is congruent with reality are not examples of transpersonal insight. Thought-disordered, paranoid, magical, or even mythical thinking processes do not connote a special "awareness," as many phenomenologists seem prone to believe these days. The goal of psychotherapy for schizophrenia is above all not to provoke the underlying cognitive and affective vulnerabilities (particularly disattention and hyperarousal), but rather with the aid of modern psychopharmacology to reestablish homeoresis and to enhance compensatory adaptive strategies. Insight or greater awareness is most welcomed when and if it evolves, but a prescription for survival without psychosis as well as the acquisition of strategies for achieving common human needs related to personal comfort, social connectedness, and the performance of important instrumental roles seem far more fundamental to attaining a basic quality of life than "insight" per se. Speculations from self psychology might well provide the grist for hypothesis *generating*, but the practice of psychosocial therapy for schizophrenia continues to lack broad implementation and development in part due to the absence of hypothesis *testing*. Modern epistemological relativism that attributes clinical authority to each practitioner's unique experience and interpretive wisdom holds great danger of becoming the cancer of clinical practice when it demeans systematic inquiry regarding the commonalties among cases, confuses the public with anecdotal claims of expertise and efficacy, fosters interdisciplinary warfare, provokes skepticism among insurers and government funding agencies, and ultimately deprives patients of the more demonstrably effective forms of care. We recall the admonition that funding agencies can hardly rally to the cause of psychological treatment while the mental health professions continue to disagree among themselves about the nature, cause, and treatment of mental disorders.

Some Caveats

A few issues should be addressed concerning the style of this volume as well as the delivery of PT, issues that might be a cause of concern among some readers. In an era when books on psychotherapy have greatly outnumbered the valid studies of psychotherapy, there was a desire throughout the writing of this text to avoid its becoming yet another *derivative* statement on psychological treatment. For this reason, the better-known and routinely implemented practice principles such as psychological support, basic skills training, or aspects of relaxation training have been deliberately made concise, given the wide dissemination of these interventions. On the other hand, clinical techniques or areas that are less well known or utilized have been discussed in detail. These include the process for accessing Social Security benefits for patients, facilitating adjustment to disability, providing information on contemporary psychopharmacology, and the essential elements of prodrome identification and management. Even a primer on the basic statistical methods used for understanding clinical trial results is included (in Appendix A), admittedly not offered in the typical psychotherapy text.

Otherwise, the "fillers" found in most clinical volumes (i.e., the dramatized individual case report) will clearly be deemphasized in this text and preference will be given to the more common concerns of patients.

The reasons for a departure from the traditional clinical text are many. First, a truly accurate portrayal of representative cases would need to be lengthy if not boring. When the response of an individual patient has been truly "dramatic," its description runs the risk of compromising anonymity and hence violating confidentiality. In an era of increased concern about the confidentiality of patient records, this possibility needs to be avoided. A more compelling reason has been the desire not to raise *unreasonable* clinical expectations among therapists, patients, or families. The dramatized (or more likely fanciful) case report too often suggests a certain "magic" that is associated with a specific form of communication or acquired skill. (When applied appropriately, it is implied that these techniques should inevitably lead to blinding insight or a radical change in patient behavior.) In practice, the positive change observed among responsive patients is often painfully slow, akin at times to "watching the grass grow." In our experience, when a beginning therapist's efforts do not parallel the outcomes of the dramatized case reports, this reality can often lead to a demoralizing and false conclusion regarding one's own personal effectiveness. For the more experienced clinician, patient outcomes that do not approximate the "success" of the dramatized case can be interpreted as evidence that the therapy itself is less effective than advertised. Neither extreme, of course, represents a valid conclusion, and an otherwise worthwhile therapeutic experience might be denied to future patients. Finally, case reports too often result in the false assumption of therapeutic cause and effect. Rarely has it been demonstrated that any one component of a treatment process has a rapid and direct linear effect on broad aspects of personal and social adjustment. Dismantling studies have essentially shown that the parts do not equal the whole. (At best, some contemporary behavioral treatments seem to approximate this ideal with regard to highly specific symptoms or behaviors [e.g., Falloon, Lindley, McDonald, & Marks, 1977], but these attempts rarely show evidence of generalization.) In reality, a better case could be made for chaos theory as a way to explain long-term recovery, that is, macro-level improvement following a series of unpredictable micro events. Our own preference leans more and more to developmental models which suggest that behavior change is a dynamic and progressive process that *interacts* with diverse treatment components that *also* change as the patient advances cognitively, emotionally, and behaviorally (Donenberg, 1999). For us, PT became a "transitional" treatment that tried to accommodate aspects of both behavioral and developmental approaches, perhaps more of the former than the latter. (The fullness of the developmental approach is better realized in our newer studies of cognitive enhancement therapy [Hogarty & Flesher, 1999a, 1999b].) As such, case material will be kept to a minimum.

Similarly, the reader will not find graphs and flowcharts that imply a tidy progression through the PT strategies. Patients will more often return to earlier introduced techniques than progressively move to new ones, especially in times of crisis or a therapeutic impasse. This ebb and flow, when coupled with blending strategies within and between phases, would be inappropriately reflected in the customary clinical diagram, in our opinion.

Also high on our list of caveats is an appreciation of the enduring antipathy among some therapists to the "manual-guided" form of clinical practice, such as this volume aspires to represent. More than one clinician has felt that evidence-based practice manuals subordinate individual patient needs to impersonal theory. Clearly there is and perhaps always will be an inevitable tension between science-based theory that is rich in hypotheses (but often thin on applications) and atheoretical forms of intuitively driven care. But in the last analysis we rely on theory-based practice not for its confirmatory value but once again as a way to provide practitioners with an understanding of schizophrenia that systematically, comfortably, and effectively guides practice. We are reminded of the quip that "even a wrong theory is better than chaos." Each new patient does not need to become a unique mental disorder that calls for a reformulation of one's understanding of the illness and a novel approach to its treatment. In our experience, a manual-guided, disorder-based intervention bestows a certain confidence and legitimacy on the practitioner and provides hope, assurance, and comfort to the patient. Again, we think of the treatment manual not as a rigid list of therapeutic prescriptions, but more as a "guardian angel" that offers direction and security to the practitioner.

We also need to remind the reader that most of our research team whose contributions are reported in this volume are not physicians. If recent commentary is any indication, esteemed psychiatrists have at times decried an alleged physician abandonment of psychotherapy to the "allied" professions and might view the nonphysician therapist as an unwanted intrusion into the patient–doctor relationship. Unlike many nonpsychotic disorders, schizophrenia and other psychotic conditions invariably require a prescribing physician. Aside from the fact that many empirically tested, nonsomatic interventions in the last half-century were equally developed by nonphysicians, we nevertheless view a *psychosociobiological* approach as being indispensable to the effective treatment of schizophrenia. Whether this therapeutic triad best remains in the hands of the psychiatrist alone or is shared with the appropriately trained and experienced nonphysician (who carefully integrates needed medical assessment and medication) is an empirical question itself. In today's managed care environment, it would seem economically unfeasible, if not practically impossible, for the circumscribed number of clinical psychiatrists in the public or private sectors to comprehensively minister to the extensive biological *and* psychosocial needs of the millions who suffer schizophrenia and other psychotic conditions. High caseloads and the restrictions on therapy sessions imposed by managed care organizations further constrain the psychiatrist's availability. In our opinion, each profession has its own perspective and approach to offer, and the systemic integration of PT attempts to accommodate these essential contributions.

Having said that, some *non*physicians might take exception to the use of medical terminology throughout this volume. This is particularly so when an individual is referred to who has experienced schizophrenia. Rather than use the vernacular and increasingly popular designations such as "client," "consumer," or worse yet "schizophrenic," the term "patient" is preferred here. Once again, that choice is as personal as it is etymologically appropriate, and one that is apparently preferred by most patients (Sharma, Whitney, Kazarian, & Manchanda, 2000). "Client" is a legal term derived from the Elizabethan Poor Law (and the Latin word *clinare*, meaning to "lean on"), which refers to "one who petitions for his rights," an often fair but inaccurate characterization of a person afflicted with a medically responsive brain disorder. So, too, "consumer" (from the Latin *consumere*, meaning to "take," "destroy," or "spend wastefully") is a term coined by the 18th-century economist Adam Smith, who saw the consumer as the market force responsible for a needed balance between demand and the orderly production of goods and services. If the PORT (patient outcomes research team) surveys are any indication (Lehman & Steinwach, 1998; Dixon et al., 1999), schizophrenia patients have had little influence on the production of needed services appropriate to demand. While a circumscribed number of high service users might well "consume" without apparent benefit, the majority has either had little opportunity to do so or is often reluctant to use the treatments that are available. "Schizophrenic" is an adjective descriptive of selected behaviors and should not be used as a noun that carries with it both the inference of a depersonalized if not dehumanized identity and the sentence of a poor prognosis. (Pinel–Halsam syndrome would be a much preferred alternative.) "Patient," on the other hand, is a term of late French (*pacient*) and early Latin (*patiens*) origin that refers narrowly to "one who suffers" and more broadly to an individual who is "awaiting or under medical care and treatment." People who experience schizophrenia do suffer and are clearly in need of medical care and treatment. These are the "patients" for whom the psychosocial *treatment* PT is intended.

The remainder of this chapter reviews the background of evidence and then its implicit rationale that led to the development of PT. Whether the theory is correct or incorrect, it did, as mentioned earlier, consistently provide PT therapists with a cognitive mastery when attempting to respond to the heterogeneity of an enigmatic disorder that varies in its precipitants, onset, symptom presentation, treatment response, course, and outcome. Chapter 2 provides an overview of PT results among two diverse samples of patients: an older population who lived on their own, and a younger group that resided with family. Both the limitations and advantages of PT are described, and attempts are made to identify those who might best profit from PT. Chapter 3 lays the foundation for the application of PT and reviews the fundamentals of good care, both those principles that are familiar and those that are less appreciated but essential to good practice. Chapters 4, 5, and 6 describe the substantive principles of PT practice and the process of their application. These chapters reflect the basic, intermediate, and advanced phases of PT, including the clinical criteria that need to be met prior to exposure of a patient to a specific phase of treatment. Finally, a proposed psychosocial treatment algorithm that places PT in its proper position within the armamentarium of contemporary treatment is presented in Chapter 7.

BACKGROUND

Speaking in a distinctly different voice, the practice of formal psychotherapy with schizophrenia patients remains alive but limping as it emerges from an empirical attack suffered at the hands of late 20th-century research and the proponents of "managed cost," as alluded to by McGlashan (1994) at the beginning of this chapter. The language now has many dialects: the repetitive tone of behavioral skills training; the less familiar accent of cognitive approaches; the soothing drawl of supportive therapy; the didactic rhythm of family and individual psychoeducation; and even the familiar lilt of more analytical forms of therapy, the last of these having endured with a persistence that only the most jaundiced would not admire.

Until recently (e.g., Fenton, 2000; Garety, Fowler, & Kuipers 2000), the *negative* reviews of formal psychotherapy studies exponentially outnumbered the relatively few controlled trials available. It will therefore serve no useful purpose to further beat upon what many consider to be the "dead horse" of early psychotherapy studies. Rather, in this introductory chapter, we focus upon a few concerns that might have conspired against the *appropriate* test of psychotherapy, followed by a brief overview of contemporary alternatives to analytically oriented approaches that have served to renew interest in the psychological treatment of schizophrenia patients. When we conclude our review of the benefits and limitations that characterize these alternatives, the rationale for our disorder-relevant PT should, we hope, be reasonably well established.

Battered and Bruised in America

In order to better appreciate the ebb and flow of psychotherapeutic interest in schizophrenia, a brief historical perspective might prove helpful. From the early to middle 19th century, the locus of care for schizophrenia patients shifted from the jails and alms houses of America to the newly established state-supported (but not owned), quasi-private asylums (Morrison, 1992). The efforts of Dorothea Dix in this evolution are now legendary. Moral treatment became the prominent therapy, influenced by the phrenological concept of specific "faculties" that could be found in discrete regions of the brain as well as by American Protestantism (Taubes, 1998). While the emphasis on a "strengths model" of treatment and recovery seems innovative today, its origin was clearly rooted in moral treatment. (The dilemma of the strengths model is discussed in the section entitled *Adjustment to Disability* in Chapter 5.) A person might have been deemed "insane" or a "lunatic," but premorbid talents could be preserved and activated according to the tenets of moral treatment. In dramatic cases, otherwise disorganized and behaviorally dysregulated patients were often observed to become well mannered and attentive during religious services. The notion developed that the healthy part of the brain could achieve dominance if the patient were only provided a sufficiently strong "motive" to behave normally, primarily a motive that was religious in nature (Taubes, 1998). Unfortunately, moral treatment appeared to have had its greatest effect on "involutional melancholia" (Morrison, 1992).

When state and local governments observed that these asylums were not only self-sufficient but profitable, they assumed ownership and management. The patient population quickly changed in diagnostic composition, severity, forms of treatment, and cost—and hence in loss of profitability. The milieu of a rural Italianate setting (and a self-contained enterprise) was deemed to be of great therapeutic benefit, and conveniently it became a way to shelter the general population from the view of severe mental illness as well (Morrison, 1992). For schizophrenia patients at the turn of the 20th century, such biological remedies as teeth extraction, daily enemas, leeching, and purges as well as an array of baths, restraints, and opiates constituted the therapeutic armamentarium, followed in the pre-World War II era by electroshock and insulin coma therapy. But throughout America's public policy toward the severely mentally ill, the driving force was and continues to this day to be cost containment, primarily focused on the least expensive setting where psychotic patients could be managed. The motives of dedicated, compassionate and skillful physicians and staff in the state institutions stood at times in bold contrast to the fiscal motivations of state legislatures, an impasse that eventually gave way to a "deinstitutionalization" that occurred in the absence of needed community services and psychosocial treatments. However, the money saved by closing state hospitals has infrequently followed patients into the community, as mentioned earlier. For the present author, an early 5-year training and work experience in one of Maryland's state hospitals provided an appreciation of what genuine quality of care for schizophrenia patients could be—*comprehensive* care that has rarely been equaled in contemporary community psychiatry.

Prior to the introduction of antipsychotic medication, the contributions of prominent psychoanalytically trained students of Sigmund Freud became a principal alternative to the custodial care and marginally effective "somatic" therapies for an illness that had largely defied common understanding and definitive management. Applications of psychoanalytic psychotherapy to schizophrenia patients proliferated in the 1930s, '40s, and '50s, especially in the private asylums that served well-to-do patients, and sometimes despite warnings by the psychiatric leadership at the time (Nemiah, 1984). Developmental theories of schizophrenia offered in the second quarter of the 20th century that stimulated this growth now seem as much a reflection of societal and political change as they did objective scientific observation. For example, it has recently been argued that the labeling of a patient's mother as "schizophrenogenic" could well have represented an abreaction to the increasing assertiveness of capable women who sought identities in a labor market that extended far beyond the traditional family roles of wife and mother (Hartwell, 1996). As something of the Cadillac of treatment, however, analytically oriented psychotherapy appeared to remain immune to systematic scrutiny until the advent of modern neuropsychopharmacology in the mid-1950s. Following the introduction of antipsychotic medication, a continuing study that compared analytically oriented psychotherapy and a placebo to psychoanalytic psychotherapy and antipsychotic medication among chronically hospitalized schizophrenia patients failed to show an advantage for psychotherapy alone (Grinspoon, Ewalt, & Shader, 1968, 1972). The rather dismal results were subsequently confirmed, in large part, by the uninspiring long-term outcomes of schizophrenia patients who had previously been treated with psychoanalytically oriented psychotherapy during very lengthy inpatient stays (McGlashan, 1984; Stone, 1986). It would be fair, however, to note that many of these patients likely suffered the more malignant forms of schizophrenia.

Close upon the heels of the negative inpatient study that addressed *chronically* hospitalized patients were a number of similar studies involving *newly* admitted schizophrenia inpatients—studies that variably compared dynamic or "uncovering" psychotherapy alone to medication alone and/or to their combination, and at times to "milieu" or electroshock treatment. (Today, most would concur that the psychotherapy of schizophrenia requires a systemic approach that accommodates practical and biological needs as much as those in the psychological realm.) The picture regarding newly admitted patients was decidedly mixed, with the better-controlled trials (e.g., May, 1968; Walsh & Kelley, 1963) showing neither an advantage for psychotherapy alone nor even an advantage of medication plus psychotherapy over medication alone. However, the trials of Karon and VandenBos (1972) and Mosher and Menn (1978) sought to argue otherwise. The first indicated that two applications of psychoanalytic psychotherapy, including one without medication, produced better results than medication and support, especially in the hands of experienced therapists. But important methodological issues were raised, principally those that indicated a failure to document the medication experience of study subjects as well as the subsequent disposition and experience of control subjects (May & Tuma, 1970). The other trial demonstrated greater independent living and employment for patients treated in a psychotherapeutically oriented community program that used minimal amounts of medication (Soteria House), compared to medication and a general hospital experience. However, the absence of randomization provided fuel for critics of the formal psychotherapy of schizophrenia.

Nonetheless, provocative questions continue to linger from these trials and have recently reemerged during the justifications offered for placebo-controlled studies in selected schizophrenia samples (Carpenter, Schooler, & Kane, 1997). Among these is the important question of whether the few patients who can "recover" with formal psychotherapy alone ultimately have a more complete and enduring remission than those whose recovery is dependent upon the receipt of antipsychotic medication. A very early maintenance study of ours, for example, showed that while only 10% of patients could survive without relapse for up to 30 months when receiving only a placebo, their adjustment was superior in many ways to the larger number of patients whose survival without re lapse was dependent on medication (Hogarty, Goldberg, & Schooler, 1974; Hogarty, Goldberg, Schooler, & Ulrich, 1974). The issue, however, has and remains one of being able to identify *beforehand* just who these rare individuals are that do not require medication, rather than only doing so *after the fact*. The inability to make this prediction when the acutely ill patient first presents ultimately places the majority of patients at risk for an unjustified decompensation should medication be withheld, and raises the possibility, at least, that serious neurotoxic sequelae might follow upon the prolonged absence of medication (Wyatt & Henter, 1998). Today, were one to routinely withhold medication from a first-episode patient (beyond the appropriate time needed to establish diagnosis or a possible spontaneous remission), the process would better qualify as "pharmacological roulette" than informed practice in the absence of valid clinical and psychobiological predictors of a good outcome *without* medication. The reader will shortly come to appreciate that without an ability to identify beforehand the few schizophrenia patients that might not require medication, the vast majority of these patients will have a very poor outcome in the absence of maintenance antipsychotic treatment. The largest controlled outpatient trial to date (Hogarty, Goldberg, Schooler, & Ulrich, 1974) has clearly indicated that no advantage accrued to the group of patients who were treated exclusively with a psychosocial treatment, despite a continuing implication that the latter might provide a holding action for medication-refusing or placebo-substituted patients. Maintenance medication, used judiciously, is the cornerstone for demonstrating the unequivocal additive and/or interactive effects of psychosocial interventions, *including* PT (see Chapters 2 and 3). We have no evidence that any of the individual, family, or group approaches developed and tested by us are a substitute for maintenance antipsychotic medication for the vast majority of patients. Contemporary authors (e.g., Breggin, 1997) that continue to decry the use of antipsychotic medications for schizophrenia appear to either ignore the unequivocal evidence from nearly 50 years of controlled studies, or forget the plight of schizophrenia patients in the predrug era.

At best then, the inpatient experience with psychoanalytically oriented psychotherapy proved to be equivocal if not discouraging. For the proponents of such approaches the negative findings nonetheless provided the methodological fodder for a counterattack, responses that variably included the citation of inappropriate designs, inexperienced therapists, at times the absence of appropriate controls, high attrition, equivocal diagnoses, small samples, the conceptual relevance to schizophrenia of the therapies chosen, failures to access needed entitlements or to control for dose, type, and route of concurrent medication, and the appropriateness and comprehensiveness of assessment (see Hogarty, Kornblith, et al., 1995, 1997, for review). It now seems true that the author of the most complete inpatient study thus far conducted had it correct when he suggested that the "action" regarding psychotherapy effectiveness might be better found in long-term clinical trials among recovering *outpatients*, rather than in studies of acutely psychotic *inpatients* (May, 1975). The suggestion echoes a similar position advanced by Leff (1981) some years ago, namely, that the "asylum" of the hospital constituted such a protected, stimulus-controlled holding environment in its own right that little outcome variance would likely remain which could be explained by concurrently applied psychotherapies. With inpatient stays now being measured in days and weeks rather than months and years, the application and test of formal psychotherapeutic procedures of appropriate length among inpatients would be practically impossible to achieve, or at best reserved to a very small and unrepresentative sample of the most impaired, treatment refractory, and chronically hospitalized patients.

And so it was that nearly a decade followed the May suggestion until the first comparative *outpatient* study of insight-oriented psychotherapy for schizophrenia patients was undertaken and published in 1984 by Gunderson et al. Unfortunately, the results were not an affirmation of investigative therapy. Important insights descriptive of useful practice principles were identified, but inferior outcomes relative to the control condition predominated. Thrice-weekly sessions of exploratory insight-oriented psychotherapy (EIO) were compared to a once-weekly reality-adaptive supportive psychotherapy (RAS) among 164 randomly assigned patients treated at three facilities. Not only were effects different than predicted, but the RAS group had significantly *better* outcomes, including fewer days hospitalized, improved functioning in the home, fewer job changes, and less dependence on family. A few "nonsignificant advantages" of EIO were found on measures of cognitive and ego functioning. Perhaps the most striking outcome of the study, however, was the small number of patients who actually complied with treatment over the 2 years of study: just 58% for 6 months and only 31% for the full 2 years. While it might be convenient to assign negative attributions to a treatment where patients seemed to have voted its value with their feet, there is some evidence that these "dropouts" were better functioning than those who remained under care; that is, study participants were likely a more difficult group to treat (H. M. Katz, Frank, Gunderson, & Hamm, 1984). As bleak as the case for an insight-oriented approach appeared, the dispassionate student of psychotherapy was at least informed that important principles embodied in the therapeutic relationship were likely to foster valued outcomes, (see A. F. Frank & Gunderson, 1990; Glass et al., 1989; Fenton, 2000). Between the mid-1980s and 1990s, however, numerous review articles served to provide something of an obituary for "dynamic," analytically oriented forms of psychotherapy, in general (Andrews, 1993), and for schizophrenia patients, in particular (Drake & Sederer, 1986). In fact, a "moratorium" on the study of dynamic psychotherapies among schizophrenia patients was invoked (Mueser & Berenbaum, 1990). Fenton (2000) has referred to the decade 1985–1995 as the "reappraisal" period. While the biological nature of schizophrenia and its pharmacological treatment became prominent, nevertheless, limitations in relapse prevention and the restoration of functioning provided new indications for psychological therapies (see Hogarty & Ulrich, 1998).

Thus, another decade passed before we were to offer a description of a new psychotherapeutic approach that we deliberately labeled "personal therapy" (Hogarty, Kornblith, et al., 1995). (In the environment of the mid-1980s, asking support for the study of a "psychotherapy" for schizophrenia was an invitation to criticism.) It was late 1997 before the results of this formal psychotherapy were published, results that demonstrated selected effects on relapse and unequivocally positive effects on the social adjustment of schizophrenia patients (Hogarty, Greenwald, et al., 1997; Hogarty, Kornblith, et al., 1997). These findings are discussed in Chapter 2. But first we describe the reconceptualization of a psychotherapy for schizophrenia that ultimately transformed largely negative effects into more positive outcomes.

Different Tongues

As insight-oriented psychotherapy weakened under the assault of empirical scrutiny, concurrent attempts to treat schizophrenia with other "nonsomatic" therapies were being developed, most often in the context of the newly introduced antipsychotic medications. Literally hundreds of brief, small-sample inpatient studies of behavioral modification, the token economy, and social skills training targeted to specific behaviors were of-fered. Improvement in discrete symptoms or social behaviors became con-sistently reported effects (Corrigan, 1991). Community studies of skills training also showed important but time-limited effects of skills training (Heinssen, Liberman, & Kopelowicz, 2000). The more inspiring of the inpatient studies was a 17-week trial among 52 of the "lowest-functioning," chronically hospitalized, and medication refractory schizophrenia inpa-tients (Paul, Tobias, & Holly 1972). In the context of a "therapeutic com-munity" ward and a "social learning" token economy ward, two random-ized groups of patients were blindly treated with either supplemental antipsychotic medication or placebo. In this population, there was no sig-nificant disadvantage and even some positive advantage that accrued to placebo-substituted patients. These results, however, when viewed in the context of placebo substitution among recovering *neuroleptic-responsive* outpatients (Hogarty, Goldberg, & Schooler, 1974; Hogarty, Goldberg, Schooler, & Ulrich, 1974), clearly needed to be reserved for a special group of custodial neuroleptic-refractory schizophrenia inpatients. Yet the observations remain relevant today for chronically hospitalized patients who are unsuccessfully treated with high doses of antipsychotic medica-tion. Elsewhere, the most definitive of the group therapy approaches (Malm, 1982) also demonstrated superior outcomes among schizophre-nia outpatients who additionally received skills training. (Remaining stud-ies of group therapy have yielded mixed, equivocal, or disappointing re-sults [see Kanas, 1986; Schooler & Keith, 1993], although a new wave of small-group cognitive approaches is yielding very promising results [e.g., Spaulding, Reed, Sullivan, Richardson, & Weiler, 1999; Hogarty & Flesher, 1999b].)

Across the Atlantic, the field turned in a promising direction during the 1980s with the development of integrated psychological treatment (IPT), a systemic approach that included training in basic cognitive func-tions and social problem solving (Brenner, Hodel, Roder, & Corrigan, 1992). Although published effects to date have been limited to selected aspects of cognition (e.g., attention) and social behavior, little evidence of generalization to broad areas of social adjustment in the community have been reported (Hodel & Brenner, 1994), an understandable outcome given that most recipients of IPT were hospitalized inpatients treated for 4 months or less. We note appreciatively that a recent application of three IPT subprograms, in an appropriately designed study, has shown evi-dence of generalization to interpersonal problem-solving abilities among severely impaired inpatients (Spaulding et al., 1999). The stimulus provided by IPT led to a largely European rebirth of interest in variants of cognitive-behavioral therapy (CBT) for schizophrenia patients, with growing evidence of broad efficacy regarding drug-resistant positive symptoms, particularly delusions and hallucinations (see Garety et al., 2000; Fenton, 2000). The results seem reminiscent of the earlier trial of Paul et al. (1972). An ongoing effort of ours (cognitive enhancement therapy [CET]) has also been influenced by IPT. It is an integrated approach to the enhancement of both nonsocial cognition (neuropsychological competence) and *social* cognition (the ability to act "wisely") among recovering outpatients (Hogarty & Flesher, 1999a, 1999b). Less behavioral in focus and method than IPT or CBT, CET is our first attempt at a developmental approach to an apparent delay in the acquisition of social cognitive competence among many patients. But with interventions that are specifically addressed to cognitive disabilities still in their infancy and, we believe, more likely to have their greatest effect in the *recovery* phase of illness, there remains a clear and persistent need for a cost-effective individualized approach to achieving postepisode clinical *stabilization* and the improvement of broad instrumental and expressive roles. These outcomes might not only be within the capacity of most patients to acquire but are within the skill level of most clinicians to achieve without extensive training. PT, we feel, not only responds to this need but would likely prepare patients for an optimal exposure to the more targeted cognitive rehabilitation approaches once the latter are fully developed and readily available.

Many other psychosocial interventions also emerged as our own schizophrenia research program evolved, but they could more properly be characterized as "service systems" rather than psychosocial treatments. Because it was often difficult to draw specific inferences regarding schizophrenia patients and their response to selected program components, these service system approaches are not discussed in detail. The service programs are best represented by the highly valued and effective Program for Assertive Community Treatment (PACT), as well as case management, foster home care, the day treatment center, and the psychosocial or vocational rehabilitation centers. (We shall comment further on case management in Chapter 3 because it did represent a fundamental element of service offered to PT recipients.) PACT and case management are the most widely documented systems approaches in terms of efficacy but are, by design, strategies that would have the greatest application among the subpopulation of schizophrenia patients that is characterized as being the most severely impaired "high users" of service (see Baronet & Gerber,

1998, for a review). The generic nature of "services" also renders these interventions less theoretical insofar as principles of practice often bear little or no relationship to an assumed pathophysiology. Patient samples that have been studied in these service system approaches have been diagnostically mixed, outcomes have not been comprehensively described, and antipsychotic medication has neither been controlled nor adequately assessed in most investigations. Service system evaluations *did* often show reductions in hospital use if not relapse, equivalent or reduced cost relative to standard care, and at times greater patient participation in supervised vocational activities, although the independent functioning of patients has not been well established. The reader can find reviews of these effective service systems in the comprehensive reports provided by Lehman (1995), Baronet and Gerber (1998), and Mueser, Bond, Drake, and Resnick (1998).

Obviously, services are *essential* for meeting the basic human needs of the severely mentally ill, be they in the areas of securing food, clothing, housing, financial assistance, or even social, vocational, educational, and recreational opportunities. It would seem intuitively feasible, appropriate, and—if empirical study is any indicator—more effective for mental health service providers to integrate psychosocial *treatments* into the service systems that respond to the needs of those with severe mental disorders. Beyond medication, service systems certainly are *necessary*, but it appears that psychosocial treatments might ultimately constitute the *sufficient* program components that are required for a successful recovery and maintenance of function. The distinction between services and treatment that is often made today is something of a false dichotomy. Both components need to be *integrated* if comprehensive care for schizophrenia patients is to become something more than a promise. We strongly believe that the optimal effects of PT would be best realized in the context of an appropriate and effective service delivery system. For example, we routinely observed that PT recipients more appropriately and efficiently used mental health services than did controls. Not only could patients better identify their own needs, but they were more able to communicate these needs to service providers, particularly intensive case managers. We propose a model of integration at the conclusion of this volume.

Supporting evidence regarding psychosocial treatment effects on the relapse and adjustment of schizophrenia patients is to be found in the controlled studies of individual and family therapy, as well as modern cognitive rehabilitation approaches that are applicable to the great majority of schizophrenia patients. Since recent reviews of this treatment literature are extensive and complete (e.g., Bellack & Mueser, 1993; Schooler & Keith, 1993; Scott & Dixon, 1995; Dixon & Lehman, 1995; Fenton, 2000; Fenton & Cole, 1995; Garety et al., 2000; Dixon, Adams, & Lucksted, 2000; Wykes, 2000; Pitschel-Walz, Leucht, Bauml, Kissling, & Engel, 2001), our focus below on the precursor treatments to PT will be more narrowly drawn to the examples and lessons that were derived from our own work that is often representative of these broad therapeutic efforts.

The Past as Prologue

The late Harry S. Truman mused that the only thing that is really new is the history with which one is unfamiliar. This wisdom seems particularly appropriate today since the life expectancy of a well-designed and well-executed study scarcely extends beyond a year of its publication. "Reviews" inevitably follow the publication of a new psychosocial treatment study and subsequently appear to be the primary source of information for clinicians, summaries that are *rarely* accurate in our experience. When compressed through meta-analyses, such reviews often draw conclusions that can be greatly influenced by the inferior studies (e.g., see Hogarty, 1989, for a critique, as well as Appendix A). In our case, PT did not arise from some creative access to a Platonic "world of ideas." Rather, in many ways its evolution derived more from a systematically acquired knowledge of what *not* to do as it did from inspiring positive findings. Insights for us have been hard won, and schizophrenia has remained the most formidable adversary, only yielding a legitimate psychosocial treatment effect (from appropriately controlled studies at least) once every decade or so (Schooler & Hogarty, 1987). We now comment on this personal history of empirical study as the basis for the rationale that led to our formulation of PT. Although a very extensive anecdotal literature supports many of our concepts, we shall primarily depend on the results of controlled studies, since this is both our public trust and our practice.

During the same period of the 1960s that saw the emergence of behavioral and service system approaches, our own research program was born in Baltimore and subsequently transplanted to Pittsburgh during 1974. For more than 30 years, we have tried to systematically improve upon the psychosocial treatment of schizophrenia by incrementally refining the components of clinical care as insights regarding the pathophysiology of schizophrenia became better elaborated by the neurobiological and behavioral sciences. In the "neuroleptic" era, at least prior to the introduction of atypical antipsychotic drugs, the development and testing of novel individual, family, and, more recently, cognitive group approaches (including studies of optimal neuroleptic dosing and supplemental thymoleptics) were offered by our program. Viewed in their historical context, these psychosocial treatment studies serve as a convenient frame of reference within which the contributions of many other investigators can be considered.

Table 1.1 illustrates the historical sequence of our psychosocial trials as well as an important characteristic that describes the relative theoretical foundation of each progressive intervention. Treatment effects have clearly increased as practice principles have more completely and accurately reflected aspects of pathophysiology. The conceptual bases have grown from an atheoretical, altruistic form of caring (major role therapy [MRT]) to a theoretically driven attempt to developmentally enhance social cognitive functioning (cognitive enhancement therapy). Within this idiosyncratic march of history, one can identify the emergence of PT. The reader will come to learn that both positive and negative effects of a given intervention served to identify potential rate-limiting factors to a fuller recovery. These limitations subsequently influenced the content and process

TABLE 1.1. Evolution of Psychosocial Treatment in Schizophrenia (Pittsburgh Program)

Treatment type	Process	Theoretical relationship to pathophysiology
Major role therapy 1968–1976	Psychosocial help for people with schizophrenia (early case management?)	Unrelated
Social skills training 1978–1986	Secondary environmental stress modification via correction of provocative behavioral deficits or excesses	Indirect
Family psychoeducation 1978–1986	Primary environmental stress modification via education and management	Indirect
Personal therapy 1987–1995	Identification and adaptive control of psychotic prodromes	Partially direct
Cognitive enhancement therapy 1996–2001	"Gistful" social cognition related to context appraisal and perspective taking using developmental secondary socialization	Entirely direct

of the next intervention. For us, the experience has been much like peeling the rings from an onion, slowly over many years of continuing study. The effort would not have been possible without the generosity of the taxpayers of this country and its science agency, the National Institute of Mental Health (NIMH).

Our goals have been reasonably consistent throughout the decades: delay of psychotic relapse and the enhancement of interepisodic personal and social adjustment. The process, however, has changed over time: from a problem-solving, case management approach of the 1960s, through the repetitive learning models of behavioral skills training; to the cognitive mastery and control of external stress embodied in the family psychoeducation approach; to a better understanding and regulation of the patients' internal world through PT, now concluding with an ongoing attempt to develop interpersonal "wisdom" by means of a computer-assisted small-group developmental approach for enhancing social cognition. In our psychosocial treatment studies, medication has either been experimentally controlled or carefully documented, outcomes have been operationally defined, and diagnoses have been reserved to well-characterized samples of schizophrenia and schizoaffective disorder patients who met explicit diagnostic criteria.

While naïveté is hardly a recommended qualification for the young investigator, it did require a certain innocence if not ignorance in order to launch the first (and as it turns out the last) controlled multicenter maintenance study that compared antipsychotic medication, a psychosocial treatment, and a combination of these treatments to their respective "placebos" among schizophrenia outpatients. But such was the case when the studies of antipsychotic medication and MRT were implemented in the late 1960s. The state of the art at the time was controversial to say the least. Maintenance antipsychotic trials were still in their clinical childhood. While the unequivocal efficacy of medication had been firmly established for the treatment of acute schizophrenia episodes, widely disparate findings characterized the prophylactic effect of medication following hospital discharge. The extent to which maintenance antipsychotic medication could serve the same purpose for schizophrenia as insulin did for diabetes remained a driving question. Among the more psychologically minded clinicians of the late 1950s and early 1960s, these medications were at times subtlely disparaged as being little more than "tranquilizers" or "symptom covers" that likely deterred patients from dealing with their "real" problems. In fact, during the author's own training immediately following the introduction of antipsychotic medications, it was often assumed that the task of therapy was to "wean" patients from their "oral dependency" on pills. The tragic consequences of this bit of purported practice wisdom served his own professional maturation well, ultimately leading to the firm conviction that empiricism was the best assurance of treatment efficacy and the foremost guardian of patient welfare.

The prophylactic effects of psychosocial treatment were even less encouraging, and the largely uncontrolled studies available in the literature best served as testimonials to the opinions of their authors. They were, according to one commentator, more akin to uncritical movie reviews than scientific reports. Following his comprehensive analysis of the treatment studies available at that time, May (1975, p. 956) concluded that "with the exception of drug effect studies, the abundance of opinion and prejudice was equaled only by the dearth of scientific evidence." No outpatient maintenance study had controlled both medication and a psychosocial treatment. With this bit of historical whimsy as background, the two studies of MRT are now briefly described.

Following discharge from the three state hospitals that served Baltimore, Maryland, 374 medicated patients with schizophrenia were randomly assigned either to MRT, a problem-solving approach that comprised social casework and vocational rehabilitation counseling, or to a less intensive form of supportive therapy. Today, one could characterize MRT as a form of clinical case management. Patients were treated in one of three outpatient clinics associated with these state hospitals for 2–3 years. Again at 2 months following discharge, patients were further randomized, on a double-blind basis, to either chlorpromazine (Thorazine) tablets or to identical looking placebo tablets. While the prevailing belief at the time was that "love would be enough," the outcome of patients who did not receive medication was sobering.

As Figure 1.1 indicates, there was no main effect of a psychosocial treatment on reducing relapse. By 2 years only 48% of patients had relapsed on medication (many were presumed to have done so following covert noncompliance), but over 80% of patients had relapsed on MRT and placebo. In fact, relapse on MRT and placebo was essentially identical to that observed in the placebo alone condition! There was a suggestion that the combination of MRT and medication might forestall relapse better than the use of drug alone, but differences among the three clinics rendered this conclusion suspect. Contrary to contemporary reviews (e.g., Gilbert, Harris, McAdams, & Jeste, 1995) that underestimate relapse rates on medication and placebo (alleged to be only 16% and 53%, respectively), the average relapse rates derived from the drug and MRT

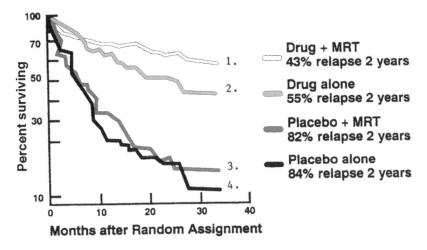

FIGURE 1.1. Drug and major role therapy study (Baltimore: 1974; $N = 374$). Data from Hogarty, Goldberg, Schooler, and Ulrich (1974).

study revealed substantially higher relapse rates on drug and placebo (Hogarty & Ulrich, 1977) than those derived from meta-analytic procedures that included inappropriate inpatient studies. Further, these "averages" were themselves misleading. For example, a recent reevaluation of relapse from the first MRT study, made according to the patients' psychiatric history (Hogarty & Ulrich, 1998), revealed that the rate of relapse *on medication* for first-episode patients was only 27% in the first year and 43% by 2 years, but for those with five or more prior episodes the rate was 48% after 1 year and 63% after two years! The *placebo* rates at 2 years ranged from 64% among first-episode patients to 85% among those who had one to four prior episodes, and it was 95% among patients with five or more prior episodes! Thus, relapse rates on medication remained unacceptably high, but the risk of relapse without medication was greater by an exponential factor of 2, a relative risk that continued to characterize placebo-substituted patients who had managed to survive even 2 years in the community without medication (Hogarty & Ulrich, 1977).

Regarding the patient's adjustment, a provocative yet consistent interaction between medication and MRT was found at all three clinics, one that was initially observed at 18 months and more completely confirmed at 2 years (Hogarty, Goldberg, & Schooler, 1974). This complex (disordinal) interaction was interpreted as follows: among medication-maintained patients who did not relapse, the addition of MRT greatly *im-*

proved the adjustment of these patients relative to those who were maintained on medication alone, much as we had predicted. However, among the relatively few who could survive on placebo without relapse, the adjustment of those who received a psychosocial therapy and no active medication was significantly and consistently *worse* than those who received placebo alone! This was *not* an expected finding. The observation was both disheartening and encouraging: disheartening in that we were not prepared at the time for "side effects" of a psychological treatment, yet encouraging in that psychosocial interventions were sufficiently powerful to dramatically alter the course of the disorder, either positively or negatively. It became very clear that psychosocial treatment for a broad population of schizophrenia patients should not be applied in the absence of medication, nor applied intensively without being timed, graduated, and titrated to the patient's apparent vulnerability and clinical state. The latter is a "process" issue that some treatment programs appear not to fully appreciate even today (see McEvoy, Scheifler, & Frances, 1999, p. 71).

Faced with the question why some patients prospered and others did poorly on a well intended psychosocial intervention, an (unpublished) analysis of literally thousands of process recordings indicated that the poor outcome of certain MRT recipients did *not* follow upon a qualitatively different form of treatment than that received by patients who made a good response to MRT. Later, a detailed predictor analysis of outcome (Goldberg, Schooler, Hogarty, & Roper, 1977) did show that it was the *type* of patient, within a specific treatment experience, that accounted for differences in outcome. Those who appeared more withdrawn, disorganized, anxious, and less insightful at the start of treatment were the ones that fared worse when exposed to a high-expectation social therapy compared to similar patients who had not received the social therapy. Better-remitted patients differentially improved with MRT, especially those maintained on antipsychotic medication. These observations subsequently found some support from the outpatient studies of the Day Treatment Center and Foster Home Care conducted by Linn, Caffey, Klett, Hogarty, and Lamb, 1979; Linn, Klett, Caffey, & Hogarty, 1977; Linn, Klett, & Caffey, 1980. These and the MRT results were also reminiscent of earlier inpatient studies (see Van Putten & May, 1976; Wing & Brown, 1970) that pointed to an emergence of dormant psychotic symptoms among some patients if they were exposed to an "enriched" or "total push" inpatient program.

With the implications of this first MRT study still poorly digested, primarily an inability to fully understand the unexpected adverse effects of a psychosocial treatment, we proceeded to address a more plausible explanation of these provocative findings, namely, that many patients might simply have failed to take their oral medication (tablets) as prescribed and thus the results of medication and MRT might have been confounded, since covert medication noncompliance might have contributed to negative findings. A subsequent study of oral and depot fluphenazine thus followed, one in which patients were, on a double-blind basis, randomly assigned to either the injectible fluphenazine decanoate (and a placebo tablet) or active fluphenazine hydrochloride tablets (and an injection of inert sesame oil). Patients were further randomized to MRT or no MRT. If a poor outcome was exclusively caused by covert noncompliance, then the relapse rate would have been less and adjustment improved among those patients whose medication was guaranteed by means of biweekly injections of fluphenazine compared to those who received an oral medication and thus had the opportunity to covertly noncomply with this route of medication. Such, as it turned out, was not always the case.

Table 1.2 describes the relapse rates associated with fluphenazine and MRT over 2 years. In the first year, relapse on the "oral" form of medication was nearly 40%, an expected rate that was similar to the medication relapse average of all published outpatient maintenance studies (Hogarty, 1984). However, relapse was *also* 35% (41% if terminations because of side effects were included) for those who were maintained on the depot form of medication! By 2 years, relapse increased to 65% for oral medication and to 40% (49% including terminations because of side effects) for fluphenazine decanoate. In year 1, the addition of MRT had no appreciable effect on forestalling relapse, but in year 2 the combination of MRT and fluphenazine decanoate did serve to protect all surviving patients from a further relapse; that is, no patient relapsed on the combination of

TABLE 1.2. Relapse among Patients Maintained on Oral or Depot Fluphenazine with or without Major Role Therapy

	N	1-year relapse	2-year relapse
Depot fluphenazine and MRT	28	29%	29%
Depot fluphenazine alone	27	41%	53%
Oral fluphenazine and MRT	25	46%	68%
Oral fluphenazine alone	25	35%	61%
All depot fluphenazine	55	35% (41%)	40% (49%)
All oral fluphenazine	50	40%	65%

Note. Percentages are rounded and based on data from Hogarty et al. (1979). Percentages in parentheses indicate terminations that included side effects.

fluphenazine decanoate and MRT between 9 and 24 months. But relapse continued unabated in the MRT plus oral fluphenazine group, again suggesting that psychosocial treatment effects were nil in the presence of medication noncompliance among those prescribed an oral medication. Without a "placebo alone" condition, however, interactive treatment effects on the *adjustment* of patients were difficult to detect. Relapsed patients who had received fluphenazine decanoate were more affectively impaired but had fewer positive symptoms of schizophrenia than those who relapsed on oral medication, another indication of covert medication noncompliance. The best single predictor of relapse in this study was the "degree of contention" in the patient's home prior to treatment! Fluphenazine decanoate tended to forestall relapse among more chronically ill patients, and overall relapse was associated with poor levels of pre-treatment psychosocial adjustment. However, no specific effects of MRT on adjustment were found. A more complete description of this study and its findings can be found elsewhere (Hogarty et al., 1979). Reassuringly, another multicenter study of oral and depot fluphenazine published shortly thereafter reported the absence of differences in relapse rates as well (Schooler et al., 1980).

Aside from our having relocated to Pittsburgh, it took a period of considerable reflection in order to determine "where we were" following the two MRT studies. Clearly, a psychosocial treatment was no substitute for medication, yet relapse associated with medication, even when the drug was administered by long-acting depot injection, remained distressingly high. However, for a substantial number of patients, maintenance chemotherapy was clearly prophylactic. Similarly, a psychosocial intervention could prove toxic to some patients yet represented a facilitator of recovery for others, especially those maintained on antipsychotic medication. Since the treatment experience of successfully treated and unsuccessfully treated patients was similar, something else was operating that had to explain a seeming interaction, so to speak, between the vulnerabilities of certain patients and the stress arising from the therapeutic environment (e.g., MRT) or the natural environment, (e.g., one's household).

As it turned out, decades of neuropsychological study had pointed to diffuse if not global impairments in such capacities as attention and arousal, working memory, and the problem-solving executive functions of many patients. (A recent overview of the relevant literature can be found in Carter & Barch, 2000.) These impairments seemed likely to be exploited in the form of a new episode by various forms of environmental press, stressors that ranged from different aspects of family life to the characteristics of one's own culture (see Leff, 2001, for recent examples). On the other hand, more benign environments seemed protective, findings similar to the observations made among "vulnerable" nonhuman primates (Suomi, 1997). The influence of stress from the external environment on schizophrenia relapse has been summarized by us elsewhere (Anderson, Reiss, & Hogarty, 1986). As such, we reasoned that if environmental demands or underlying impairments were sufficiently severe, then these variables alone or more likely together could represent a sufficient cause of schizophrenia relapse even when the receipt of medication was ensured. Conversely, regulation of attention and arousal by appropriately used medication and the provision of a more benign, stimuli-controlled environment could possibly result in a reduction or delay of schizophrenia relapse. Atheoretical altruism would no longer characterize our treatment efforts. For us, a new era had begun.

In 1977 we moved to formulate our first theoretically based psychosocial approach to managing schizophrenia (family psychoeducation), one that had been influenced by empirically sound studies from the fields of neuropsychology and environmental psychology. In retrospect, the theory behind our family psychoeducation approach now seems simplistic, but at the time it represented a clear departure from the unconfirmed speculation about poor parenting (see Hirsh & Leff, 1975, for a review), as well as from the atheoretical forms of caring (e.g., MRT) that could often do as much harm as good, depending on the patient.

Taking a cue from the studies of expressed emotion (EE; Vaughn & Leff, 1976), we narrowed our focus on aspects of family life such as "criticism" or "emotional overinvolvement" that might precipitate relapse following hospital discharge, even among patients who were being maintained on medication. It was *not* that we believed that families "caused" schizophrenia relapse; rather, the construct of EE served as a convenient measurement of one (*of many*) aspects of environmental stress. Given that our subsequent work (Hogarty, 1985) suggested that the EE measures of critical comments and emotional overinvolvement might have served as suppressor variables for dissatisfaction with role performance and a reduction of warmth, we came to view EE as a set of attitudes (often understandable reactions to a loved one who had failed to thrive) that could just as likely characterize the response of therapists (e.g., MRT), teachers, friends, or even caretakers (Ball, Moore, & Kuipers, 1992) as much as family members. Not only did patients seem to survive longer without relapse in "low-EE" households, but the outcomes were similar to those of patients who happened to have become ill in the less-demanding "developing" countries as opposed to the high expectations for performance in the more-demanding industrialized nations (Warner, 1983; Leff, 2001).

We chose to address environmental stress both directly and indirectly. Were we to engage families as allies, work to reduce their anxiety, self-blame, guilt, and feelings of helplessness and hopelessness, provide them with information on the nature, course, and treatment of schizophrenia, teach practical survival skills needed to normalize daily life, and collaboratively form a step-by-step plan of recovery, perhaps the emotional temperature of the home could be diminished and a safe, predictable, stimuli-controlled environment ensured. "Therapy" would perhaps be too strong a term to describe this psychoeducation/management process, and we have come to view the approach as something of an exercise in "environmental engineering." In 1978, we obtained grant support for this family approach and coined the term "psychoeducation" (Anderson, Hogarty, & Reiss, 1980), a movement that has led to a number of studies that quickly confirmed the effectiveness of this new approach (see Dixon & Lehman, 1995; Dixon et al., 2000; Pitschel-Walz et al., 2001, for reviews). Our treatment manual describes this form of family intervention in detail (Anderson et al., 1986). Except for the now somewhat dated information on the nature of schizophrenia, this volume continues to provide effective guidelines for joining and working with families of schizophrenia patients.

Otherwise, it seemed that if social skills training could be reconceptualized as a long-term, more "dynamic" maintenance strategy (rather than a relatively brief, didactic attempt to modify motoric or topographic behaviors), one might also be able to indirectly modify the external environment. Our skills-training approach focused on the behaviors (derived from audiotaped Camberwell Family Interviews of Expressed Emotion) that seemed to precipitate the critical comments and overinvolvement of family members. If patient behaviors could be modified, particularly those that most likely drove families to despair, perhaps indirectly the edge would come off the "high-EE" atmosphere of a household.

As Table 1.3 indicates, the family approach was clearly effective over the 2 years of controlled study. All patients in all treatment conditions were prescribed an antipsychotic medication and all resided in households characterized as high in expressed emotion. Among those randomized to the family psychoeducational treatment approach (FPT), only 19% experienced a relapse by 1 year, 20% relapsed on social skills training (SST) alone, and 0% relapsed on the combination of FPT and SST. Among those treated with medication and support (the control condition), the

TABLE 1.3. Relapse Rates for Family
Psychoeducation Treatment (FPT), Social Skills
Training (SST), and Supportive Therapy (Control)

	N	Year 1 relapse	Year 2 relapse
FPT + drug	21	19%	29%
SST + drug	20	20%	50%
FPT + SST + drug	20	0%	25%
Support + drug	29	38%	62%

Note. Data from Hogarty et al. (1991).

characteristic 38% relapse rate was once again observed. By 2 years, relapse among patients assigned to FPT alone rose to 29%, but among those receiving only SST, 50% had experienced another decompensation, often in the last months of study. The latter was a likely reaction to the pending termination of skills training. (Family clinicians had been trained elsewhere in our institution, thus reducing the threat of an interrupted FPT, but opportunities for continued skills training were not available.) In the combined treatment condition, relapse rates rose from 0% to 25%, and "control" patients assigned to medication and support experienced a 62% relapse rate by 2 years. As such, a very convincing long-term prophylactic effect of family psychoeducation was demonstrated ($\chi^2 = 8.20, p = .004$), but the *individual* SST approach proved to only have short-term benefits. Support plus medication also seemed minimally effective for these high-risk patients. Clearly a more effective individual approach to maintaining schizophrenia patients was needed. These results contributed greatly to our resolve to develop an individual PT for schizophrenia patients that would be more effective and enduring.

On a positive note, we were finally able to address a long-standing criticism of psychosocial interventions, namely, that the primary effect of a "psychological" therapy was simply to enhance medication compliance. If true, the prophylactic effect of psychosocial treatment would be better interpreted as an indirect effect of medication. Such was not the case with the family approach. When outcomes for the 75 patients who were unequivocally medication compliant were analyzed (nearly all maintained on fluphenazine decanoate), only 18% of the family treated subjects and 25% of the family plus skills training recipients had experienced a relapse, but 41% of the skills training alone and 48% of the medication controls had relapsed by 2 years. An independent effect of FPT, beyond medication taking, was thus clearly established (χ^2 = 4.56, p = .03). While many other family educational approaches have also documented a significant effect on forestalling relapse (see Dixon & Lehman, 1995; Dixon et al., 2000; Pitschel-Walz et al., 2001, for reviews), the recently completed multicenter study of NIMH failed to show a difference in relapse between *two* family approaches (Schooler et al., 1997). However, the design did not provide a control (no family treatment) condition, and the outcomes for patients in both family conditions were quite similar to the relapse rates observed in the family condition among studies that did include appropriate controls. Further, as we note in Appendix A, maintenance studies that rule out patients who failed to make a good response to medication in the acute phase tend not to show a relapse rate difference for psychosocial treatment.

A likely mechanism of action for our own FPT approach was suggested by an analysis addressed to changes in EE status from intake to 1 year. Across treatment conditions, 30% of all households changed from high to low EE and not one patient relapsed in these households! The observation was particularly true for criticism, but emotional over-involvement seemed to be a less important construct (perhaps better conceptualized as "love"). There was some evidence that EE changes were more likely to occur in the FPT cells (39% of families) than in the no-FPT cells (25% of families), a confirmation of the earlier observation provided by Leff, Kuipers, Berkowitz, and Sturgeon (1985) and one that has subsequently been supported in other studies (see Pitschel-Walz et al., 2001). However, similar rates of EE change for the SST-alone condition and the medication control condition indicated that the first-year effect of skills training could not be interpreted as having followed upon "indirectly" influencing household EE. It must be noted, however, that the persistence of high EE in many households could just as well have been a *response* to patient relapse, not its provocation.

Turning to the effects of the FPT and SST approaches on the personal and social adjustment of patients, once again without an appropriate placebo condition the magnitude of interactive effects could not be detected. The effects of our psychosocial interventions that could be documented were very modest indeed. In fact, as was the case with the MRT and fluphenazine study, these effects seemed to be not worth more than a passing reference (Hogarty et al., 1991). If anything, the few adjustment effects observed at year 1 favored those patients who had been treated with an SST approach exclusively, and 2-year effects accrued to patients who participated in the two family conditions, a likely reflection of the greater survivorship of these family-treated subjects.

While it is not our intent to induce unconsciousness in the reader by means of a heavy methodological club, the failure to have clearly detected the adjustment effects of contemporary psychosocial interventions is a serious problem that not only militates against a greater understanding of specific treatments but fuels the rationale for cost containment should treatment effects be largely limited to forestalling relapse. (A new, "atypical" antipsychotic medication that could more effectively reduce relapse, for example, would clearly become a more cost-effective approach to care, should independent effects on adjustment not be realized by an additional psychosocial intervention.) If we were to correctly assess the effects of PT on adjustment, the methodological issue that operated against a "best" test of its efficacy would have to be addressed directly and appropriately, especially when long-term placebo-controlled studies were no longer feasible or warranted.

We believed that the absence of clear adjustment findings that could be directly attributed to psychosocial treatment had more to do with the design of previous studies than with any essential flaw in the psychosocial interventions themselves. In point of fact, outcomes other than symptom status and relapse rate have rarely been assessed (Lehman et al., 1995). Prior to the PT studies, all of the important long-term maintenance trials (both in schizophrenia and other severe mental disorders) had, to our knowledge, approached the analysis of adjustment in one of two entirely inadequate ways. To begin, most longitudinal studies, our own included, had chosen to terminate patients from follow-up observation once the patient experienced a relapse or recurrence of symptoms. As such, investigators had the option of including all assessments in an analysis that were available at each follow-up period, including the assessments of relapsed patients. If a patient had relapsed early in the course of treatment, then these relapse assessments would be carried along to future periods as well. The practice is often called "endpoint analysis," or "the last observation carried forward" (LOCF) method. The major constraint against inference making in such analyses is that "adjustment" effects tend to become redundant statements of the earlier-described prophylactic (relapse) effect, a result that inevitably occurs when the treatments differ greatly in their ability to forestall relapse, as they most often did. The other option, one historically used by us, was to limit the analysis of adjustment to only those patients who survived without a relapse, a somewhat better solution but one that also remained seriously flawed. In this case, not only does the treatment condition that has the greatest number of relapses have the fewest number of patients available for analysis, but these hardy souls are scarcely representative of the original sample and make subsequent comparisons to the larger and more representative subsamples very difficult when one is attempting to detect adjustment effects. More often than not, in the face of long-term relapse rates that ranged between 40% to more than 80% for a given treatment condition, the statistical "power" to reliably detect even large effects was difficult if not impossible to achieve with the small number of surviving patients available. Borrowing from the recent Treatment Strategies in Schizophrenia Collaborative Study (see Schooler et al., 1997), which was in the planning stage at the time, the PT studies chose to reenter relapsed patients into their respective treatment cell once they recovered from an interim relapse. All patients except for dropouts would be available for analysis, thus correcting for the problems associated with survivor analysis. It was also reasoned that even though different rates of relapse might characterize treatment conditions over many years of study, the absolute number of relapsed patients at any 6-month assessment, for example, would be smaller than the total number of relapses over 3 years of treatment, thus avoiding the methodologic contaminant of endpoint analysis. The new method would also exclude "between-rating period" relapsed patients, and at any specific semiannual assessment the number of relapsed patients would be minimally different between treatment conditions. This was the first design modification that was made for the PT studies long before they were implemented.

Before summarizing the conclusions and inferences that were drawn from the investigations that served to support the rationale for PT, corollary results that arose from our study of drug dose and environment also provided important pieces to the treatment puzzle. Stable neuroleptic-responsive and -remitted patients who were randomly and blindly assigned to a standard maintenance dose of fluphenazine decanoate (about 25 mg every 2 weeks) did not have an increased rate of relapse compared to patients assigned to an 80% dose reduction over 2 years of treatment (Hogarty et al., 1988). This was an important observation for psychosocial therapists, since unwanted extrapyramidal side effects that were associated with higher doses of typical neuroleptic medication had often conspired against the best test of a psychosocial treatment. Nonetheless, "minor" symptom exacerbations were observed among low-dose subjects in the second treatment year, miniepisodes that were largely explained by the fact that these also were the patients who resided in more stressful households. As the stores of fluphenazine that had cumulated in fatty tissue were likely to have been depleted over time (as also suggested elsewhere by Marder et al., 1994), the interface between stress and the reversal of a positive drug effect became more clear. In the clinical management of outpatients, one option, of course, would be to increase the maintenance dose of medication in the presence of a minor exacerbation, a strategy that has proven useful (Marder et al., 1994). But a supplementary option, if the family treatment results could be believed, would be to also work with families to reduce the emotional climate of the household, thus limiting the period of supplemental medication. These findings are noted here only to reinforce the consistent observation that the effective management of medication and psychosocial factors (in the natural or therapeutic environments) *always* go hand in hand.

RATIONALE

So let us now take a moment to review what had been learned before we sat down in 1985 to formulate the premises for a PT of schizophrenia. Clearly, if external stress was sufficiently severe, then the protective effects of medication could easily be overwhelmed. Such stress could just as likely arise in the clinic (e.g., during MRT) as it did in the home or the workplace. Our attempt to modify the natural environment of the high-EE household was certainly effective, but the adjustment of patients in these environments that had lowered expectations for performance left much to be desired. Conversely, an individual approach such as SST had relatively short-term effects on forestalling relapse and did not appear to indirectly influence the origins of household stress. Nor did the effects of SST appear to generalize to broad areas of community adjustment. An ongoing monitoring of the subsequent course of the "successfully" treated patients also led to an equally disheartening conclusion. Given sufficient time, most patients eventually succumbed to another episode of schizophrenia once formal treatment ended, a long-recognized outcome of schizophrenia treatment studies in the absence of an enduring "verbal decanoate." Once patients attempted to leave the protected setting of the home or clinic and ventured into independent living, work, school, or even vocational training, the roof seemed to eventually collapse and nearly all of our FPT and SST patients experienced another psychotic episode over the 1–7 years that followed termination of the study (Hogarty et al., 1991). Even during the second year of the study, most late relapses occurred in the setting of a collaborating vocational rehabilitation agency. The increased expectations for patients that "looked normal" ultimately provoked both a negative feedback from rehabilitation counselors when patients failed to respond as expected (a likely form of therapist high EE) and a decompensation for the patient. During the study itself, we frequently removed patients from different rehabilitation settings when inappropriate expectations for performance and the patient's failure to meet these expectations appeared to precipitate a destabilization.

If the triggers of decompensation were to be found in the external environment, most certainly we could not manipulate each and every community setting to which patients were drawn. Nor did the individual approaches provided (whether MRT, FPT, SST, or supportive therapy) seem to have helped patients to negotiate environments outside the home on their own. More often than not, patients appeared to be dependent on the "problem-solving ego" of the therapist. Thus, we concluded that there was a great need to address the *internal* subjective sequelae of stress, the natural consequences of external demands that served to destabilize a recovering patient. If patients could only learn to identify the deeply *personal* effects of stress, then once they were equipped with adequate strategies that were tailored to individual need and clinical state, perhaps control of the cognitive, physiological, and emotional effects of stress could be possible. Something of an "inoculation" against relapse might occur, and the resulting comfort might enable patients to pursue a more fulfilling social and vocational life. In turn, these coping strategies might travel better with each patient wherever he or she went, with or without an omnipresent problem-solving therapist. The seed of PT had thus been planted.

A Reformulation

We began our conceptualization of PT with an appraisal of what might be called the "anatomy" of psychotic decompensation. In the years prior to the development of PT, an extensive literature had been devoted to exploring the processes of psychosis onset and recovery (e.g., Searles, 1965; Arieti, 1974; Carr, 1983; Braden, 1984; Donlon & Blacker, 1973; Breier & Strauss, 1983; Carlson & Goodwin, 1973). These concepts have continued to evolve in more recent years (Strauss, 1989; Takai, Ulmatsu, Kaiza, Inoue, & Velki, 1990; Dittman & Schuttler, 1990). Whether described in terms of "stages" or as a "continuum," various models acknowledged the central role of psychomotor and affective activation as the precursors of psychotic symptoms, the latter including mania, schizoaffective disorder, and schizophrenia itself. Hyperreactivity was seen as a continuously distributed vulnerability with important genetic, age-related, neurobiological, and environmental contributions to the severity and frequency of episodes (Braden, 1984). (This reactivity has recently been described as a biochemical "sensitization" to life experience [Lieberman, Sheitman, & Kinon, 1997], which we explore in the *Psychoeducation* section of Chapter

4.) More important, other studies of psychotic prodromes had served to reinforce the central role of affectivity as the likely herald of a new episode among patients with an established diagnosis of schizophrenia (e.g., Herz, 1985; Herz & Melville, 1980). Not infrequently, insomnia, restlessness, excitement, fearfulness and depression and its associated affects preceded the more widely acknowledged cognitive disruptions associated with the acute schizophrenia presentation (e.g., altered perceptions, attention deficits, disorganized thinking or language, and identity crises [Hatfield, 1989], including such positive symptoms as hallucinations and delusions). These models of psychotic decompensation and recovery bore a striking similarity to the theoretical speculation regarding "symptom formation" among nonpsychotic states. More analytical in conceptualization, these historical accounts have ranged from the four-stage theory of Sigmund Freud to the novel eight-stage formulation described by Luborsky (1996). The models variably included the elements of perceived threat or danger, an associated fear, anxiety or dread, followed by helplessness, lack of control, hopelessness, and ultimately the formation of a psycho-physiological symptom complex. Interepisodically, impairments of affect have also seemed ubiquitous among schizophrenia patients, a "pathological lingering of affect" according to Eugen Bleuler. As we have reviewed elsewhere (Hogarty, McEvoy, et al., 1995), such persistent affectivity could not only serve to precipitate a new psychotic exacerbation but could also contribute to profound handicaps in personal and social adjustment, treatment noncompliance, and even suicide.

PT thus included internal coping as a methodological centerpiece, a way to elicit and subsequently address the earliest indicators of affect dys-regulation. However, internal coping clearly pales in contrast to the voluminous literature on "stress management," the latter now employed as a strategy deemed to be effective for the management of many human ailments ranging from back pain to burnout, cancer to cardiovascular disease, and even clinical anxiety or depression. PT differs in the identification and control of the *earliest* cues of distress and its ability to disrupt a chain of events that ends not with a painful emotion or two in the stress management sense but with psychosis in neurobiologically compromised individuals.

Some have commented that PT thus appears to be a variant of formal cognitive-behavioral therapy (CBT). We feel that an important theoretical premise distinguishes the cognitive elements of PT from formal CBT. McKay, Davis, and Fanney (1981) usefully described two theoretical models of distressing affects. In the first, an environmental trigger leads to physiological arousal that in turn precipitates negative thoughts which result in troubling affects. In the second model, more akin to that which supports formal CBT, the environmental stimulus is believed to first trigger negative thoughts, which then lead to arousal and disordered affect. The internal coping component of PT, for better or worse, more closely aligned with the first premise, one that found support in the early work of Schacter and Singer (1962). Their studies in *attribution* (or labeling) *theory*, for example, focused on the common human process of making attributions to nonspecific states of arousal, a process that allows emotions to be identified or "labeled." In one study, subjects who were injected with a physiologically arousing substance (epinephrine [adrenaline]) subsequently "labeled" their state of arousal as *either* anger *or* euphoria depending on the modeling provided by an actor who feigned having received epinephrine. A person's search for emotional labels that correspond to psychophysiological arousal thus seemed quite dependent on context and did not necessarily result in negative thoughts initially.

Since PT, through its internal coping technique, essentially involves identifying and labeling the self-perceived "cues of distress," the critic might argue that labeling indications of arousal as *positive* affects might have been more to the patient's benefit than attributing "distress" to these subjective states. For example, one PT patient identified muscle tension as a precursor cue to joining any family celebration. It is conceivable that a therapist's attribution of "joyful anticipation" to this psychophysiological state might have served a better purpose than the label of "distress" that we preferred. Our choice of labels arose from the reality that the schizophrenia patient's propensity toward affective dysregulation (of either positive or negative emotions) held the potential for serious consequences, and that an intuitively sensible labeling of the subjective states that patients often tended to view as "upsetting" would ultimately provide the cognitive mastery and ultimate management skill that we sought. Further, as mentioned above, the stages of psychotic decompensation consistently implicated poorly regulated indicators of negative rather than positive affects. It is of course theoretically possible that had we directly addressed the negative thoughts provoked by environmentally stimuli, as opposed to the affective cues of distress that possibly led to negative thoughts, we might have provided relief to patients using this approach as well, as recent studies of formal CBT applications among schizophrenia patients suggest (see Fowler, Garety, & Kuipers, 1995; Garety et al., 2000). However, PT was not a strategy designed to directly address the positive symptoms of psychosis. We have historically relied on psychopharmacology to produce this effect. Rather, PT's focus would be on the containment of re-mitted symptoms and the prevention of exacerbations among medication-responsive patients. (About 7% of patients in the PT studies had severe drug-refractory symptoms, and these patients failed to advance beyond the basic phase of PT.) Clearly CBT is becoming a necessary intervention that prepares the persistently psychotic patient for a more comprehensive psychosocial treatment experience (Garety et al., 2000).

Affect dysregulation and the cues of distress thus became important "points of entry" for a personal psychotherapy that sought to forestall psy-chotic relapse and to enhance personal and social adjustment. The concept of affect dysregulation, of course, is as old as modern psychiatry itself, dat-ing at least to the work of P. M. F. Janet at the Salpêtrière in Paris in the late 19th century (see van der Kolk, Pelcovitz, Roth, & Mandel, 1996, for a recent review). Used initially to describe the automatic, stereotyped, un-controlled, and often dramatic response to stress among "hysterics," the concept evolved to include somatization and dissociation, primarily the separation of emotional states from cognition and perception. In the ex-treme, affect dysregulation was the disassociation of will and behavior. Such disruptions were believed to represent catastrophic reactions to the memory of past traumatic events, theoretical formulations that currently find favor in the various DSM-IV diagnoses of posttraumatic stress disor-der (PTSD), somatization disorder, and a variety of dissociative reactions (American Psychiatric Association, 1994). Central to a definition of disso-ciation was an alleged loss of both awareness and voluntary control of one's behavior. In PTSD (Barlow, Chorpita, & Turovsky, 1986), the defi-nition had been extended to include overarousal, hypervigilence and a nar-rowing of attention, that is, the cognitive components of dysregulated af-fect that are also common among many presentations of schizophrenia. While the dissociation of affect and cognition is clearly useful if not central to an understanding of schizophrenia itself, we do not at all imply that schizophrenia is a variant of dissociative disorder, including severe "loss of awareness" or alexithymia (the inability to identify or describe affect). Rather, a personal psychotherapy for schizophrenia would essentially seek to refine and enhance the patient's *existing* awareness of the affective, so-matic, and cognitive prodromes that most patients could broadly, albeit incompletely, describe when asked. The systematic identification of these disturbing affects, their temporal emergence in relationship to stress and their potential association with relapse, when coupled with coping strate-gies appropriate to their intensity and the patient's clinical state, seemed to be a reasonable approach to the mastery of possible psychotic prodromes.

While recommended for the treatment of PTSD and associated disorders, the use of "emotions as signals," their systematic identification and labeling, as well as the utilization of self-control techniques (see McKay et al., 1987; van der Kolk et al., 1996) seem eminently worthwhile strategies for treating schizophrenia patients as well.

If mistakes of the past were to be avoided, the treatment process would also need to accommodate the patient's stage of clinical recovery, as well as the constraints against the "executive" control of behavior that existed in the form of pervasive neuropsychological deficits (see Carter & Barch, 2000). Foremost among the latter were the following: the well-characterized problems of disattention (often involving irrelevant stimuli), primarily the influence of information-processing demands on a limited capacity system; difficulty in holding the details of any self-regulating adaptive strategy in "working" memory; and the abiding ambivalence, limitations in abstraction, and an often laborious cognitive effort that was required to initiate behaviors appropriate to solving interpersonal problems. "Bridging the gap" between instruction and application would also need to be accomplished through real-life experiences that were clinically guided. Fortunately, the literature provided a rich description and often empirical support regarding the stages of reintegration and recovery from psychosis, together with associated coping strategies from the fields of SST and supportive psychotherapy, including the self-protective techniques volunteered by patients themselves, as well as psychoeducation and medication management. (Relaxation training also seemed useful to a comprehensive approach even though empirical studies among schizophrenia patients were few.) Clinical insights that were potentially helpful for regulating affect were consolidated and labeled by us as "internal coping," an essential clinical element of our new psychotherapeutic approach. Efficacy studies of these diverse treatment strategies had the greatest influence on the selection of PT components.

We thus shifted focus from the management of the *external* environment to the regulation of the patient's *internal* subjective state through a graduated repetitive learning model that featured an amalgam of techniques useful for the probing, subsequent learning, and control of vulnerable affects. We reasoned that a greater awareness and management of dysregulated affect would enable the schizophrenia patient to maintain a remission of psychotic symptoms and foster recovery and generalization in a manner that could well be more beneficial than previous psychosocial interventions. This conceptualization of PT was finally completed in 1985 and shortly thereafter underwent its first application.

CHAPTER TWO

Personal Therapy and Evidence-Based Practice

There is a rather outrageous quote from the 18th-century Scottish philosopher David Hume that has clear relevance for the contemporary struggle between the advocates of empiricism and practice wisdom: "If we take in our hand any volume, let us ask, Does it contain any abstract reasoning concerning quantity? No. Does it contain any experimental reasoning concerning matter of fact and existence? No. Commit it then to the flames; for it can contain nothing but sophistry and illusion!" (cited in Garrett & Woodworth, 1953, p. ii).

Since this distinctly provocative and extreme position regarding the alleged value of empiricism has not immediately precipitated page turning (or book burning), we shall take the opportunity to comment on the abiding if not growing ill will between the proponents of clinical research findings and traditional clinical practice. These few comments are offered with the hope that the empirical foundations of PT will become more understandable and thus acceptable. On one hand, it is hard to argue against the value of an experimental intervention that has produced superior outcomes under carefully controlled conditions when compared to "treatment as usual" or even to a previously tested, formal intervention. As mentioned earlier, this approach to establishing treatment efficacy has characterized our own program throughout its existence. On the other hand, some see practice traditions being "superseded, even extinguished"

(Cloward, 1998) by a quantitatively driven research movement that is alleged to be dominated by intellectually conceited, academic elitists who venture into the clinical arena largely to collect data that become the empirical club used to beat traditional practitioners into submission. Others decry evidence-based practice itself (Witken, 1998). In our opinion, both perspectives are in need of modification if we are to ever implement the better-informed and more effective treatments for schizophrenia patients that are now available.

After we consider these different belief systems, the remainder of this chapter describes many of the treatment outcomes that were found between the groups of patients that were treated with either PT or contrasting interventions over a period of 3 years. With these major effects reviewed, we then attempt to move toward identifying the outcomes of distinct subgroups of patients with the goal of ultimately associating treatment effects as closely as possible to the individual patient.

EVIDENCE-BASED PRACTICE

For many decades, it seems that at least one force behind the clinical antipathy toward empiricism has been a love affair with epistomological relativism, or "the many ways of knowing," particularly idiosyncratic practice experience. At professional meetings, how often has the latest therapy guru disclaimed theory, facts and findings and embraced his or her own intuition, insight, and unique experience as the exclusive foundation for an effective practice? This preference for subjective practice wisdom seems clearly understandable. After all, clinical scientists have yet to prove much of anything when it comes to the human psyche, including consciousness, the meaning of personal experience, and spirituality. Some scientists fail to consider the possible errors in their analyses, and wide individual differences in treatment outcome clearly make extrapolation from group averages difficult indeed. In point of fact, the significance of group differences most often rests on probability theory. In fairness, however, little in life has really been proven, but clinical theory that is supported by consistent results from appropriately designed experiments conducted among a large number of patients from the same population does stand somewhere beyond a gut feeling or a special insight. Individual experience can certainly inform practice, but too often it seems that if one case provides evidence, a second similar case constitutes certainty in the minds of some practitioners. Nearly 20 years ago, the renowned psychologist Paul E. Meehl

(1973) wrote an article on why he no longer attended clinical case presentations in psychiatry. It often seemed that the results of large, well-conducted treatment studies could be easily dismissed by the single-case outcome that departed from the research-based evidence—while those in attendance nodded approvingly.

One might certainly identify with some characteristics of an individual case, but rarely will even two similar cases be identical on other important characteristics. Large, controlled studies give the clinician a better handle, for example, on the obvious and not so obvious shared characteristics or treatment components that are associated with a desirable outcome across many, many cases. Proponents of the single-case design method often confidently claim a superior base for inference making, but the approach has its limits. (It is good for *generating* a hypothesis but limited for *testing* a hypothesis.) If patient A, for example, has been exposed to a specific intervention and achieved a discrete outcome, and patient B has achieved another outcome with the same intervention, and C yet another, and so forth, then the single cases quickly pile up. Quite soon an understanding of the intervention's major effects will require some organization of the various outcomes, let alone whether the outcomes differ in any meaningful way from the equally diverse outcomes of a contrasting intervention. From innumerable conversations with practicing clinicians as well as students from the ranks of psychiatry residency and master's-level social work, counseling, and nursing, we have often felt that a personal comfort with and preference for a qualitatively based understanding of human behavior might have developed as an abreaction to seemingly impersonal quantitative approaches, particularly those embodied in *biostatistics*. With the exception of psychologists, it is not at all uncommon to encounter mental health professionals, across disciplines, who have never been exposed to the rudimentary concepts that characterize the statistical methods used to evaluate treatment outcome. Thus, it is easily understandable that a professional person might not warm to the empirical evidence that supports an intervention when the statistical methods themselves are a mystery and the findings are largely uninterpretable. For people who pride themselves on being critical thinkers, as skilled clinicians invariably are, it is unlikely that an empirically based practice will find acceptance when the methods for analyzing clinical outcomes are difficult to understand and the resulting findings difficult to evaluate. Before scientific journal editors completely succumb to the pressure for more "qualitative" reports (NIMH Consortium of Editors, 1999), we offer clarifying statements on the quantitative methods used in clinical research, in gen-

eral, and in the PT studies, in particular. This overview can be found in
Appendix A.

We are aware that there is a risk of appearing to be presumptuous,
but if the clinician finds the treatment literature more comprehensible and
less intimidating after reviewing Appendix A, the effort will have been
worthwhile. We have often agreed with our clinical colleagues that the
representation of statistical methods and test results in most clinical jour-
nals are very often incomprehensible, sometimes to other statisticians as
well! In Appendix A, we try to clearly describe what statistical tests are
trying to accomplish, give a detailed description of a basic parametric and
nonparametric test or two, and then briefly allude to the more sophisticated extensions of these primary methods. Along the way, we share a few
recurrent problems in the analysis of treatment studies that might well
help the clinician make a more informed judgment when approaching the
evidence-based clinical literature. Without a basic understanding of biostatistics, a judgment regarding the *validity* of clinical research findings
will likely be left to the opinion of others. However, reviewers of the literature, even better informed or professional colleagues, will often "get it
wrong," if history is any indication. Worse yet, many clinicians will come
to rely on the unsupported testimonials of the latest therapy proponents,
presentations that are too often represented in the expanding but marginally useful business venture that we have euphemistically come to call
"continuing education." Thus, we encourage the reader who might be unfamiliar with statistical methods at least to peruse Appendix A as a way to
better understand the evidence base to PT.

THE STUDIES OF PT

Design

As described in Chapter 1, the goals of PT were to reduce the relapse rate
and enhance the adjustment of schizophrenia patients beyond that observed with available psychosocial interventions. Further, we wanted to
specifically learn more about the effects of PT on adjustment that might
be independent of the relapse effect. Even in the face of these few objectives, the design of the studies would need to be carefully tailored to these
major hypotheses. First, we would need to select patients with schizophrenia or schizoaffective disorder who met widely recognized diagnostic
standards (in our case, the RDC [Research Diagnostic Criteria] and the

DSM-III-R criteria [American Psychiatric Association, 1987]) and whose schizophrenia would not be obscured or worse yet confounded by coexisting disorders for which a treatment other than PT might be indicated. Otherwise, we would want to include the widest representation of adult patients in terms of age, gender, race, marital status, social class, and psychiatric history, for example, in order to generalize to the largest population of schizophrenia patients possible. Next, all eligible patients should, at the start of outpatient treatment, be as similar as possible in their clinical state, especially if relapse were to be an important outcome (Hogarty & Ulrich, 1977). Selecting recently admitted inpatients who were experiencing an acute episode of schizophrenia seemed a reasonable way to ensure this clinical state similarity at hospital discharge. Third, we would want to treat patients for a sufficient period of time (3 years) such that clinicians could move past the "crisis of the day" and have an opportunity to apply (and patients a chance to learn) the adaptive strategies of PT. Fourth, we would want to contrast PT to the best psychosocial treatment approach available to us at the time (family psychoeducation treatment, FPT) in a way that accounted for the independent effects of PT alone, FPT alone, and their combination, compared to an excellent form of standard care (supportive therapy). Without comparing PT to the best available psychosocial treatment and standard clinical care, we could run the risk of simply developing another "me too" psychosocial treatment. Fifth, we wanted to include a significant minority of patients (about 45% of all schizophrenia patients [Tessler, Bernstein, Rosen, & Goldman, 1982]) who no longer lived with their families and who essentially had been excluded from contemporary trials of psychosocial treatment during the era of family psychoeducation that had been popular in the 1980s.

Finally, unlike what was done in most outcome studies, we wanted to randomly assign patients to the various treatment options. Patients are randomized to treatment for very important reasons, not the least of which is that should treatment outcomes differ, we would be assured that the difference was in fact due to the treatment itself and not due to differences in the patient groups at the start of treatment. Today, "real-world" researchers who conduct effectiveness studies will often not randomize patients to treatment, and justify the decision by saying that a comparison of "important" characteristics revealed that the treatment groups "were not statistically different" at the beginning of treatment and/or that groups were "matched" on these important characteristics. While such assurances are comforting regarding the particular characteristics in question, there are often other crucial, covert differences operating, primarily the clinical (or intuitive) reasons that led the treating clinician to provide one treatment rather than another to a given patient in the first place! One rarely ever learns about these reasons in the published report. Otherwise, samples of patients will inevitably differ on numerous dimensions that are either unknown, as is often the case with important neurobiological factors, or judged to be "less important," although both types of characteristics could very well influence outcome *independent* of the treatment received. Random assignment is thus the best option available for legitimate inference making because it offers an assurance that these unidentified or nonspecific factors have been equalized to some extent between groups prior to treatment. Even when randomization fails to assure equality on important characteristics at the start of treatment, as is sometimes the case with relatively small treatment groups, the investigator can often legitimately "control" for these initial differences statistically, since they are believed to have been random and not real. (We describe this rationale further in the discussion of analysis of covariance [ANCOVA] in Appendix A).

Those who do not look on random assignment favorably often contend that random assignment to treatment is, once again, not a "real-world" condition in that patients might be randomized to a treatment not otherwise routinely available (obviously true in the case of an experimental treatment) or to one that is not indicated. Rarely, however, will this latter concern be the case in schizophrenia treatment studies if all patients were initially selected as being appropriate and eligible for the various treatments being tested, as they should have been. Without randomization the clinician can never be sure whether the association between treatment and outcome is *causal* or simply an example of antecedent and consequence, as described in our discussion of correlation (Appendix A). Unfortunately, the clinical literature continues to give as much if not more exposure to the results of nonrandomized treatment contrasts as it does to well-controlled studies, with only a caveat or two regarding the constraints that exist when drawing conclusions. The late Philip R. A. May said it best in his comprehensive review of the treatment literature some years ago: "One excellently controlled, carefully measured and adequately analyzed comparison is worth 10 or even 100 other attempts" (1975, p. 965).

In designing our studies, we also needed to rule out patients for whom PT (by design) would not likely be the treatment of choice. First, those with untreated alcohol and/or drug abuse that seriously compromised recent adjustment and/or diagnosis composed the largest group of patients whom we excluded from study (about 60% of those ruled out).

Many have questioned the value of efficacy studies that allegedly do not "reflect the real clinical world" by excluding these comorbid patients. We have countered by saying that in the real clinical world, schizophrenia patients who are regularly intoxicated or whose cognitive functioning is seriously impaired by illicit drugs clearly need a different psychosocial intervention that extends beyond PT, given the psychology that leads to addiction and/or the neurobiological consequences that follow. (As we shall see below, PT did have surprising effects on a subsample (20%) of substance-misusing patients that managed to enter the PT studies by disclaiming a serious effect of substance misuse on their lives). We have dealt with this "efficacy versus effectiveness" controversy elsewhere (Hogarty, Schooler, & Baker, 1997; Hogarty, 1998) and concluded that the subpopulations of schizophrenia patients that are typically excluded from efficacy studies clearly require specifically formulated psychosocial treatments that address their special treatments needs, that, in turn, could subsequently be tested for their own efficacy. There are no somatic treatments in medicine that do not contain indications and contraindications for their use. We feel that the same condition should apply to psychosocial treatments as well. Our sample also excluded patients who were unequivocally and historically rejecting of available treatments (the seriously noncompliant), as well as those under the age of 16 since their developmentally based treatment needs were unquestionably distinct. Finally, we excluded a number of patients who were characterized by clear organic brain syndrome, with or without mental insufficiency (IQ below 75). We have often felt that the unfortunate, Kraepelinean-like "therapeutic nihilism" that remains associated with schizophrenia outcomes might be due to misdiagnosed organic brain syndromes rather than to schizophrenia itself. The treatment needs of those with organic brain syndrome or mild retardation are once again very different from those who suffer from a primary schizophrenia disorder, and their "cognitive" deficits are not those that otherwise characterize schizophrenia.

We determined that 186 patients admitted to our adult schizophrenia inpatient unit met criteria for study admission during the period of intake. Somewhat older patients, typically those above the age of 60, were most often referred to a geriatric unit and thereby excluded from consideration. Ultimately, 151 of the 186 patients entered the actual study, with 25 patients never connecting with our outpatient clinic, 6 terminated for administrative reasons such as relocation, and 4 subsequently diagnosed with organic brain syndrome upon further evaluation. Table 2.1 illustrates the experimental design of the study and how these 151 patients were

TABLE 2.1. Study Design of the Personal Therapy Trials

		Approximate active patients during:			
		Year 1	Year 2	Year 3	Treatment terminations
	Trial 1 randomized to:				
Living with family (N = 97)	Support (control)	24	18	16	(8)
	Family psychoeducation treatment (FPT)	24	22	19	(5)
	Personal treatment (PT)	23	23	21	(1)
	PT + FPT	26	25	24	(1)

		Approximate active patients during:			
		Year 1	Year 2	Year 3	Treatment terminations
	Trial 2 randomized to:				
Living alone (N = 54)	Support (control)	29	25	23	(5)
	Personal treatment	25	22	21	(4)

treated. The first important observation drawn from this table is that the PT study was, in fact, two concurrent investigations that we have identified as trial 1 and trial 2. Trial 1 included 97 of the 151 patients who currently resided with their families, typically in a parental household, while trial 2 included 54 patients who lived alone or, in a few instances, with nonrelatives. Within these trials, patients were randomly assigned to one of the available treatment conditions. Using a table of random numbers, we assigned patients in trial 1 to either supportive therapy (the control condition), family psychoeducation treatment (FPT), PT, or the combination of PT and FPT. Patients in trial 2 were randomly assigned to either supportive psychotherapy or PT. All patients in both trials received maintenance antipsychotic medication, primarily the long-acting, injectible form of fluphenazine decanoate prescribed at the minimum effective dose (see Chapter 3), since the first-line atypical antipsychotic drugs were not available.

The second observation of note is that only 27 (or 18%) of these 151 patients failed to complete all 3 years of treatment: 3 patients were administratively terminated (they moved away), and 24 were terminated for reasons related to treatment, such as noncompliance or voluntary withdrawal. Most of these latter patients went on to relapse. Remarkably, only 2 of 15 treatment-related terminations in trial 1 occurred in the PT conditions.

Definitions of Treatment

Medication

The majority of patients received biweekly injections of long-acting medication (primarily fluphenazine and less often haloperidol decanoate): 72% in year 1, 62% in year 2, and 59% in year 3. Injected medication thus ensured that any differences in relapse or adjustment observed among treatments were not due to medication noncompliance for most patients. The remaining patients were typically faithful takers of oral medication, which increasingly included clozapine during year 3 (18%), following its introduction in 1990. The weekly doses of medication, prescribed in fluphenazine decanoate equivalents, ranged from 7.16 mg in year 1 to 6.93 mg in year 3, with standard deviations of about 6.3 mg, thus reflecting our goal of maintaining patients on the lowest dose needed to keep patients well, with minimum side effects (see Chapter 3). Medication compliance was also quite high: 76% of patients received their scheduled injections as prescribed, and only 21% were late by one to six weeks; 89% appeared to take their oral medications as prescribed and only 9% was judged to have been noncompliant for 1–6 weeks. About 50% of all patients received an anticholinergic medication for side effects at some time during the study, and patients were prescribed supplemental thymoleptics for concurrent anxiety or depression as needed. The bottom line regarding medication was that there were no systematic or significant differences in drug type, dose, or route of administration between the treatment conditions *within* a specific trial and therefore no apparent artifacts of medication use that could account for the psychosocial treatment outcomes observed! There were, however, two medication differences *between* trial 1 and trial 2, but these did not affect tests of outcome. Trial 2 patients, being older and more chronically impaired, received somewhat higher doses of medication and over time were more likely to receive clozapine than patients in trial 1. (Clozapine was introduced midway through the study.) Overall, the dose of antipsychotic medication was lower than that used in any controlled psychosocial maintenance study of schizophrenia reported in the literature, to our knowledge.

Family Psychoeducation Treatment

The three-staged approach of our FPT program has been described in detail elsewhere (Anderson et al., 1986) and included joining and survival skills training, reintegration within the home, and reintegration within the community. The intervention attempted to reduce the common emotional responses of family members when coping with severe mental illness in another family member, such as anxiety and fear, guilt, frustration, anger, sadness, and hopelessness. It also addressed unhelpful coping strategies such as accommodating or normalizing psychotic behavior, debating or rationalizing psychotic content, ignoring intolerable behaviors and the needs of others, or "doing everything" for the patient. Families were encouraged to temporarily revise expectations while the patient recovered and to use an "internal yardstick" to judge progress. Strategies designed to create barriers to overstimulation were also taught. These techniques were provided in the context of an ongoing psychoeducation program regarding the nature and treatment of schizophrenia as described in Chapter 4 (the section on *Psychoeducation*), supplemented with a formal, all-day psychoeducation workshop offered in the early months of treatment.

Supportive Therapy

The principles of supportive therapy (ST) exceeded that of any control treatment used in our past psychosocial treatment studies. *All* patients in *both* trials received ST, but the control condition in each trial *only* received ST and no additional FPT or FPT interventions. ST included needed case management services as well as the provision of both psychological and material support, medication management and basic psychoeducation. (The details of these strategies are described in Chapter 3 as the prerequisites for PT.) It is again worthwhile noting that the frequency and content of ST was at least equivalent to the best routine care that one might find for schizophrenia patients. Thus, our ultimate test of PT was not only quite difficult but also the observed effects of PT are probably an underestimate of the effectiveness likely to be found had the comparison been made to "routine" clinical practice.

Personal Therapy

The three phases of PT are, of course, the substance of this volume and are described in detail in Chapters 4, 5, and 6.

Frequency of Treatment Sessions

The studies of PT have at times been criticized on the grounds that significant differences in session frequency existed between PT and the FPT and ST conditions. This is quite true—by intent. Our goal was to closely approximate, as much as possible, what the proponents of each treatment would judge to have been a faithful "real world" application of the respective interventions. If the frequency of weekly 30- to 45-minute PT sessions were to be the same for recipients of FPT and ST, then the latter interventions would not have reflected what is customarily available to patients or intended by the developers of these treatments. This assumed relationship between session frequency and greater improvement does not appear to have strong support from evidenced-based studies, although it is intuitively sensible to think that more of an intervention would achieve better results than less. Our earliest study, for example, compared intensive psychiatric day center treatment to once per week medication management sessions among mixed diagnostic patients who would otherwise have been hospitalized (Guy, Gross, & Hogarty, 1969). There were no differences in subsequent hospitalization (except that the length of hospitalization was shorter for day center patients than for outpatient relapsed patients, hardly a direct effect of earlier session frequency). Further, there were no overall treatment differences on personal and social adjustment across diagnostic groups, although schizophrenia patients did show a differential response on selected measures. If therapy hours were *the* important determinant of improvement and good outcome, then posthospital day care facilities, clubhouses, and psychiatric rehabilitation centers should have uniformly demonstrated better outcomes than the less encumbrance outpatient treatment approaches (e.g., family psychoeducation treatment [FPT], social skills training [SST],or even PT). Such evidence does not exist to our knowledge. In fact, in the Boston Collaborative Study of Psychotherapy, the 3 hours per week insight-oriented treatment had worse outcomes than the 1 hour per week supportive approach (Gunderson et al., 1984). More recently, a 9-month study that matched therapist hours plus standard treatment to an experimental treatment and standard treatment alone had relapse rates of 69% for the matched hour group, 33% for the standard care group, and only 13% for the experimental group (Velligan et al., 2000). Increasing control hours but not treatment might simply alert clinicians to the psychopathology and unmet needs of patients.

Our earlier study of patients receiving major role therapy (MRT), drug, and placebo was more related to the question, but the influence of session frequency was equally inconclusive (Hogarty, Goldberg, Schooler, & Ulrich, 1974). MRT patients received 2.0 sessions each month and no-MRT controls received 1.44 sessions, a clear but not a profound difference. However, MRT had no *main* effect on either relapse or adjustment. Moreover the excess of MRT sessions was largely accounted for by the recipients of MRT plus placebo (2.43 sessions) and not the MRT plus drug recipients (1.78 sessions). MRT plus placebo, however, had the same relapse rate as the fewer session plus placebo alone group (1.60 sessions), and MRT actually led to a *deterioration* in adjustment among those who survived on placebo compared to those maintained on placebo alone. (Placebo-treated patients had more sessions than drug-treated patients because of more crises.) Only in combination with drug did MRT have a positive effect on adjustment, as described in Chapter 1. Thus, there was little or no support for a "session frequency" effect in this most carefully controlled study. Our FPT and SST study (Hogarty et al., 1991) did show a superior effect for the combined treatment (which had the most sessions) in forestalling 1-year relapse but *not* 2-year relapse. Further, there were no important effects of the combined treatment on adjustment relative to the effects of either treatment alone. Finally, the treatment cell with the most sessions in the PT study (the combined FPT and PT condition) did not have the best outcome. Thus, we are inclined to conclude that it is the nature of therapy sessions that has more to do with the outcome than the frequency of sessions. Otherwise, intensive, psychoanalytically based psychotherapy would likely have achieved a demonstrable superiority over other psychologically based interventions many years ago.

FPT and ST were designed to provide biweekly sessions during the first year and less frequent contacts as patients stabilized and achieved the goals of treatment in subsequent years. For example, standard care in the better outpatient facilities equals or slightly exceeds 16 visits a year for schizophrenia patients (Narrow, Regier, Rae, Mandersheid, & Locke, 1993). Our ST patients received approximately 21 visits annually, on average. Increasing the frequency of FPT sessions (as we had determined earlier) tends to raise unrealistic expectations of families regarding the association between session frequency and incremental advances in patient adjustment. In practice, PT recipients received about three sessions per month in year 1 that declined to about two sessions per month by year 3. (We originally intended four sessions per month in year 1, with a decline in year 3 as patients met treatment objectives.) Both FPT and ST recipients received about two sessions per month in year 1, as designed, and approximately 1.5 sessions per month in year 3, somewhat more than originally anticipated. Further, the PT and FPT sessions were also supplemented by approximately two brief (15-minute) medication sessions per month in years 1 and 2, and 1.3 such sessions in year 3. These medication sessions, however, were an integral part of the SST received by control patients. Thus, PT sessions were significantly more frequent than FPT and ST sessions, but the latter two conditions did not differ from each other in session frequency. We were entirely satisfied that each treatment had been given a faithful and competent application, which is an important distinguishing characteristic of the often-maligned "efficacy" study.

Description of Patients

Characteristics that differed between trial 1 and trial 2 patients are presented in Table 2.2 and a summary of other patient characteristics that were *not* different between trials is presented in Table 2.3. Overall, what is apparent from these tables is that the 151 patients are, for the most part, quite familiar to the practicing clinician, a reality that stands in some contrast to the alleged "uniqueness" or "atypicality" that is often critically directed toward efficacy studies. By definition, patients who lived independent of their families should have differed in terms of residence, but somewhat unexpectedly these trial 2 patients were also better represented with women, those of African American ethnicity, and those who were previously but not currently married. Given their more prolonged psychiatric history (four prior hospitalizations on average) and a length of illness that exceeded 10 years, these patients were also older than trial 1 patients (33 vs. 29 years old).

As seen in Table 2.3, patients in the two trials were not different on many other important characteristics: 95 (63%) of the 151 patients met RDC for definite schizophrenia, and 7% for "probable" schizophrenia. Of the 30% diagnosed as having a schizoaffective disorder, 87% (39 patients) were judged to be of the "mainly schizophrenia" subtype; 3 patients, of the "affective" subtype; and 3 patients could not be classified. Also, 126 patients (83%) met DSM-III-R criteria during hospitalization for the index episode. Eleven other patients judged at that time to have "schizophreniform" disorder ultimately met DSM-III-R criteria with the passage of time following hospital discharge. Fourteen patients who carried a nonschizophrenia DSM-III-R hospital diagnosis (but who met

TABLE 2.2. Different Characteristics between Patients in Trial 1 and Trial 2

	Patients living with family (N = 97) (trial 1)		Patients living independent of family (N = 54) (trial 2)	
	N	%	N	%
Gender				
Male	56	58	24	44
Female	41	42	30	56
Race				
Caucasian	78	80	32	59
African American	19	20	22	41
Marital status				
Married	22	23	0	0
Separated or divorced	7	7	19	35
Never married	68	70	35	65
Residence				
In parental home	74	76	0	0
In conjugal home	19	20	0	0
With other relatives	4	4	0	0
With nonrelatives	0	0	5	9
Alone	0	0	49	91
	Mean	SD	Mean	SD
Age	28.6	7.5	33.0	7.6
Number of previous hospitalizations (excluding index hospitalization)	2.7	2.6	4.0	2.6
Number of years ill	6.2	6.5	10.0	8.2

Note. $p < .05$ from chi-square or analysis of variance.

RDC criteria) subsequently either had an unequivocal schizophrenia episode during the course of study or clearly manifest positive schizophrenia symptoms at various times. A most difficult challenge to our outpatient clinicians was the decreasing length of inpatient stay for a schizophrenia episode (less than 4 weeks on average $\pm$ 10 days) relative to what we observed in our past studies. Decades ago it was not unusual to have patients hospitalized for 3 months or longer during their index hospitalization (e.g., Hogarty & Goldberg 1973). Since we reported elsewhere that it takes 4–6 months to symptomatically stabilize 75% of patients and 7–10 months to stabilize an additional 17% (Hogarty et al., 1988), the culture of our outpatient clinic during the PT studies resembled the increasingly popular "intensive outpatient treatment program" that characterizes many

**TABLE 2.3. Similar Characteristics
of Patients in Trials 1 and 2**

RDC criteria
  Definite schizophrenia = 63%
  Definite schizoaffective = 30%
  Probable schizophrenia = 7%

Length of index hospitalization
  3.9 + 1.5 weeks

Age first psychosis
  22.5 ± 5.7 years

Drug abuse (any)
  11.3%

Alcohol abuse (moderate–severe)
  13.2%

Expected major role
  Wage earner = 61%
  Student = 17%
  Homemaker (unemployed) = 14%
  Homemaker (employed) = 8%

Education
  College graduate = 24%
  Attended college = 39%
  High school graduate = 27%
  Attended high school or less = 10%

Highest occupation
  Manager/administrative = 14%
  Clerical = 20%
  Semiskilled = 17%
  Unskilled = 21%
  Homemaker/student (never worked) = 28%

facilities in the United States, thus further extending the generalizability of our results.

While we had tried to rule out the more serious alcohol- and drug-abusing patients, 20% of patients was found to be abusers of these substances (approximately half the rate one might otherwise encounter in the larger population of schizophrenia patients). These patients were included in recognition of their motivation to maintain the treatment contract. For most patients, their expected instrumental role in life was that of a wage earner, given that three-quarters of patients had some prior employment history. If the sample of 151 patients departed in any significant way from schizophrenia patients who are routinely encountered in community mental health programs, it was that this sample had a somewhat higher education level than prior samples—with 24% graduating college and 39% having attended college. We suspect that these percentages reflect the increasing education level among younger adults in the general population and will become a more common characteristic of acutely ill young adult patients in future studies as well.

Finally, we should note that the strategy designed to establish a therapeutic alliance (see Chapter 4) seemed successful in that 90% of all 760 patient assessments of "treatment connectedness" indicated at least a moderately high alliance over the 3 years of study, as did 80% of the 124 family assessments. However, patients who participated in the combined FPT + PT condition were less connected than patients who received other treatments, and the family members in the FPT alone condition were less connected at times than family members in the FPT + PT condition. This difference in "connectedness" is also reflected in the judgments made by patients at the end of the study regarding their satisfaction with treatment (Table 2.4). Two-thirds of patients found PT alone to be "very helpful" but only one-third of patients who participated with their families in the FPT condition (with or without PT) judged their experience to be "very helpful." While one-half of the ST patients also rated their treatment experience quite high, a quarter felt that ST alone was of "little or no help," possibly reflecting their disappointment with not having been randomly assigned to either the PT or FPT condition. Clearly families seek and value the information and practical assistance provided through FPT (Anderson et al., 1986), but it does seem that the adult patient might not always warm as readily to this condition as to one that provides an individual psychotherapy alone. In this context, we are reminded of the personal value that schizophrenia patients tend to place on their individual psychotherapeutic experience (Coursey, Keller, & Farrell, 1995).

TABLE 2.4. Patient Satisfaction with Treatment

	Very helpful % (N)	Moderately helpful % (N)	Little or no help[a] % (N)
Personal therapy alone (2 cells: N = 48)	67% (32)	21% (10)	12% (6)
Supportive therapy (2 cells: N = 53)	51% (27)	23% (12)	26% (14)
Family therapy alone, and FPT + PT (2 cells: N = 50)	36% (18)	46% (23)	18% (9)

[a]Includes five no responses.

TREATMENT GROUP RESULTS

We begin our overview of PT effects with a description of results that were obtained from parametric testing of the mean differences between PT and other treatment groups, or from nonparametric testing of the difference between observed and expected proportional outcomes, as described in Appendix A. A more detailed presentation of these major findings can be found elsewhere (Hogarty, Greenwald, et al., 1997; Hogarty, Kornblith, et al., 1997). At the outset, we should recall that the distributions of outcome scores around the different treatment means being contrasted provide no real clues as to what the likely outcome would be for an individual patient that would be exposed to PT in the future. Would he or she be at the mean of the earlier PT group? Would the new patient be a better responder than the "average" PT recipient of the past? Or, for that matter, would the patient's outcome fall in the negative "tail" of the PT scores and become more similar to the average outcome of the control treatment group? Group contrasts are therefore limited in the information they can offer regarding the likely outcome to be expected for the individual patient, but they do provide very important information about the outcome one could expect "on average." Thus, we shall summarize the more significant group differences before moving on to ever-decreasing subsamples that might bring us closer to the likely outcome of individual patients. In our analyses of the PT results, we analyzed data by treatment trial and then, in order to derive more reliable means as well as to assess the magnitude of PT effects across two different samples, we combined trials 1 and 2 in a search for the most robust and consistent effects of PT.

Relapse Rates

Relapse rates were analyzed by a survivorship method that relied on the nonparametric Wilcoxon (Gehan) statistic which, as described in Appendix A, is essentially a chi-square that examines rank differences in the proportions of patients surviving without relapse by treatment group each month. Thus the speed of relapse, adjusting for patients who terminated from treatment prior to 3 years, was also tested by this approach. For ease of presentation, we shall present the percentages of patients who relapsed that are based on these analyses and cite the relevant chi-square values when appropriate. As with all analyses, the reader might want to return to the statistical methods section of Appendix A when further clarification of the analytical approach used is desired.

Table 2.5 describes the numbers and percentages of patients who had an adverse outcome over the 3 years of treatment. Regarding trial 1, the adverse outcome associated with PT (i.e., psychotic relapse, affective relapse, and treatment-related termination) was significantly less than that of patients who did not receive PT. The difference between PT and ST is noteworthy. When we specifically examined the rates for psychotic relapse, it was seen that PT alone, for example, was better at forestalling the speed and rate of relapse than ST alone ($\chi^2 = 2.74$, $df = 1$, $p = .10$), although this is only a marginally significant difference. The superiority of PT was more clear in the contrast to FPT alone ($\chi^2 = 5.33$, $df = 1$, $p = .02$). The principal reason why the effects of PT are not more "dramatic" is largely due to the surprisingly good outcome of our control patients! For example, if we recall the outcomes from our earlier study of FPT and SST (Table 1.3), about 68% of the ST control patients in that study had a psychotic relapse by 2 years, whereas approximately 29% of the ST patients in the present study had a relapse by 2 years. (Also noteworthy: 50% of patients who received our previous individual treatment alone [SST] had a relapse by 2 years compared to only 13% of patients after 3 years who received PT alone.) So too with the FPT conditions: whereas the relapse rates associated with FPT were similar in the previous and present studies, the FPT relapse rate was significantly lower than that of controls in the previous study but not so in the present study.

TABLE 2.5. Adverse Outcome (Psychotic Relapse, Affective Relapse, and Treatment Termination) by Treatment Condition

	Adverse outcomes over 3 years		
	Psychotic relapse (N)	Affective relapse (N)	Treatment terms (N)
Trial 1 (with family)[a]			
Supportive therapy (N = 24)	29% (7)	17% (4)	33% (8)
Personal therapy (N = 23)[b]	13% (3)	13% (3)	4% (1)
Family therapy (N = 24)	42% (10)	8% (2)	21% (5)
Personal therapy + family therapy (N = 26)	35% (9)	23% (6)	4% (1)
Trial 2 (without family)[c]			
Supportive therapy (N = 29)	14% (4)	24% (7)	17% (5)
Personal therapy (N = 25)	44% (11)	8% (2)	16% (4)

[a]PT better than no PT: $\chi^2 = 3.64$, $df = 1$, $p = .06$ for adverse outcomes.
[b]PT better than ST: $\chi^2 = 6.62$, $df = 1$, $p = .01$ for adverse outcomes.
[c]PT worse than ST: $\chi^2 = 5.63$, $df = 1$, $p = .02$ for psychotic relapse.

Why would outcomes, especially for controls, have improved so much with the passage of time? First, our earlier study of family and individual treatment, much like most early family studies, contained patients who were at a very elevated risk of relapse; that is, all patients lived in high-EE households. The present study contained both high- *and* low-EE households. Second, as mentioned above, the supportive therapy provided to our control patients was a state-of-the-art standard treatment. Third, medication management with traditional neuroleptics had been finely tuned by us following various studies of the minimum effective dose (see Chapter 3). Fourth, we allocated between $6,000 and $7,000 per year (total cost) simply to transport patients to our clinic when cost was a constraint against attendance, a seeming extravagance at one level, but clearly less than the cost of a single typical rehospitalization. And, finally, the treatment team itself was considerably more experienced and wise in the ways of managing schizophrenia patients.

The relapse experience of patients in (trial 2) was quite different, as can be seen in the lower ledger of Table 2.5. While there was no overall difference in adverse outcome between the two treatment groups in trial 2, clearly the psychotic relapse rate for PT recipients who lived alone was considerably greater than for patients who received ST. (Eleven PT patients experienced 27 psychotic episodes, but only 4 ST patients had a single episode.) As alluded to earlier, the reason for this unexpected outcome might have been that we simply failed to specify stabilization criteria that should have been met *prior to* the introduction of basic phase PT techniques. Our sensitivity to "therapeutic overload" had led to the stipulation of clinical criteria that needed to be met before a patient could move to the intermediate and advanced phases of PT, but we overlooked this important consideration for the basic phase, a serious oversight since these patients lacked the resources of an available and supportive family. While ST and PT recipients in trial 2 were not different at intake on an array of important personal and clinical characteristics, the possibility does remain that the PT patients that relapsed might have been different on other risk measures that were not assessed (e.g., neurobiological indicators) in spite of random assignment.

Nevertheless, our analysis of the 11 (trial 2) PT patients who had one or more psychotic relapses was revealing. At study intake, these patients were experiencing more problems in securing food and clothing than those PT recipients who ultimately remained well. Over the course of study, they also had more persistent arguments and conflicts with landlords and/or community residential or transitional living staff than did PT patients who had no relapse. Psychotic relapse only declined significantly when appropriate supported housing was finally secured. Given the occasionally adverse outcomes that had characterized our earlier efforts, as well as a decidedly disappointing outcome for patients treated with more investigative psychotherapeutic procedures (see Chapter 1), we have wondered whether these historical negative effects of psychotherapy might have had less to do with the intervention per se and more with the cognitively overwhelming life experiences that were ongoing for selected patients and/or the absence of family support. Thus, we have adopted a general principle prior to introducing the basic phase of PT (see Chapter 3) that might also be fruitfully implemented for any treatment intervention that makes demands on a limited information-processing capacity among symptomatically unstable schizophrenia patients. It is a common-sense approach offered in the spirit of doing "first things first," namely, that the basic and common human needs for food, clothing, medical care, and—most important—residential stability be secured prior to the introduction of learning-based approaches that place demands on the patient's attention, memory, and problem-solving abilities! ST that has a strong case management component, such as the approach we describe in Chapter 3, seems a good way to start given the remarkable outcome of ST patients. Fortunately for most patients, these basic necessities are frequently provided by family, often at great financial and emotional cost. But it is critically important that clinicians remain attuned to the constraints on families, being especially vigilant that the family itself not be forced to become the primary provider of services.

Otherwise, PT recipients in trial 2 did have fewer "affective" episodes than ST patients, but this difference is not likely to be clinically important if, in fact, most PT decompensations were of a psychotic nature. As uninspiring as the psychotic relapse outcome was for PT recipients in trial 2, the effects of PT on interepisodic adjustment were reassuring not only for trial 1 participants but also for those who lived alone (trial 2). We now turn to a brief description of these important adjustment outcomes.

Effects on Adjustment

"Adjustment" is a broad and often confusing concept. We make various distinctions in our definition of the term, the first being the difference between *personal* and *social* adjustment. The former reflects diverse aspects of symptomatic behavior, such as the positive and negative symptoms of schizophrenia, as well as associated impairments of mood, primarily anxiety and depression. Social adjustment, on the other hand, is quite different, as it refers to the performance of expected social roles that are further defined in the traditional sociological sense of being *instrumental* or *expressive* in nature. Instrumental role performance refers to tasks, whether they be those associated with one's customary employment or with the activities of daily living, including leisure pursuits. Expressive role performance is characterized by the quality and quantity of interpersonal relationships within one's immediate family as well as those with friends and other relatives outside the home. Sometimes the domains of personal and social adjustment overlap, but when such issues as sensitivity, emotional distance, or friction arise in the context of interpersonal relationships, we feel that they are better classified as aspects of expressive role performance rather than symptomatic expressions of personal adjustment.

The studies of PT had as many as 44 outcome measures of personal and social adjustment, represented by global clinical judgments, total scores from standard rating scales, and specific parameters of adjustment derived from factor analyses. The outcome measures represented the reports of clinician raters, patients, and family members. Were we to have analyzed each item from these various assessments at each assessment period, the outcomes would have numbered in the hundreds, if not thousands, and the chance of random findings from multiple testing would have increased dramatically, as described in Appendix A. Given the number of outcome measures that we did use, as well as the unusually large number of assessment periods made at baseline and at 6 semiannual intervals over 3 years, there was a clear need to reduce data in order to make conceptual sense of the results and to avoid the problems associated with multiple testing. We were also aware of the need to increase the reliability of the primary outcomes of interest as a way to avoid type I and II errors, as described in Appendix A. (The reliability of an outcome measure would increase, for example, when the standard errors of our means were reduced through a very large number of assessments and when correlated scores were combined as a single measure that reflected shared common variance.)

Thus, we began our approach to the analysis of adjustment by conducting a "super" factor analysis, literally a factor analysis of total rating scale scores, existing factor scores, and global clinical judgments, aware that many outcomes were themselves highly intercorrelated. Two major and one minor composite scores were generated. The first represented a *personal adjustment composite* that initially had encompassed 22 outcomes such as the Raskin Depression Scale, the Covi Anxiety Scale and the Wing Negative Symptom Scale, and the minor symptom factor from the Brief

Psychiatric Rating Scale (all completed by clinical raters), as well as measures from the patient self-report called the Subjective Response Questionnaire, which captured various aspects of mood. The *social adjustment composite* initially accommodated 18 outcome measures primarily drawn from the Major Role Adjustment Inventory (a clinician rating) and the Social Adjustment Scale II, a structured interview that attempted to faithfully record the patient's own report of instrumental and expressive role performance. (This latter scale would contain our primary outcomes of interest in the univariate tests if the social adjustment composite were significantly different between groups.) A third composite was ultimately scored as a single item and represented a close family member's description of the patient's *performance of expected social role activities* as rated on the Katz Adjustment Scale (R2) (M. M. Katz & Warren, 1999). When we ultimately generated the personal and social adjustment composite scores for each patient at each period, we did not include measures that were minimally associated with a given composite (i.e., which did not "load" highly in the factor analysis) or that were highly redundant measures of other outcomes in the composite (see Hogarty, Greenwald, et al., 1997).

At this point, and prior to any analysis of the individual outcome measures themselves, we made a decision that we would not proceed to the interpretation of all 44 individual outcomes unless we had some evidence that a treatment had an effect on one or more of the composite measures that contained the corresponding individual outcome measures. Next, in order to further guide against overanalysis and the possible misinterpretation of effects (particularly type I errors), we established stringent criteria that would guide our inference making. An effect on any individual outcome that had been protected with a significant composite measure effect not only had to be significant in the "overall" analysis of change scores across all six rating periods but also had to be statistically significant ($p < .05$) for at least two of the six semiannual rating periods themselves. In point of fact, the treatment effects that were judged to be important most often occurred at *four* periods of time and at p values that usually exceeded the .01 level. The latter criterion offered assurance that a significant outcome was not a random effect, but rather once it appeared it usually remained consistent and clinically important over time. Statistical testing primarily relied on a version of the t test, as described in Appendix A, namely, a t test of the beta coefficients or slopes derived from regression analysis. In the analyses that combined both trials, as well as the separate analyses of trial 1 that had the larger sample, we wanted to account for (i.e., covary) any random differences between treatment groups at the beginning of treatment as well as the possible effects of the independent variables represented by gender, age, race, chronicity, and (in trial 1) household EE that might influence outcome independent of treatment. (As shown in our discussion of parametric testing [Appendix A], by removing the variance attributable to independent variables we would be reducing the standard error [the denominator] when testing the difference [the numerator] between treatment means or slopes.) Unfortunately, the small trial 2 sample precluded the control of independent variables other than the initial level difference of the outcome measure itself. For example, when treatment (PT vs. ST) was analyzed according to a measure of chronicity (more vs. less) in trial 2, the majority of these patients had been "more" chronically ill, thus leaving a small and unequal number of patients in the "less" chronically ill categories, a clear invitation to erroneous testing.

The analysis of outcome in which we had the most confidence was that which combined the two trials and tested the difference between the three PT treatment cells (PT alone in trials 1 and 2, plus the PT + FPT condition in trial 1) and the three treatment cells that did not receive PT (the two ST conditions and the FPT alone condition). These two samples were therefore the largest available for statistical testing (N's of 74 and 77), and thus the means would be more reliable and the standard errors smaller, as discussed in Appendix A. The first observation made (see Hogarty, Greenwald, et al., 1997) was perhaps the most important for clinicians and policy analysts. With a single exception noted at month 12, all of the significant treatment effects occurred at 18 months and thereafter, particularly at 36 months. This observation provides very strong evidence that optimal recovery of function from an episode of schizophrenia takes both time and a disorder appropriate treatment, a belief long held by experienced psychotherapists, but for which little empirical support had been available. We shall return to the practice and policy implications of this observation shortly, but first offer a note of caution in order to avoid a common misinterpretation of this observation. Some clinicians might feel that their own psychotherapeutic efforts are "observable" following a year or less of treatment. (Why labor for effects that take 2 or more years?) As we shall soon see, *all* patients, both PT and no-PT recipients, also improved significantly in the first year, dramatically so regarding symptom remission! But there were no differences in this impressive improvement *between* treatments in the first year. The point we wish to underscore is that the unique and *differential* effects of PT take time before their statistical and clinical significance are clearly established, that is, after a second and third year of treatment.

Regarding specific positive outcomes derived from the combined trial analyses, the requisite criteria for detailed testing was first satisfied by a highly significant effect for PT that was observed on the multivariate social adjustment composite. The significant (univariate) outcomes, most of these embodied in the composite score, included an improvement in relationships outside the home, an overall normalization of behavior and adjustment, enhanced work performance (including the number of hours employed), and an improvement in leisure pursuits that represented both the frequency and depth of these activities. The most robust improvement was found on a measure of decreased interpersonal anguish, a factor derived from the Social Adjustment Scale II (SAS). This summary measure reflects a reduction in friction and distress associated with the performance of major role obligations (as a wage earner, student, or homemaker), as well as a decrease in sensitivity, loneliness, self-abasement, worry, guilt, and feelings of being wronged that were associated with familial relationships, either in or out of the home. So too with the SAS factors of self-care and social relations, the latter including improved leisure activities as well as a decrease in conflict, communication difficulties, and friction associated with these social activities. Consistently improved over time were both negative symptoms (the Wing Negative Symptom Scale) and the withdraw/retardation factor derived from the Brief Psychiatric Rating Scale. However, as mentioned above, a note of caution is necessary regarding these latter personal adjustment outcomes since PT had no overall effect on the personal adjustment composite. From a somewhat different perspective, the global degree of illness and the SAS factors of interpersonal anguish and social relations also remained significantly improved when the two trials were analyzed separately, even though the respective sample sizes had decreased. Overall, the magnitude of these PT main effects observed from the combined trials analyses was represented by a median effect size of 0.45 at 36 months (range = 0.37–0.71 among the individual outcomes). Figure 2.1 is also revealing. In terms of paid employment, there were no differences among treatments prior to study intake, but after 3 years of treatment 43% of PT alone recipients and only 20% of ST alone recipients were working part- or full-time in the open labor market ($\chi^2 = 4.63$, $df = 1$, $p = .03$).

Otherwise there were important effects that accrued to PT recipients in one or the other (but not both) trials. A normalization of role functioning and an increase in social leisure activities as well as self-care were more

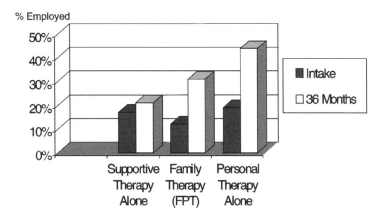

FIGURE 2.1. Employment (part- or full-time) at intake and 36 months by treatment.

characteristic of PT recipients in trial 1 than trial 2; in addition, trial 1 PT recipients showed greater improvement in the affective symptoms of anxiety and depression as well as withdraw/retardation and negative symptoms. (The latter findings once again are measures of personal adjustment and should be interpreted cautiously.) Most reassuring was the confirmation provided by the families themselves of increased performance of expected social roles for PT recipients in trial 1. In trial 2, only relationships outside the home and overall work performance preferentially characterized PT recipients. Again, the median effect size at 3 years for PT, by separate trial, was 0.57 (range = 0.43–1.05), a compelling clinical effect.

Worthy of note was the outcome of patients who participated in the FPT condition. As we recall from Chapter 1, the effects of family psychoeducation on the adjustment of patients in our earlier trial were meager, with the strongest effects observed in forestalling relapse. The same conclusion is now reflected in the trial 1 results. Positive adjustment effects for FPT were few and limited primarily to gains in personal adjustment. (In fact, only a single outcome measure of social adjustment differentially improved, but this occurred in the absence of any effect on the social adjustment composite.) Not only was the personal adjustment composite significantly improved for FPT recipients, but specific measures of anxiety (the Covi Anxiety Scale) as well as existential and major worries reported by the patient (the Everyday Worry Scale) decreased significantly for FPT recipients. FPT did not improve the social role performance of patients, and in fact such performance actually declined (according to the families' own report) compared to that of patients whose families did not receive FPT. A subsequent test of interactions led to the following conclusions: male patients who received PT significantly increased their social adjustment, but they did so in the presence of persistent anxiety; female patients who received FPT had a decrease in their social adjustment, but their feelings of personal comfort increased. A possible explanation for this interaction can be found in early sociological theory suggesting a positive correlation between expectations and role performance. (In schizophrenia, however, inappropriately high expectations can at times lead to symptomatic exacerbation, as described earlier.) Appropriate clinical expectations for patient role performance were clearly embodied in PT, but an attempt was made to temporarily revise familial expectations, as is the custom when using the FPT approach. Thus, there seems to be a price that is paid for one's clinical value system: high expectations might lead to increased performance but at the price of concurrent anxiety; low expectations might increase personal comfort, but little is gained in the way of social role performance.

Not to be ignored were other negative effects of PT. As mentioned above, there was a general increase in observed anxiety (Covi Anxiety Scale) as well as self-reported anxiety (Everyday Worry Scale) that characterized the recipients of PT; also, there was a tendency for PT recipients (presumably those who were doing well) to periodically noncomply with medication after 2 years of treatment. The observation of increased anxiety has, in different reviews of our work, been interpreted as a contraindication for PT. We disagree and simply wish to state that the absolute degree of "anxiety" measured was not at all indicative of clinical psychopathology or an anxiety disorder per se. Rather, the low but different level of anxiety that did characterize PT recipients likely represented an appropriate and expected increase in arousal that typically accompanies the resumption of a more normal social and vocational life. (It takes a bit of angst to get out of bed in the morning for most people.)

Finally, we conclude our discussion of group effects by returning to the earlier-promised implications contained in the timing of PT effects. Ignoring the definitive cross-sectional effects just described, we next sought to identify each of the 44 outcome measures that improved significantly between the beginning and the end of treatment, even though they may not have been significantly different between treatments in the cross-sectional (period) analyses. In this longitudinal analysis, improvement was calculated as an effect size expressed in standard deviation units (described in Appendix A), and in this case we chose to select each measure of symptom state and social adjustment that improved at least 0.50 *SD* between intake and 36 months. An effect size of 0.50 should not only be obvious, as indicated in Appendix A, but of considerable clinical importance. We then calculated the effect sizes year by year for the 74 patients who received PT and the 77 patients who did not.

Figures 2.2 and 2.3 graphically illustrate the results. Regarding the 11 symptom outcomes (Figure 2.2), it is clear that both groups of patients significantly improved at the same dramatic level in the first treatment year, an improvement that slightly exceeded 0.50 *SD*. A small increment in continuing improvement is noted at 24 months. These observations were largely to be expected given that all patients were managed on an individually tailored dose of antipsychotic medication and historically psychosocial treatment had not been expected to primarily improve manifest symptoms. These observations essentially reflect the results of our previous 2-year trials of MRT and the later study of FPT and SST. However, the unprecedented opportunity to observe residual symptoms through a third treatment year did surprisingly reveal a further and significant improvement in symptoms, but *only* among PT recipients! Symptomatic improvement among no-PT patients essentially leveled off after 2 years.

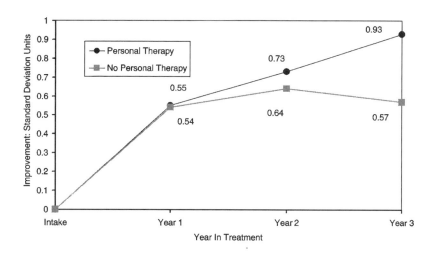

FIGURE 2.2. Cumulative effect sizes: 11 symptom outcomes.

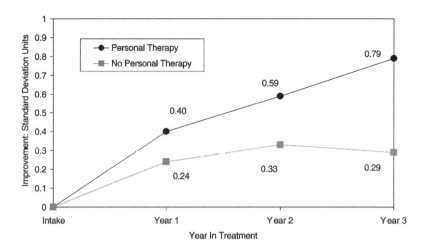

FIGURE 2.3. Cumulative effect sizes: 12 adjustment outcomes.

The 12 social adjustment outcomes were even more revealing (Figure 2.3). Once again, as in our past studies, little difference could be found between a psychosocial treatment (PT) and its control treatment at 1 year, but by 24 months clear and clinically important differences could be found. In a manner not previously studied, improvement among PT recipients *continued* to increase in the third treatment year, whereas the very modest gains in social adjustment among controls essentially remained unchanged from the first to the third years. Moreover, there was no indication that the effects of PT had plateaued by 3 years, while we were able to confidently state that the small improvement that followed ST and FPT alone was essentially the same at 36 months as that observed at 12 months. In fact, by 3 years the difference in effect size between PT and no-PT conditions was itself 0.50 *SD*, a highly significant difference.

If these observations are validated by others, the implications that can be drawn from them are compelling. Clinically, a specific psychosocial intervention that accommodates the reality of schizophrenia does lead to a differential enhancement of recovery if prescribed at the proper "dose" and for a sufficient length of time, much like the argument used to justify maintenance chemotherapy. From a policy perspective, managed care systems that either ration or preclude a definitive psychosocial treatment or that rely primarily on supportive approaches and "warm" medication can look forward to results that achieve an adequate clinical stabilization (accompanied by residual symptoms), but only minimal improvement in social and vocational functioning, a recovery that does not change substantially after 1 year of maintenance treatment. On the other hand, recovery continues to increase with PT for at least 3 years, if not longer. This is an issue, in our opinion, that extends far beyond financial considerations. For us, these data represent a moral imperative to provide an efficacious psychosocial treatment for those who suffer persistent mental disorders. Eventually, we hope sooner rather than later, the price of not treating schizophrenia appropriately will need to be factored into the cost–benefit equation.

TOWARD INDIVIDUAL OUTCOMES

Instead of writing a treatise on each of the 151 patients and 97 families that participated in the studies of PT, we opted for a description of patient characteristics that reflected subsamples of interest together with their various outcomes. The results were often surprising, if not provocative.

Our search for more individualized outcomes centered on the "gold standard" outcome just described; namely, the standardized score (*z* score) for each patient derived from the 12 social adjustment measures that changed by 0.50 *SD* or more from study intake through the 3 years of continuing treatment. Most of these measures had also proven to be sensitive to the effects of PT in the cross-sectional analyses as well. The pooled measures were based on standardized scores (raw scores converted to the same *SD* scale) from the social adjustment composite: the Social Adjustment Scale's global judgments of work performance; the quality of relationships within and outside the home; overall adjustment; and the specific factors of interpersonal anguish and social relations. The global judgments of major role performance and functioning compared to the normal person in the community were drawn from the Major Role Adjustment Inventory. Scores reflecting the degree of improvement between intake and 3 years on the Global Assessment Scale completed the pooled estimate.

Quite surprising to us was the difficulty we encountered when simply trying to define "outcome," a challenge that we dare say has escaped the attention of many policy analysts who are concerned with efficacy and effectiveness studies. By "outcome" did we mean the amount of improvement over time, or did we mean "final status" (i.e., the specific functional level of recovery)? As it turned out, patient characteristics (i.e., predictors) that were associated with these outcomes differed greatly depending upon which criterion was used. As we shall see below, patients that were most symptomatic at the beginning of treatment were often those that improved the most on PT (and the least on no PT), even though their absolute level of functioning might not have been at the highest level after 3 years of treatment. Conversely, those with the highest level of functioning posttreatment likely had the best absolute levels of functioning pretreatment, even though many might not have improved much over time. (Our cross-sectional analyses, published elsewhere [Hogarty et al., 1997b] and summarized above, tended to "walk the line" between these two criteria, both by regressing scores toward the general improvement mean and by adjusting the final levels of adjustment in terms of initial levels; see Appendix A.)

Thus, in our effort to identify and describe individual patients who were most responsive to treatment there was a question as to which definition of outcome would be more clinically important. In the following descriptive analyses we favor the "improvement" criterion over "final status" for a number of reasons. First, we had a measure of improvement for each of the 151 study subjects, a score that reflected the patient's time in treatment even though some might have prematurely terminated prior to 3 years. The final 3-year status analysis was, by definition, reserved to those subjects who survived 3 years of treatment. Second, there were more numerous and clinically interesting "interactions" among patient characteristics, the treatment received, and improvement. Finally, in clinical terms the therapist is probably more interested in determining whether a potential patient would respond to PT than in learning whether PT would enable the patient to become a corporate executive, for example.

The post hoc analyses that we now describe are essentially descriptive and rely largely on the important correlations between a specific patient characteristic and outcome. (For some truly dichotomous variables, such as gender or marital status, we relied on the chi-square statistic or a different test of linear relationship than the Pearson r.) We first examine characteristics that are associated with good or poor outcome in general, that is, independent of a specific treatment. Next, and clearly of more clinical significance, we examine the characteristics of patients that predict outcome for a specific treatment condition, be it PT or no PT (i.e., an interaction). The subsamples of patients that we describe are defined in terms of *quartiles* that are grouped according to improvement scores expressed in standard deviation units (i.e., the z scores): those in the worst quartile contain the lowest 25% of standard scores; those in the interquartile range comprise the middle 25% to 75% of scores, and those in the upper quartile, between the 75th and 100th percentile, contains the highest scores and best outcomes. This three-way classification permitted a good test of the two extreme groups, that is, the subsamples of interest in our clinical search for whom PT helped the most and for whom there was no positive and even a negative effect. To our good fortune, the upper and lower cut-off (*z*) scores for the extreme quartiles of improvement fell approximately at zero or below for the lowest quartile, and at 1 or more *SD*'s for the upper quartile. In the following discussion we shall refer to the lowest quartile of patients (group 1) as the subsample that showed "no improvement" since no patient improved over the course of study. In fact, most patients deteriorated in the range of –0.25 *SD* among PT recipients and –0.50 *SD* among no-PT recipients. The 50% of patients in group 2 are described as the sample who showed "some improvement," given that each patient manifested modest gains from 0 up to 1 *SD*, effect sizes that averaged 0.33 *SD* for no-PT recipients and 0.50 *SD* for PT subjects. Our best subsample of responders, Group 3, is labeled "large improvement," since it includes only patients who improved at least 1 *SD* and on average 1.35 ± 0.31 *SD*'s, an unequivocal and formidable amount of positive change.

Table 2.6 clearly illustrates the superiority of PT both in terms of improvement and with respect to the number of patients who either improved dramatically or deteriorated. About 74% of patients in the large-improvement group are recipients of PT, and only 26% of those that did not improve or deteriorated are PT recipients. (It will help to keep these particular numbers in mind when we consider the quartile improvement by treatment condition for each of the significant "predictors.") It is worthwhile noting that the proportions of the best and worst responders by treatment were similar for *both* trials, a reassuring form of validity.

TABLE 2.6. Improvement by Treatment Group

	No improvement Group 1: $N = 35$ Lowest quartile	Some improvement Group 2: $N = 81$ Interquartile range	Large improvement Group 3: $N = 35$ Highest quartile
PT ($N = 74$)	$N = 9$ Mean deterioration = $-0.25 \pm 0.21\ SD$	$N = 39$ Mean improve – $0.52 \pm 0.28\ SD$	$N = 26$ Mean improve = $1.39 \pm 0.28\ SD$
No PT ($N = 77$)	$N = 26$ Mean deterioration = $-0.52 \pm 0.38\ SD$	$N = 42$ Mean improve = $0.36 \pm 0.29\ SD$	$N = 9$ Mean improve $1.45 \pm 0.32\ SD$

Note. Group 1 = ≤ 0 *SD* change; group 2 = > 0, < 1 *SD* change; group 3 = > 1 *SD* change.

General Predictors of Improvement

First, we shall note the general predictors that are associated with this outcome criterion for all treatment conditions. Unless otherwise indicated, all p values are .05. We examined 47 history characteristics and 46 clinical state variables descriptive of patients at baseline, many of which also served as outcome measures. In addition, 11 measures descriptive of the family, or provided by the family, were also evaluated. Many variables, especially the clinical state measures, are at times highly intercorrelated and thus are not independent predictors of outcome. At this juncture, however, our goal is an admittedly post hoc descriptive statement rather than a definite predictor analysis. Sometimes, for example, a clinician might have only a few but highly intercorrelated variables available when attempting to determine a patient's suitability for a given treatment.

The historical characteristics related to improvement were few: patients with a shorter index hospitalization (3.4 weeks) did better ($p = .06$) than those who had a longer index hospitalization (4.67 weeks). (However, as we shall see below, PT patients with good outcomes were also more ill at the beginning of treatment.) Otherwise, those with a higher-skilled occupation at the time of their last employment tended to improve more than others. Most of the general predictors of outcome were baseline measures of clinical state, and (as alluded to above) all these measures uniformly indicated that those who were *more* impaired or symptomatic at baseline improved the most, although there are important interactions with a specific treatment that will be described below. These baseline measures included the following: the social adjustment composite and to a lesser extent the personal adjustment composite ($p = .08$); the quality of relationships both in and out of the home; the performance of obligations associated with the individual's major occupational role; the patient's Global Adjustment Scale rating (a mean of 52 for those who did poorly, but only 42 for those who did well); a global measure of illness severity (*mildly ill* for those who did poorly, but *moderately* ill for those who improved the most); and associated symptoms such as residual psychoticism and anxious depression.

Finally, two family ratings (obviously applicable only to trial 1 participants) were also related to outcome: less family dissatisfaction with the patient's expressive (relationship) role performance prior to treatment as rated by clinicians correlated with good outcome. Similarly, the family's own report that indicated less of a discrepancy between the patient's overall role performance and their own expectations ($p = .09$) was associated with ultimate improvement.

As such, there are only a few descriptors that would aid the clinician in determining who might improve, independent of treatment condition, and these suggest something more than what immediately meets the eye. Patients with a shorter index hospitalization and a higher occupational functioning might ultimately do best, yet paradoxically these are often the most symptomatic patients following hospital discharge; however, they generally live in families where dissatisfaction with performance is low and acceptance is apparently high. While this "snapshot" is interesting, the interactions between patient characteristics and the specific treatment received provide far more revealing insights into the question of relative improvement and pretreatment status.

Predictors of Specific Treatment Improvement

When clinicians inquire about the characteristics of patients who might be good candidates for a specific treatment, their seemingly straightforward question often precludes an easy or valid response. For example, the simple question "Do young males do better on PT?" requires a set of contingency tables (i.e., cross-tabulated categories described in Appendix A) that only an extraordinarily large sample would satisfy. This simple question would necessitate large and ideally equal numbers of (1) older and younger patients, (2) patients who are male and female, (3) patients with good and bad outcomes, and (4) patients following assignment to either PT or no PT (i.e., a contingency table represented by $2 \times 2 \times 2 \times 2$, or 16, separate categories). If one were to add the qualifier "premorbid history" to the question of gender, age, and treatment condition, the cells would quickly jump to 32 (16×2, the latter representing good or poor premorbid background). With an ideal sample of 20 patients per cell, one can readily see that a sample of 640 would be both unlikely and, from the perspective of equal distribution among categories, nearly impossible to achieve given the confound between the prevalence of schizophrenia and its distribution by age and gender. Thus, in the discussion of outcome, we shall of necessity limit ourselves to the simple interactions between a characteristic of interest and the treatment received. Even here, the numbers become precariously small as can be seen from Table 2.4, which includes only a treatment × improvement table (6 categories). The flag of caution is therefore raised, as it must be in any exploration of unprotected univariate findings.

Historical variables provide the first clue to differential treatment improvement. Educational level is illustrative. In terms of a large improvement among patients with a high school education or less, no PT proved to be as effective as PT (6 of 32 among no-PT recipients, and 5 of 24 among PT recipients who had a high school education or less). It was only among patients with college attendance or graduation that PT showed its differential superiority: 21 of 50 PT recipients showing a large improvement, compared to only 3 of 45 no-PT recipients. Similarly, 5 of 9 no-PT recipients with a superior outcome had been hospitalized one or more times in the year prior to the index study hospitalization, as had 4 of 7 PT high responders. However, except for the index hospitalization, 22 (or 85%) of the best PT responders had no other hospital admission in the previous year, but only 4 (or 44%) of the no-PT best responders were without hospitalization in the preceding year ($p = .07$). (Notably missing from the list of demographic predictors was any contribution of race and age to outcome.)

Perhaps the most revealing of demographic characteristics is the patient's sex (Table 2.7). As suggested earlier in the cross-sectional analysis, males are *over*represented and females *under*represented in the PT group having a large improvement. An opposite trend is noted for the no-PT condition, where females are found in proportionately greater numbers in the best-outcome group and males in the poorest-outcome group. The relative's ratings are also of interest. The best outcome among PT recipients was achieved among patients who lived in low-hostility families, but the fewer non-PT high improvers came from higher-hostility households (again reserved to trial 1 participants). The same could be said for the family's dissatisfaction with instrumental role performance: low pretreatment dissatisfaction among PT high responders, and higher dissatisfaction among no-PT high responders. The observation supports a long-standing belief of ours that family support contributes greatly to the success of more demanding psychosocial treatments that require continuing effort on the part of the patient. In fact, the absence of an intact family likely contributed greatly to the high relapse of trial 2 PT recipients, as de-

TABLE 2.7. Improvement by Sex and Treatment

	No improvement		Some improvement		Large improvement	
	PT	No PT	PT	No PT	PT	No PT
Males ($N = 80$)	5	16	19	19	18	3
Females ($N = 71$)	4	10	20	23	8	6

scribed earlier. While alcohol and drug abuse (as well as medication non-compliance) were relatively infrequent prior to study, PT responders surprisingly scored higher on these measures and no-PT responders scored considerably lower on these measures at study intake. This observation was quite intriguing—a suggestion that PT produced a larger degree of improvement than no PT among substance abusers. Briefly, the outcome of 36 no-PT patients who used any alcohol tended to be worse than the outcome of 33 PT recipients who used alcohol ($\chi^2 = 3.6$, $df = 2$, $p = .16$). More significantly, Table 2.8 illustrates that among the 20 patients who used alcohol excessively (7 drinks a day), PT recipients had the same superior outcomes as PT recipients that did not drink. No-PT patients who drank heavily had a significantly worse outcome ($\chi^2 = 7.4$, $df = 2$, $p = .02$). The same is true for the few patients who used cannabis. However, given the exclusion criterion that ruled out the more serious drug and alcohol abusers and the relatively small number of patients so affected, these observations must await further testing among more representative patients.

Prestudy clinical assessments are the most provocative and revealing of predictors, and nearly all these significant interactions with treatment follow a consistent pattern. The observation made for the general clinical predictors—that those patients who were most symptomatic at baseline improved the most over time—becomes highly qualified when we describe patients by their specific treatment condition. On these clinical measures, *it is the most symptomatic patient at baseline that responds best to PT and the least symptomatic patient that improves the most with no PT!* This disordinal interaction occurs on the total score derived from the BPRS at

TABLE 2.8. Heavy Alcohol and Any Cannabis Use and Outcome

	Deteriorated	Some improvement	Large improvement
Heavy alcohol use ($N = 20$)			
PT (8)	2 (25%)	3 (37.5%)	3 (37.5%)
No PT (12)	8 (66%)	3 (25%)	1 (9%)
Any cannabis use ($N = 17$)			
PT (8)	0 (0%)	5 (63%)	3 (37%)
No PT (9)	5 (56%)	4 (44%)	0 (0%)

TABLE 2.9. Treatment Outcomes According to Baseline Mean Scores on the BPRS Psychotic Symptom Cluster

Outcome	Baseline Psychotic Symptom Score	
	No PT ($N = 77$)	PT ($N = 74$)
No improvement	1.84	1.75
Some improvement	1.97	1.88
Large improvement	1.58	2.24

baseline, as well as the minor symptom and major symptom ($p = .06$) clusters and the hostility factor. So too with the patient's own self-report of anxious mood and euthymia derived from the Subjective Response Questionnaire, as well as the family's report of symptomatic behavior (the Katz Adjustment Scale R1 revision, $p = .08$). Table 2.9 illustrates this pattern using the major (psychotic) symptom cluster derived from the Brief Psychiatric Rating Scale.

Thus, good candidates for PT are not necessarily those that are in the best clinical remission; rather, one can more easily conclude that those who eventually improve most with PT are somewhat more anxious, willful, socially dysfunctional, and residually psychotic at baseline, particularly males, who nonetheless might have achieved more premorbidly and who often live with supportive families. Good responders to supportive therapy tend to be less clinically impaired and more often women, but include patients who were less successful premorbidly and who had a less supportive environment. Before we conclude this portrait of the appropriate treatment candidate, we need to note the interesting predictors of functional level that were observed independent of improvement.

Predictors of Functional Level

As mentioned above, when the outcome of interest is overall functional level, those who had functioned well in the past, including performance immediately prior to study intake, tended to function best at the end of treatment. Approximately 50% of all the variables analyzed support this observation, that is, very strong correlations between baseline and 3-year status. A detailed presentation of each variable would be redundant. It should be emphasized however, that nearly twice the number of PT recipients (33%) achieved the highest functional (group 3) outcome status compared to no-PT participants (17%). Thus, evidence of PT efficacy extends beyond the degree of improvement per se, and often includes patients whose functional level increased significantly even though the amount of improvement might have been less than 1 *SD*. This conclusion is supported by the observation that only 41% of patients who met one of the best-outcome criteria (large improvement or highest functional level) also met *both* outcome criteria. For example, only 14 (or 18%) of no-PT recipients achieved a superior (group 3) outcome, 6 meeting both improvement and final state criteria and 8 meeting only one criterion, whereas 34 (or 46%) of all PT recipients met one ($N = 20$) or both ($N = 14$) of these group 3 criteria. There are two variables (other than premorbid clinical status or psychiatric history) that are also informative: (1) a low level of pretreatment household EE was associated with high functional status at 3 years for both the PT and no-PT conditions; (2) the number of persons dependent on available family income was related to the highest functional level posttreatment, likely an indirect measure of expectations.

Otherwise, there are a few interactions with treatment that are informative. A baseline measure of locus of control, essentially a personal conviction as to whether one's future is dependent on chance or individual effort, shows that high internalizers (individual effort) eventually achieved a higher status while externalizers (chance) achieved a lower status with PT. (A trend in the opposite direction characterized the outcome status of no-PT recipients.) This observation was complemented by a more "realistic work attitude" and "adjustment to disability" among PT higher achievers. Elsewhere, two family reports were of interest. Much like the improvement previously associated with low familial dissatisfaction with expressive role performance, a low level of family dissatisfaction with instrumental role performance was associated with high functional status for PT recipients but a low functional status for no-PT patients. Family reports of actual performance also indicated that high PT achievers were doing best at baseline. Thus, family level of satisfaction or expectation is not always linearly related to outcome, but rather has an influence on ultimate status as a function of the treatment experience of the patient (i.e., a disordinal interaction). In a similar fashion, the highest-achieving PT recipients had *fewer* prior hospitalizations (2.0) but the best-achieving no-PT patients had the most prior hospitalizations (7.8), $p = .06$. The former were also less likely and the latter more likely to have carried a previous diagnosis of depression.

In sum, finding the right treatment for the right patient is easier said than done. The specific characteristics that we identify can only be considered suggestive, given the small numbers of patients often observed in one or more of the descriptive categories. But we can more confidently draw a few overarching conclusions related to outcome, preferred treatment, and patient characteristics. The first is something of a confirmation regarding a long-held suspicion of ours, namely, that it is the patient who is relatively "rich" in premorbid functioning and resources that tends to become "richer" with psychosocial treatment. However, no one should conclude that this represents a therapeutic bias. To the contrary, *a relevant psychosocial treatment appears absolutely necessary in order to realize the outcome potential of a good premorbid endowment!* As we comment upon in Chapter 7, the prevailing opinion of psychosocial treatment experts tends to ignore, if not disenfranchise, these less-disabled patients (who appear to do relatively well) by simply recommending outpatient checkups for the most part and tends to allocate most resources (essentially an array of necessary social services) to those who struggle to survive in the community (McEvoy et al., 1999). From our past review of psychosocial treatment studies (Schooler & Hogarty, 1987) as well as current experience, it seems that substantial reductions in morbidity and significant advances in functioning can indeed accrue to this relatively large population of better endowed patients provided they are offered a relevant psychosocial treatment. If anything, this population will likely increase in the future as the newer atypical antipsychotic medications find wider patient acceptance, with fewer subsequent relapses, rehospitalizations, side effects, and perhaps negative symptoms or progressive impairment. One might conclude from the above analyses that the best-outcome PT patients are literally "anxious" to get on with their lives, often seek shorter hospital stays at the expense of continuing symptoms, and otherwise embrace their individual psychosocial treatment experience.

Finally, there seems to be an important lesson that can be drawn from the improvement analyses for clinical consumers of the evidenced-based literature, as well as for those who actually design and execute these studies. Many maintenance studies of combined medication and psychosocial treatment show no differential effect of this combination over that achieved with medication alone, in studies of both affective disorder (e.g., E. Frank et al., 1990) and schizophrenia (e.g., Schooler et al., 1997). Uniformly, these investigators required that the patient either unequivocally respond to medication during treatment of the index episode (in the case of depression studies) or be able to survive a period of time without medication following the successful treatment of the index episode (in the case of the highly regarded schizophrenia collaborative study) prior to entering the maintenance study. If our PT predictors of improvement are any indication, such studies effectively exclude the very patients who would most likely show clinical improvement with combined medication and psychosocial treatment. Thus, in an evaluation of the psychosocial treatment literature, when improvement is the outcome of interest (measured in terms of personal and social adjustment, or reduced risk of relapse), it is important to note whether the more symptomatic, unstable, or dysfunctional patients have been precluded from maintenance study participation following treatment of the index episode.

Otherwise, supportive therapies are not without benefit and candidates. Those few patients who do relatively well tend to have been somewhat less accomplished in their preillness lives and carry a burden of prolonged social dysfunctioning, multiple episodes of illness, frequent hospitalizations, and reduced environmental support, yet appear to be more clinically stable at the beginning of the supportive therapy experience. Whether these characteristics speak to the nature of the schizophrenia diathesis or to the past failure of the treatment system is open to debate.

With the background, rationale, and empirical basis of PT thus reviewed, we now turn to the detailed description of the three phases that constitute PT, as well as the clinical prerequisites that support it.

CHAPTER THREE

Essential Prerequisites for Personal Therapy

While the practicing clinician might at times marvel at the published outcomes associated with novel and increasingly sophisticated psychosocial interventions for schizophrenia and other disorders, rarely (if ever) do these reports describe the substantial effort that was devoted to the clinical prerequisites that support a new therapeutic initiative. For decades our program has been guided by a silent mantra: *innovative psychosocial treatment is for naught unless the fundamentals of good care are firmly in place.* Much of the initial treatment experience provided to a recently hospitalized and often unfamiliar patient, for example, is focused on diagnostic and medication issues as well as the acquisition of material and human resources that are fundamental to a patient's survival in the community. The introduction of a novel psychosocial intervention presupposes the provision of psychological and material support, as well as the establishment of the most appropriate, safe, and effective medication program. Thus, this chapter reviews the essentials of—

- Psychological and material support
- Medication management

Our abiding philosophy has been that the recovery of function that is fostered by psychosocial treatment can be hindered or even reversed in the absence of exquisite medication management and an associated treatment

84

plan that addresses comorbid medical disorders. This is an important if not crucial distinguishing characteristic of our program; namely, that we do not aspire to treat psychologically the basic impairments of schizophrenia or associated disease states that give rise to medication-responsive symptoms, be they cognitive, affective, or behavioral in nature. Rather, our psychosocial treatment efforts build on the treatment-specific effects of medication on symptoms then move beyond the clear limitations of psychopharmacology to achieve social and vocational recovery. This includes positive and negative as well as residual symptoms (primarily those that are nonpsychotic in nature). Our psychosocial interventions will extend beyond the point where medication effects have appeared to plateau, as reviewed in Chapter 2. As we describe next, newer medications, particularly the atypical antipsychotic medications, make it possible for an ever-increasing number of patients to participate in psychosocial rehabilitation programs. A majority of our current protocol patients might never have been eligible for a novel rehabilitation program as recently as the early 1990s. Medication that reverses persistent psychosis (e.g., clozapine) as well as the new "first-line," atypical antipsychotic drugs no longer burden patients with such (extrapyramidal) side effects as those that impact on volition, motivation, stamina, and psychomotor retardation or excess (e.g., akinesia or akathisia). Nor is anticholinergic medication routinely required for such patients in this new medication era, thus reducing such anticholinergic side effects as those that adversely affect verbal memory (McEvoy & Freter, 1989) that is fundamental to learning-based rehabilitation programs. In short, never before have the conditions been as favorable for a successful psychosocial treatment experience for schizophrenia patients as they are today.

It might appear to be cognitively dissonant to suggest that maintenance medication is the cornerstone of a new psychotherapy—or that the well-known and widely endorsed principles of supportive therapy (ST) that had been prescribed for decades, long before the conceptualization of PT was attempted, are central to its practice. For this reason we have elected to take the process of what is commonly referred to as "warm medication" and to describe these components of support and chemotherapy as the sine qua non of PT implementation. By reserving these fundamentals to a separate chapter, we hope to underscore their importance as the primary ingredients of good care, a basic (though not sufficient) standard of care that has traditionally stood on its own. In fact, psychological and material support and medication management (together with the fundamentals of a therapeutic alliance and the provision of a generic form of psychoeducation) constituted the successful ST experience of control subjects during the PT studies, as previously described.

Given the relative neglect of psychopharmacology fundamentals during the training of most nonpsychiatrists, a relatively greater elaboration of this topic is provided in this chapter. Regarding the principles of supportive therapy, we shall only touch on the techniques that characterize psychological support, since these have been the substance of innumerable volumes and articles over the years. For recent and past reviews, including the application of supportive psychotherapy among schizophrenia patients, the reader can consult the following reports: Wasylenki (1992); Forrest (1994); Fenton and McGlashan (1999); Eaton (1996); Buckley and Lys (1996); Kates and Rockland (1994); Mace and Margison (2000); Winston, Pinsker, and McCullough (1986); McGlashan (1983); Gomes-Schwartz (1984); Weiden and Havens (1994); Coursey (1989); and Sarti and Cournos (1990). Less frequently reported, and often neglected because of unfamiliarity or because of ambivalence about dependency issues, is the provision of material support, a necessary form of care that has too often assumed a secondary role in the office-based treatment of schizophrenia and other severe mental illnesses. Although some may consider it more a social service than a part of therapy, we devote considerable attention below to the acquisition of selected types of material support, particularly the method and process of accessing Social Security benefits.

Finally, while additional fundamentals of good care also stand independent of PT (such as joining with the patient, conducting a needs assessment, and establishing the treatment contract), we have chosen to address these practice principles in Chapter 4 as elements of basic phase PT, since the substance of the therapeutic alliance and the treatment plan dictates the application of PT strategies. In practice, of course, the distinction between PT and the independent fundamentals of good care are more logical than real. We present them separately both for convenience and as a way to describe more concisely and clearly the specific techniques as well as the process that are embodied in PT.

PSYCHOLOGICAL AND MATERIAL SUPPORT

Psychological Support

In both its forms, "support" is directed toward facilitating day-to-day functioning rather than skill acquisition. (Some have referred to PT as simply a form of "supportive psychotherapy," ignoring the active participation of patients in developing awareness and acquiring coping strategies.) Psychological support, however, is a clinical response that will permeate each PT session in all three phases. It includes *attending to*, *observing*, *listening to*, and *responding to* the patient's personal accounts and descriptions of subjective state. Closely associated with this "therapeutic" listening (Wasylenki, 1992) is a *correct empathy* when responding, an emotional posture that leaves the patient assured that the clinician is genuinely trying to understand the reality of the patient's feelings and thinking. (Often this empathy is conveyed by temporarily suspending the established agenda of a PT session during a time of crisis.) The well-known dictum to *begin where the patient is* has particular relevance to schizophrenia, given the constraints on understanding, motivation, and performance that are imposed by persistent symptoms or residual problems in cognitive functioning. Otherwise, appropriate *reassurance* is an abiding characteristic of psychological support, one that is tempered by realistic assumptions regarding the pace of treatment and recovery as well as a recognition of the likely residual impairments, disabilities, and social handicaps that will vary within and between patients. Remaining features of psychological support include the *reinforcement* and *encouragement* of the patient's own health-promoting activities as well as the message that it is appropriate to rely on the therapist for advocacy and practical problem solving in times of crisis.

While most clinicians will readily attest that they routinely provide "supportive psychotherapy," in our experience few are able to cite a specific theoretical basis for their intervention and likely defer to an "eclectic" approach when queried. Whether the practice orientation is Rogerian, Adelerian, Jungian, or Sullivanian in nature seems of little concern. However, their supportive therapy orientation has great bearing on how clinicians will proceed with treatment, be it the modification of impaired psychosocial development, a response to defense mechanisms, or the interaction between vulnerability and environment (Gomes-Schwartz, 1984). The supportive therapy stance of PT adopts the interpersonal (rather than intrapsychic), psychosociobiological orientation. It assumes that while patients are not responsible for their biological vulnerability, they do have an active role in its management, both through the appropriate use of pharmacotherapy and the acquisition of effective coping strategies that enhance knowledge and mastery of potentially dysregulating relationships.

Independent of theory, the manner by which clinicians interact with patients in the supportive role can be characterized as personal and friendly. However, as described by Winston et al. (1986), it is a friendliness that is always governed by a purpose, namely, the goals of the treatment plan. Otherwise, the clinician runs the risk of overidentification that is more characteristic of a nonprofessional friendship, including the possibility of collusion with the patient's inappropriate construction of reality, or reinforcement of negative affect and self-disparagement. Effective support imparts an acceptance of the patient's disabilities as well as confidence in existing abilities, regardless of the length or malignancy of the psychiatric history. Catharsis and ventilation, rather than being viewed as purposeless exercises, can often provide the opportunity for attentive listening and a sensitive assessment of the patient's concerns related to important relationships, vocational aspirations, and health and economic issues. In PT, however, catharsis and ventilation are not goals per se, but rather serve as the medium within which the explicit principles of PT are provided and evaluated. Otherwise, psychological support can become an aimless (and endless) exercise in verbalization. Therapist self-disclosure can also be useful, provided that it is appropriate and does not violate personal boundaries by being too personal, intrusive, or emotionally provocative. The examples shared with the patient should not serve to trivialize the problems reported by the patient (Weiden & Havens, 1994).

In contrast to most psychoanalytically influenced approaches, we generally desist from "interpretation" as a practice principle except in rare instances when negative transference might preclude the patient's acceptance of or continuation in treatment. Even here the explanations used to clarify resistance are invariably nonthreatening and gently focus on reengaging the patient in treatment. Negative countertransference among therapists includes a wide range of often troublesome attitudes and affects concerning the patient. In our opinion the attitude most frequently encountered is a variant of "expressed emotion." Dissatisfaction and/or the withholding of warmth and regard can lead to rejection of the patient or premature termination from treatment when the patient fails to meet treatment goals in spite of months or even years of therapist effort. In these rare cases, if the therapist is an otherwise skillful clinician, reassignment of the case to a new primary clinician is often the most feasible and practical approach to take. Psychological support is also apparent in the "advice-giving" provisions of PT such as the psychoeducation curriculum and when it is necessary for the patient to rely upon the therapist's problem solving and advocacy skills. PT's response to "faulty defenses" occurs in the intermediate stage exercises addressed to communication styles, and in the advanced stage when the reciprocal relationship between the patient's affect and coping strategies and the behavioral response of others are addressed. In the last analysis, the foremost contribution of psychological support during the PT process is the comfort and reassurance provided for the patient through the presence of a consistently available, confident, respectful and attentive clinician who can skillfully negotiate the intricacies of a treatment plan, as well as husband the family and community resources needed for its successful implementation.

Material Support

While the provision of services defined as material support appears at face value to be a benign activity, it is one that has frequently fallen outside the traditional scope of psychotherapy and has sometimes represented an ethical dilemma for many clinicians. For this reason, we now describe in greater detail the components of material support that we believe are central to the patient's welfare. Beginning with the deinstitutionalization movement, case management services became the preferred response to material needs in the absence of integrated community programs (Baronet & Gerber, 1998). Many if not most forms of intensive or regular case management narrowly focused on the tasks of brokering and coordinating services, but with limited success (Mueser, Bond, Drake, & Resnick, 1998). In PT, however, the provision of services needed to meet common human needs occurs in a process that is similar to the clinical or therapeutic case management model described by Kanter (1989). Material support is thus an integral part of the PT therapeutic process, as it should be in all forms of standard care. During PT, it becomes a seamless set of services that fosters and promotes the patient's treatment plan and the goals of symptom stabilization, knowledge acquisition, skill attainment, and recovery of social and vocational functioning.

Some case management services are less controversial than others. Among the former, access to competent and comprehensive medical care is crucial. While the quantity, quality, and frequency of services might differ from one health insurance plan to another, patients are increasingly able to make a choice, especially Medicaid-eligible patients. It has become incumbent upon therapists to review the various plans available and to assist patients in making the choice that best accommodates individual health needs, both psychiatric and medical. One of the benefits for a patient that has participated in a clinical research trial, for example, has been the careful medical examinations that have often led to the detection of previously undiagnosed (or poorly managed) medical illnesses such as hypertension, diabetes, renal/hepatic disease, and the consequences of heavy smoking or obesity. (As many as 50% of the seriously mentally ill

have concurrent systemic disease [Goldman, 1999].) Psychotropic medications need to be finely coordinated with the primary-care treatment of
systemic, infectious, or contagious disease if clinical stability and recovery
are to be achieved and sustained. The competent practice of PT (and other
forms of psychiatric care) should always begin with a comprehensive medical examination and a review of the medical history, with the coordinated
management of a medical illness made with the patient's primary-care
physician.

Otherwise the acquisition of supported housing for residentially unstable patients is often necessary. While we most certainly do not recommend routine "familiectomies," as our efforts in developing family psychoeducation clearly demonstrate (Anderson et al., 1986), there does
come a time in many adult patient lives when loved ones pass on or move
away. For others, life together is acknowledged as being unfeasible or lo-
gistically impossible. Criteria for implementing *supported* housing often
include a current difficulty in maintaining independent quarters, including
medication noncompliance in the face of persistent symptoms, as well as a
destabilizing social isolation and the absence of needed social supports.
Declines in nutritional status, personal hygiene, and financial competence
are often telltale indicators that the patient cannot independently maintain
a domicile at the present time.

Initiatives needed to secure financial assistance are often more difficult for some clinicians to endorse. These include the (ever decreasing) resources of the public welfare system, and more importantly, the entitlement programs represented by Social Security Disability Income (SSDI)
and Supplemental Security Income (SSI). Unfortunately, in our opinion,
many mental health providers resist an active role in accessing these benefits because of the effort required or because of concerns related to "encouraging dependency" and/or a belief that symptomatically stable patients are able to work immediately. We have resolved whatever slight
ambivalence might have existed in this area based upon an experience with
schizophrenia that now spans several decades. First, the challenge of
achieving stabilization is practically impossible to accomplish while the
patient remains financially impoverished and uncertain as to whether
food, shelter, clothing, and utilities, for example, will be reliably available.
Second, even the most symptomatically stable patient can quickly decom-
pensate in the face of everyday life events that would not evoke such a catastrophic response among the unaffected. Unless attempts at employment
early in the recovery period are supported, structured, and constrained in
terms of hours worked, and unless job responsibilities are introduced in a

manner that accommodates the slow resolution of less-apparent cognitive deficits, then a rapid resumption of work can provoke a recurrence of symptoms in our experience (see Goldberg et al., 1977, for a relevant example). Such ideal employment opportunities have rarely been made available to schizophrenia patients in the early stages of recovery. The process of social and vocational community integration takes time (see Chapter 6), and being financially destitute in the interim clearly does not serve the goal of recovery. Third, until we unequivocally know the "cause" and the "cure" of schizophrenia and can confidently offer an assurance for continued symptom remission, we inappropriately deprive patients of their legal right to public programs by discouraging or ignoring their desire to access these entitlements. Only when the process of recovery leads to *sustained* clinical stability, employment, and a developed sense of self-sufficiency should thought be given to terminating these entitlement programs.

The "dependency" opponents cite evidence that SSDI and SSI recipients are often reluctant to compromise benefits by seeking gainful employment once they are clinically stable. Our response to this concern is that the problem rests more with the system than with the patient. For example, a 1999 increase in the monthly wage base that triggers a loss of SSDI benefits (from $500 to $780 at the moment) will likely stimulate the employment aspirations of many mentally ill patients, as would other needed modifications to the law. (This wage cap is now indexed to inflation.) Further, in December 1999, a new federal law was passed that enables states to better support disabled patients who return to work (see below). Rarely has a schizophrenia patient deliberately tried to "beat the system" in our experience, but given the limitations in our understanding of the uncertain course of schizophrenia, it is better to be safe than sorry, even in these instances. Recent evidence suggests that homeless patients, for example, that receive Social Security benefits use the money on basic necessities that improve their quality of life, rather than on drugs and alcohol, as has sometimes been claimed (Rosenheck, Dausey, Frisman, & Kasprow, 2000).

Since many patients are unfortunately deprived of Social Security benefits through the absence of therapist advocacy or because of confusion about the law and the application process, we next discuss the nature of these benefit programs and the successful strategies that we have used in accessing them for the majority of our patients. The qualifications that apply to the various benefits are sufficiently detailed that we shall simply provide a broad description of the programs. While some readers of this volume may well reside in countries other than the United States, we assume that the issues related to public benefits should be relevant elsewhere and perhaps might evoke the same clinical concerns.

Social Security Benefits

There are three important clinical considerations that need to be appreciated when accessing SSDI or SSI benefits. First, the very process of applying for such benefits requires that patients come to appreciate how they are functionally disabled, a rare event for those who might have been in denial. Inevitably, this awareness will become an important goal of the PT treatment plan itself! Second, in the process of applying (or reapplying) for Social Security benefits, the clinician needs to paint a picture of *disability* that extends well beyond symptoms or clinical state. Third, once the provisions of the law are understood by patients (e.g., the availability of trial work periods), it is our experience that patients become more (not less) likely to attempt work once they are clinically stable. Most Social Security Administration (SSA) representatives are sensitive and compassionate people who want to see the law applied in a fair and appropriate manner. Honest, candid, and nontechnical descriptions of how schizophrenia will keep the patient from working in the next year will usually serve to establish trusting and mutually respectful relationships among the Social Security adjudicator, patient, and clinician.

The SSA oversees the Title II and Title XVI programs that pay disability benefits. Mentally ill patients constitute a large percentage of the persons served by this agency, and the review and appeal of claims can draw upon valuable clinic resources and at times even threaten the clinical stability of the patient. It is not only the quantity but also the quality of information to be reported that often troubles the clinician. While the clinical record not surprisingly contains clinical information, the SSA requires information concerning *functional disability*. Beyond the symptoms that are familiar to clinicians, the SSA needs to know what the impairments, disabilities, and handicaps of the illness are and why the patient is unable to work. Impairments are the basic disruptions caused by the illness process. A person that is nearsighted, for example, has impaired eyesight. Disabilities refer to what the patients cannot do. The nearsighted person cannot see adequately without corrective lenses. And handicaps refer to the functional implications of the impairments and disabilities such as social roles that patients are unable to assume even following modification of a disability. Someone with corrected eyesight, for example, might still not see well enough to function in a previous role, such as a pilot. In schizophrenia, a basic impairment might be an impoverished cognition (with poverty of speech and thought, and a lack of motivation). The disability could present in the form of difficulty in planning and problem solving or in initiating behavior. The patient could be handicapped by having work roles precluded that require the ability to express needs or opinions, to maintain high stamina and interest, to be socially engaged, or to give a credible account of work performance and responsibilities. (See Chapter 7 for operational definitions of disability.)

The transition from reporting symptoms to thinking in terms of functional disability is a difficult one for many therapists. While the SSA is interested in symptoms such as hallucinations as proof that the patient is ill, symptoms per se do not provide evidence of disability. Why, for instance, can't someone who hears voices work? A compelling explanation is required as to how the voices lead to impaired concentration for the patient, which in turn leads to an inability to work at tasks that require attention to detail or to people and would thus disqualify a claimant from many types of work. Experienced clinicians have all known patients with residual positive symptoms who have somehow been gainfully employed. By comparison, however, many patients who appear to be in a decent remission of positive symptoms can nevertheless be functionally quite disabled by negative symptoms and/or by cognitive deficits in the reception, processing, and response to sensory input that impact upon attention, memory, and problem-solving abilities. Impoverished, disorganized, or rigid thinking are often important sources of impairment among asymptomatic patients. Over the years, millions of applications for disability benefits have been denied, and many of these might have been avoided had therapists been properly prepared. This lack of preparation is understandable given the intricacies of the law and the system.

Title II

Title II includes the SSDI program as well as the Social Security retirement program that politicians are so desperate to "save" these days. Title II is considered to be an insurance program paid from the FICA (Federal Insurance Contributions Act) premiums that most working Americans contribute from their wages. Title II is not means tested, and neither nonwage income nor the total worth of a person has any bearing whatsoever on benefit eligibility! This has significant implications, since patients can retain savings and possessions such as homes and cars and still receive

Title II benefits. The amount of the benefit depends on how much the patient had *contributed* into the system (equivalent to the retirement benefit) as well as the *date of onset* of his or her disability. The importance of establishing the correct date of onset cannot be overemphasized. The amount of the benefit, or even the approval or denial of a claim, depends on this critical piece of information. The clinician is often the most instrumental person in determining the date of onset. In principle, any adjudicator in the SSA could carefully review a record and establish a date of onset. In practice, however, most adjudicators have neither the time to review a comprehensive record nor sufficient confidence in the information available to feel comfortable with the task. Therefore, determinations are often made conservatively and patients can be denied benefits to which they are entitled. When the therapist advocates for disability benefits, it does not mean that he or she is saying that the patient can *never* work, only that the illness will likely keep the patient from working in the next 12 months.

The SSA will release to the patient a list of employment quarters and FICA contributions that will help in determining eligibility. A certain number of quarterly contributions are required immediately prior to the date of onset of the disability in order to qualify for SSDI. Younger people are given preferential treatment since they may not have had time to accumulate enough quarters before coming ill. While 40 quarters are needed for retirement, the number required for a disability benefit depends on the year of birth (e.g., six credits in the last 3 years for those born after 1975). Because the clinician's report typically sets the date of onset, great care must be taken to document the subsequent period of disability even if several decades need to be accommodated. The SSA will typically look to see whether the date of disability onset corresponds to the date last worked, a process that reflects a certain naïveté about the developmental origin of psychosis. In reality, the onset of disability often *precedes* the last work period. Take, for example, the patient who worked for 3 years until age 21, when he became acutely ill and disabled. At age 23, he recovered sufficiently such that he worked for 3 months in a convenience store, but then lost the job because he had been undercharging customers for months. The claim needs to document the onset date at age 21. Even though the patient worked for 3 months at age 23, he was clearly disabled during that time and during the preceding 2 years as well. (The 3 months of work could, however, constitute a "quarter" when determining the amount of the benefit.) The clinician should not rely solely on the clinical record. The patient and family should be interviewed in order to account for the time not described in the clinical record. The patient need not be floridly psychotic throughout the period of disability. Again, even if a patient returns to work for a period of time, he or she may still be considered disabled if work performance was considerably impaired. Accurate documentation of date of the onset is also important for another section of Title II law. The adult child of a retired, disabled, or deceased parent (who had been receiving Title II benefits) is also eligible for SSDI provided the onset of illness was before age 22, a frequent characteristic of schizophrenia. For many patients who became disabled prior to age 22 and before they accumulated enough quarters to qualify for SSDI, this little-known provision of the law can help them eventually qualify for the benefit based on a *parent's* work history! Once again, the ability of the clinician to review the patient's history and convincingly establish an age of onset and continuity of disability may mean the difference between a favorable and an unfavorable claim decision.

Once a patient has received SSDI benefits, there are two ways for him or her to return to work while maintaining benefits. The first is a 9-month "trial work" period in which there is no upper limit to what a patient can earn in any given month (the minimum needed to qualify as substantial work is about $560 per month at the moment). If the patient is unable to sustain employment, he or she can try again 60 months following an individual trial-work month. (For example, if a patient worked for 5 months 6 years ago and for 4 months 3 years ago, he or she would be eligible for a new 5-month trial work period immediately and be eligible for an additional 4 months of trial work in 2 years.) At the end of 9 months, the SSA typically allows another 3-month "grace period" if the patient has been successfully employed. The second method for continuing employment that will not compromise benefits pertains to the "substantial gainful activity" (SGA) cap. A patient can earn $780 per month (up from $500), a rate that is now indexed to inflation. Increasing the SGA, as noted above, will likely motivate many employed patients to work more hours. Again, when determining work capacity and the SGA cap, honesty is the best policy. The SSA has the authority to terminate benefits if it feels that someone is manipulating the system (e.g., keeping monthly earnings just below the cap). Also, the cap is not inflexible. If a patient needs to pay $100 per month for the management of his or her disability (e.g., for medication or psychotherapy), then this $100 can be added to the cap by the SSA representative such that the patient is allowed to earn $880 per month and not lose the benefit at the time of this writing.

Title XVI (Supplemental Security Income)

Title XVI is a means-tested program for the needy that provides approximately $545 per month at the moment, often more than public welfare. About 15 states now supplement this federal contribution. While the $545 is indexed to inflation, the state supplement is not. The section of the program for the disabled is called Supplemental Security Income (SSI). A claimant can qualify for SSI benefits without ever having contributed to FICA. However, there is a clear downside to SSI. In order for a person to qualify for SSI there are restrictions on the total value of the patient's financial and capital assets, including any source of income—typically cumulated wealth that exceeds $2,000 in value. These capital assets include not only property and bank accounts but also the cash value of whole-life insurance policies and retirement accounts. Sometimes a patient will have relatively small assets that prevent him or her from qualifying, and it will fall to the therapist to suggest liquidating some of those assets in order to qualify. For many patients, applying for SSI is a difficult experience. They are asked to come to terms in a swift and concrete manner with the fact that they are disabled. Their small assets often constitute a source of pride and are the symbols of independence. Psychologically, their loss can be far from trivial.

There are times when the SSI process works in strange ways that can confound the patient. For example, if the adjudication and appeals process for SSI had been lengthy (which it often is), a successful claimant will receive an initial payment of many thousands of dollars in back benefits, enough to make the patient fail the means test that he or she passed in order to get the benefit in the first place (i.e., "Catch 22") . Under the law, patients are required to "spend down" those benefits within a limited time. A failure to do so will result in a loss of the SSI benefits. For example, if the SSA makes a determination that an SSI beneficiary has accepted subsequent payments while his or her assets were above $2,000 (from the initial check), an overpayment judgment will be issued and the claimant could be required to repay a considerable sum of money. This places many patients in the position of having to spend a large sum of money quickly and many lack the requisite judgment and experience to do so responsibly. Once again, this becomes both a practical problem and a stressor that the therapist will need to negotiate with the patient. (Since some patients are unable to adjust to these realities, it is always essential to carefully examine the course of the illness, including the date of eligibility onset, and work history with the goal of first obtaining the *non-means-tested* Title II SSDI benefit.) Often the local welfare department will work with the clinician in order to remove a patient from welfare and become SSI eligible. However, once the patient receives the initial SSI check, the welfare department will likely demand a reimbursement for those overlapping months of SSI and welfare payments. Means-tested programs in the United States continue to be meager and often demeaning and complex despite popular myths to the contrary. If the patient receiving SSI returns to work, he or she will lose $1 for every $2 earned in excess of $85 per month at the moment.

Finally, clinicians are well advised to pay close attention to the issue of health insurance for their patients and to be aware of the ramifications associated with being a recipient of either Medicare or Medicaid. Medicaid is the state-administered but federally supported means-tested federal health insurance program. All SSI recipients are eligible (as are welfare recipients), but some SSDI recipients might not meet the means test for income and thus be ineligible for Medicaid. SSDI recipients are eligible for Medicare, but only after 2 years. While Medicare is not means tested, it provides less coverage than Medicaid and requires a monthly fee. Many patients are eligible for both SSDI and SSI, such that in instances where the SSDI payments would be lower than the SSI, the latter might in certain cases be preferable since the health insurance options are better.

On December 17, 1999, the Ticket to Work and Work Incentives Improvement Act (PL 106-170) was signed into law and addressed some of the disincentives in the disability benefit programs. Foremost, the act allows (but does not require) states to provide extended Medicare health coverage to SSDI recipients for an additional 4.5 years beyond the trial-work period even when patients earn more than the SGA cap. SSI recipients can be allowed by states to continue Medicaid coverage when they return to work (on a sliding scale) even if their income rises up to 250% of the poverty level. Further, states now have the option of offering Medicaid to employed mentally disabled individuals if such health coverage would deter patients from seeking disability benefits in the future. These programs are made more attractive to states through a Federal matching grant. In addition, there is provision for an "expedited" return to SSI or SSDI benefits if an acute exacerbation of illness prevents a person from continuing employment. Starting in 2002 patients are protected from "unscheduled" disability reviews that are often triggered when they return to work. As for the year 2001, some patients were offered "vouchers" that would enable them to choose their employment/rehab provider and to secure supportive services for as long as 5 years. (However, it appears that the provider will be paid only if the outcome is successful.) At the moment, the "ticket-to-work" program is not fully implemented. Other actions are being considered that would allow SSDI beneficiaries to more gradually reduce their benefit when their continuing employment exceeds the SGA cap. The overall effects of these changes will likely encourage more patients to seek employment and to reassure clinicians that their advocacy for disability benefits does not result in a sentence to life-long dependency.

Applying for Social Security Benefits

Any individuals who believe that they have a disability that will keep them from working in the next year can report to their local Social Security office. Some schizophrenia patients may be too ill to go on their own, and the therapist will have to make a judgment about how to get them to the SSA office to make an application. (A recent study indicates that patients who failed to apply for benefits were more impatient, disorganized, and less willing to follow the application procedures [Rosenheck et al., 2000].) If the patient is receiving public assistance, the local welfare office may have workers willing to accompany the patient, since it is in their interest to have the patient qualify for Social Security benefits. Case managers can also be enlisted to help. In some instances, it may be wise for the therapist to accompany the patient. The clinician should first try to determine whether the patient is eligible for Title II or Title XVI, or both, and then instruct the patient to specifically apply for the correct program(s). Without this assistance, the patient might well be eligible for one program but apply to the other one, for which he or she is ineligible, and thus be turned down. Sometimes patients are reluctant to apply even though they desire the benefit and believe themselves to be disabled. This reluctance can stem from residual psychosis but more often than not from fear and misinformation about the program. (More federal money is now available to correctly inform patients about the complex trial-work program.) Among the most common fears is that the patient will be required to spend down savings (a correct concern if the patient is applying to SSI, but not for SSDI), and a fear that he or she will be made to answer embarrassing questions. (While there are a large number of questions to be answered, only a small minority of patients actually experience them as embarrassing.) Finally, there is a fear that he or she will need to go through a prolonged litigation process and appear before a judge. However, if the correct information is provided, litigation can most often be avoided.

The patient should be advised whom to list as the treating doctor, an important piece of information. Licensed physicians and psychologists are recognized as treating doctors. If the request for information is mailed to a person or an office that is not connected to the treating clinician, it is unlikely that a report will be filed and the patient will be referred for an independent psychologist or physician evaluation. Since the independent evaluator does not know the patient, the chances for speedy approval of a claim are greatly reduced. If the treating clinician is not a licensed physician or psychologist, the prescribing psychiatrist can sign off on the information, including the detailed report provided by the treating clinician. In our experience, the prescribing psychiatrist might have less time available to complete a detailed disability evaluation than the nonphysician therapist. Frequently, the request for information comes to the (nondoctor) treating clinician but still requires the signature of the doctor. It is helpful if patients are instructed to share all correspondence from the SSA with the clinician so that any misunderstandings can be quickly resolved. Most correspondence has the name and phone number of a Social Security adjudicator at the bottom. Calling the adjudicator and introducing yourself as the treating clinician is advisable. Adjudicators are typically pleased to learn that they will receive an accredited report within the required time. Many prefer information from the treating clinician (doctor or not) because of the correct assumption that this is the preferred way to obtain accurate information. Adjudicators will often offer an extension to a filing deadline if they feel confident about receiving a complete report in a reasonable period of time.

The Patient and Therapist Reports

Shortly after a patient applies, he or she will receive a form in the mail with a set of questions about daily activities. The therapist should have the patient bring this form to a session where it can be completed jointly. The questions relate to how the patient spends his or her time, what sort of activities are engaged in, and how competent the patient is at managing his or her affairs. Patients will very often tend to *overestimate* what they do and how well they do it! *Therefore it is important not to take the patient's en-*

tire account at face value! For example, when one patient was asked how he spent his day, the answer was "I watch really interesting shows on TV." On further inquiry, the clinician discovered that the patient simply sat and watched the weather channel for long periods of time yet was unable to remember the forecast. These distinctions are very important since a few words can change the picture presented to the SSA from one of unqualified ability to clear disability. Again, completing the form also provides a clear opportunity to initiate the process of adjustment to disability (see Chapter 5) and the creation of the treatment plan (Chapter 4) At the time of filing, many patients are in denial about their illness. Others simply know very little about their illness, either associating it with symptoms alone or offering idiosyncratic explanations. Few know how they are disabled and why they can't work. A common reason offered for needing disability is "I can't work because I hear voices." The completion of the report is the first opportunity that many patients have to understand how they are disabled. (This understanding is frequently an added incentive to master the techniques of PT.)

Some weeks after the patient completes his or her report, a request for information will come to the treating clinician or doctor of record. Completing this report is more of a chore, yet will influence the claim decision more than the patient's report. Since information about *disability* is rarely found in the medical record, interviews with the patient and significant others are advised, as indicated earlier. Minor details that normally do not appear in the clinical record need to be carefully documented. But the report is far more than a collection of facts. Rather, a graphic image of the patient's disability can provide the foundation for a successful claim—*and* for the treatment plan itself!

Selected information bears on the determination of a claim. In many states, an outline of relevant issues will be provided to the clinician. In all states, the adjudicator will seek to form an image of the patient and why he or she is disabled. Specifically, the adjudicator will want to know (1) the impairments associated with the illness; (2) what it is that the patient cannot do as a result of these impairments (i.e., the disabilities); and (3) what major roles the patient is excluded from performing as a result of the disabilities (i.e., the handicaps). This way of thinking is foreign to many clinicians who have been trained to focus largely on clinical symptoms. Information is not routinely collected and documented in the medical record regarding the impairments, disabilities, and handicaps that are central to determining a disability claim. After reading the report, the adjudicator or any reasonable person should be able to form a vivid picture of how the claimant is disabled and what prevents him or her from working. Since *deviance from social norms* is an important aspect of disability, evidence of such deviance should be emphasized.

Many clinicians are tempted to write a "neutral" report and let the facts speak for themselves. Such motivations seem to arise from a fear of appearing too partial or adversarial, or simply reflect an ambivalence regarding "dependency." While understandable, this approach is generally unhelpful. Adjudicators are reluctant to make decisions without a clear statement on the record, and without such a statement they often choose to disallow a claim. Clinicians are well advised to gather the information and then, based on their clinical and rehabilitation judgment, answer the following question: "Is this patient really capable of working independently in the coming year?" If the answer is no, then the report should paint a clear picture of how the patient is disabled. Below are discussed some of the important areas that are included in the body of the report. This is where the "rubber hits the road," so to speak, regarding the justification of a claim.

Diagnosis and Date of Onset. The importance of a diagnosis is self-evident, and the therapist should check the medical record for all previous diagnoses. The current diagnosis should be specifically recorded, since the SSA will request information from the medical record. If there are different diagnoses, some explanation should be given. For example, the patient may have been diagnosed as suffering a bipolar disorder in the past but the recent presentation may be an unequivocal schizoaffective disorder. The importance of establishing the date of onset has already been emphasized. The therapist should be careful to document the date of the onset of *disability,* not of the current diagnosis or episode. For example, a patient may have presented initially with a diagnosis of adjustment reaction and subsequently was unable to work. Sometime later, with the appearance of frank psychotic symptoms, a diagnosis of schizophrenia was established. The SSA will often try to link the onset with the date of the schizophrenia diagnosis, thus effectively denying the patient benefits for a longer period of disability. In cases where the clinician truly believes that the onset predates the current diagnosis, this should be clearly stated. A brief justification of the rationale for the earlier date of onset should be presented and such points should be reiterated throughout the report.

Medication. Most states will ask about medications and the medication strategy. The most recent medications and their effects will be sufficient for a claim, except in the case where the therapist is attempting to establish a date of onset. In those instances, a more extensive discussion of medications dating back to the date of onset may be needed. When this information is not easily garnered from the medical record, it is often useful to ask patients and family members to provide it. The clinician should alert the adjudicator, however, regarding sources of information other than the medical record.

Hospitalizations. This information is also useful in establishing the severity of illness as well as the date of onset. When not available in the medical record (patients may have been hospitalized at institutions that might not release information quickly), it is necessary to retrieve information from the patient and family, and again the source of the information on the report should be indicated. When eliciting information about hospitalization(s), the therapist should look beyond the date of admission and the length of stay. The clinical state of the patient preceding the hospitalization as well as during the aftercare disposition are also important. Many times patients will simply say, "I lost my job because I got sick." The complex process by which people become overwhelmed with stressors and begin to experience symptoms is not captured by such a simplified account. Eliciting a more complete picture of a decompensation and hospitalization provides both vital information for the report and grist for PT. For example, the therapist might ask, "Could you give me a better picture of how you gradually became ill? After all, one is not healthy one day and sick the next." Even the more paranoid patients can recognize how environmental stress can contribute to decompensation and hospitalization. For example, one patient stated, "Yeah, they did something to my brain, implanted some kind of chip or something. But working all those hours at the mall sure didn't help. I got real run down, and I was getting nervous and forgetting things. I got that pressure again in my head and had to go back to the hospital." In one stroke the clinician can collect information needed to establish disability while also identifying specific prodromal signs of the illness.

Neuropsychological Testing. Often the medical record will contain the results of neuropsychological testing. Sometimes raw scores are available. While the results of testing are not the most important aspect of a report, they do help. For the adjudicator, test results can be tangible evidence of impairment. The utility of test results is greatest, however, when the clinician knows how to interpret the tests and how to connect them to aspects of disability. Often the test already includes an interpretation and explanation of deficits by a trained neuropsychologist, and this can be described in the report.

Current Social Situation. Establishing how independently a patient lives and how greatly he or she depends on the support of others is an important component of the disability determination. Therapists are well advised to document the degree to which patients are dependent on others for their living arrangement and social support. The material and social support a claimant receives from others is important evidence of disability (e.g., living with family or in supported housing). If the patient cannot live independently, then his or her ability to work is called into question.

Mental Status. Mental status is a multifaceted concept that extends beyond the traditional clinical account. The specific questions may vary from state to state, but the basic gist remains constant. Therapists are well advised not to answer the questions in a literal fashion, but rather to think how the patient's illness presents to the public.

1. *Appearance* need not only apply to the patient's grooming and dress but to the general visual presentation that a patient makes. A patient who is well dressed and well groomed but appears hunched over and apprehensive is likely to appear deviant at a job interview. Therefore, painting a visual picture of the patient's appearance for the adjudicator is advisable.

2. *Behavior and psychomotor activity* refers to those obvious characteristics of slowing or agitation related to symptom patterns. This is an opportunity to go beyond the brief statement that the patient appears agitated and say, for example, "The patient appears extremely restless, often standing up and leaving the room to use the toilet at least three times during an hour interview."

3. *Characteristics of speech* refer to production and content as well as organization and fluidness. Idiosyncratic language and disorganized speech should be noted as well as the contextual relevance of verbal production. Rambling or pressured speech are particularly illustrative. Offering an example is helpful: "Excuse, sir, excuse me, sir, excuse me . . . but I am . . . I don't mean to interrupt, excuse me but . . . you know . . . can I be excused?" Impoverished speech is also disabling, such as uninformative answers to inquiries about general well-being ("I dunno" or "OK, I guess").

4. *Mood*. Mood falls into a realm well known by clinicians. Evidence of impaired mood, if present, should be presented as well as the pharmacological treatment prescribed. The associated disability should be illustrated: "The patient's depressed mood keeps him from concentrating. It is therefore difficult for him to read or follow instructions."

5. *Affective expression*. Blunted, depressed, or manic affects should be described in ways that enable the adjudicator to appreciate their disabling and deviant nature: "The patient responds with the same flat affect to every question, leaving the listener without a clue to any deeper human emotion."

6. *Appropriateness*. Of all the questions, the issue of appropriateness most often requires a judgment call on the part of the clinician, as well as an example that will clearly establish the presence of disability in the mind of the adjudicator: "The patient talks to other patients nonstop in the waiting room, often seeming to intrude on their privacy against their wishes. He speaks loudly, and thus constitutes a constant distraction to the staff as well."

7. *Hallucinations*. The therapist need not confine the report of hallucinations to the current clinical presentation. Since hallucinations, particularly auditory hallucinations, can be important diagnostic markers of schizophrenia, the adjudicator is likely to be interested in the presence of these symptoms during an episode: "When psychotic, the patient hears voices screaming insults at him. Currently this symptom is in remission, although the patient will occasionally hear a voice or two when stressed."

8. *Stream of thought*. This item refers to impoverished thought as well as thinking that is disorganized or rigid, including such formal thought disorder as illogical thinking, derailment, or incoherence. Again, illustrative samples of the patient's speech can be helpful for the adjudicator.

Consideration, Reconsideration, and Appeal

They are several steps to approving a claim. A claim can be and often is approved at the first level of consideration. In this case an adjudicator works together with a government doctor to approve the claim. Sometimes the claim is turned down at this level for no other reason than that the reports and medical records were incomplete. In other cases, the adjudicator and doctor have made a judgment that the evidence in the file does not justify approval. Claimants are then given two choices: reconsideration or appeal. When available, reconsideration is always the preferable choice for several reasons. First, reconsideration is a more rapid and uncomplicated process that is completed in weeks or months (whereas an appeal can take a year or more) and never requires the legal counsel that is often necessary for an appeal. Further, a failed reconsideration can always be followed by an appeal, but the only recourse after a failed appeal is another appeal to a federal court or submitting a new claim. Finally, the clinician has more access to and influence on the adjudicator during the reconsideration process, although an appeals judge might be more likely to approve a claim that falls within the letter of the law. Reconsideration is based on two assumptions: there has either been an exacerbation of the illness, or there is additional information available that was not contained in the first report.

An unofficial reason that might have led to reconsideration includes the possibility that the report was not adequately prepared or that the clinician missed a deadline. As soon as reconsideration begins, the clinician should contact the adjudicator and promise an interim or clarifying report. Often the adjudicator will allow some leeway with deadlines if assured that a report will be forthcoming. Adjudicators do not work directly for the SSA but rather are employed by a state agency often named the Bureau of Disability Determination (or something similar). This means that state-to-state differences are to be expected in the interpretation and the administration of the law. The clinician needs to adjust to the culture of the local office. If new to disability claim issues, the clinician should take an hour or two and visit the local office well prepared with questions related to the process and the local interpretation of disability criteria.

The appeals process is conducted by an entirely different entity, a federal agency called the Office of Hearings and Appeals. These offices are very busy and appeals take a long time to be heard. The judges and lawyers who work for this agency are often more knowledgeable about the law than adjudicators at the state agency. This agency is fair and very faithful to the law, but backlogs are common and decisions can take a year or more, as already noted. While claimants often need to retain legal counsel, those with schizophrenia most often *do* win their appeals. Waiting for benefits, dealing with lawyers, and preparing to appear before a judge in court all create stress and can distract the patient from the treatment process. Thus, it is wise to urge patients to apply for reconsideration before they request an appeal. If a clinician is reasonably certain that a complete case has been made and the reconsideration period has passed, it is sometimes advisable to ask the Office of Hearings and Appeals for a "Review of the Record." Government lawyers can review an appeal and grant the claim without a hearing, thus saving time.

A successful claim will be subject to periodic review, but the "culture of denial" is less. Often one can simply cite the original application, indicating that the disability has not changed substantially. Also, if patients return to work and earn enough to terminate benefits, they can now have benefits reinstated quickly (if they relapse or become unemployed by reason of their disability) by having the treating clinician write a brief letter that describes the basis of reeligibility. As the law changes, the clinician will want to keep abreast of events by following SSA publications, many of which can be accessed on the Internet at *www.ssa.gov*. The important "ticket-to-work" program can be accessed at *www.ssa.gov./work/resourcestoolkit/html*.

MEDICATION MANAGEMENT

As stated at the outset of this chapter, *the optimal improvement that is possible with PT (or any other psychosocial treatment) is essentially dependent upon establishing the most effective and comfortable medication regimen for the individual patient.* This admittedly strong premise would apply to all but a very small number of poorly characterized schizophrenia patients. It is one that is not only based on decades of personal observation and experience but also from the results of controlled and integrated studies of medication and psychosocial treatment. Given the apparent inadequacy of medication management for all but 29% of schizophrenia patients (Lehman & Steinwachs, 1998), it is remarkable indeed that the efficacy of mental health services and psychosocial treatments has been documented at all. The studies of PT were the first to our knowledge that attempted to ensure an *optimal* medication condition for a psychosocial treatment by relying on the *minimum effective dosing strategy* (MED [Hogarty et al., 1988; McEvoy, Hogarty, & Steingard, 1991]) appropriate to the management of typical neuroleptics. With the exception of clozapine, which was introduced midway in the PT studies, all patients were maintained on typical neuroleptics, principally on a low dose of the injectable, long-acting fluphenazine (Prolixin) decanoate as described in Chapter 2.

In this section we briefly review a few principles of clinical psychopharmacology, including some remarks addressed to the nonphysician who will need to collaborate with a prescribing physician. Although many patients today will be treated with an *atypical* antipsychotic medication, we provide a review of *typical* neuroleptics as well, since some patients are precluded from receiving the newer atypical antipsychotic drugs by reason of cost, local public policy, insurer restrictions, the lack of insurance coverage and private financial resources, or (in some cases) clear indications for continuing treatment with typical neuroleptics, including failure to respond to the newer medications. Approximately one-half of schizophrenia patients continue to be treated with typical neuroleptics at the time of this writing. We comment on the central role of long-acting depot preparations for an important minority of patients. Finally, we review management approaches using the newer and often "first-line" atypical antipsychotic medications and conclude with some lessons learned from the study of *integrated* medication and psychosocial treatment. While we realize that nonphysicians are not responsible for medication management, they are often the primary source of information that influences medication decisions. Further, without a knowledge of medication issues, the nonphysician can feel that he or she is not an integral member of the treatment team. Knowledge of medication and its management clearly results in a more "complete" clinician.

Some Basic Principles

Whether or not a patient responds to a psychoactive medication depends on the correctness of the diagnosis and hence the appropriate choice of medication, on the patient's physical health and nutrition, on individual differences in pharmacokinetics (or how the body handles medication by absorption, distribution and metabolism), and to a lesser but nonetheless important extent on the patient's personal and family psychiatric history of prior medication response. The greatest contribution to suboptimal response is *medication noncompliance*, and thus repeated inquiry regarding patient beliefs, fears, personal comfort, and prior treatment response is paramount. It must be recognized that a complicated medication regimen that often might include multiple doses, cotherapy with a mood-regulating medication, supplemental medication for side effects, and as-needed prescriptions for the management of agitation, insomnia, or anxiety are formidable routines to follow for the cognitively impaired, particularly those with obvious memory deficits. Written instructions, memory props, and dispensing kits are often necessary. Ensuring access to a competent and convenient pharmacy is also essential, a growing problem in the era of "managed" pharmacies. Many nonspecific factors influence the magnitude and quality of medication response, including the *attitude* of the clinician and family toward medication, the *supportiveness* of the setting, and the *control* of psychosocial stressors. Finally, there is a "cost" involved in taking any medication, the price of which must be balanced by the known benefit derived from research and through the careful monitoring of the individual patient. For the nonphysician, there is a good overview of clinical psychopharmacology in the text of Bentley and Walsh (2000). Other texts include the comprehensive but more advanced volume by Schatzburg, Cole, and DeBallistu (1997) as well as the less expensive, easy-to-read, but more concise handbook of Pies (1998).

Typical (Conventional) Antipsychotic Drugs

While the lithium salts that are useful in the management of mania had been available since the late 1940s, the first "antipsychotic" of the modern drug era that began in the early 1950s was the rauwolfia alkaloid called reserpine (Serpasil), essentially a drug used to control high blood pressure. Its action, however, not only "emptied" or depleted the neuron of many important chemical messengers believed to be related to psychosis but also depleted neurotransmitters that were thought to be important for maintaining mood. A significant risk for depression, for example, led to the general discontinuation of reserpine as the treatment of choice for psychotic conditions, particularly among patients with a family history of depression.

In the latter part of the 19th century, the nucleus of a molecule that eventually led to the first group of antipsychotic medications, the phenothiazines, was synthesized in the search for dyes. One of the first phenothiazine drugs later developed was promethazine (Phenergan), which was observed to have antihistaminic and sedative but not antipsychotic properties. It is still used today for treating children with stuffy noses and allergies. Chlorpromazine (e.g., Thorazine) was perhaps the most significant phenothiazine derivative related to psychosis, one used initially as an anesthetic preparation for surgery by the French surgeon H. Laborit in 1950. In the early 1950s, chlorpromazine was also observed to enhance the effect of barbiturates in the treatment of psychotic patients. In 1952, Laborit encouraged the French psychiatrists J. Delay and P. Deniker to use chlorpromazine with acutely psychotic patients, and they did so with dramatic results. By 1955, the use of chlorpromazine was widespread and the effect internationally was nothing short of dramatic. In the United States, for example, the number of chronic psychotic patients who had been hospitalized for a year or longer prior to chlorpromazine exceeded one-half million. These numbers would likely have surpassed 2 million today without antipsychotic drugs. At the moment, less than 80,000 of these hospitalized patients now occupy public mental hospital beds on a continuous basis. Similar results were obtained worldwide in a relatively short period of time.

The phenothiazine structure (like that of tricyclic antidepressant medications) contains three chemical rings—hence the term "tricyclic." These are six-sided ("benzene") rings with the middle ring containing a sulfur atom and a nitrogen atom, together with a side chain of carbon atoms that ends in yet another nitrogen atom. Over two dozen phenothiazines have been synthesized (about nine of which have been commonly used) by simply substituting one atom for another, often on the side chain. Another group of conventional antipsychotics, the *thioxanthenes*, was developed by replacing the nitrogen atom on the middle ring with a carbon atom. Thiothixene (Navane) and chlorprothixene (Taractan) are the most popular drugs of this group among clinicians. Another structurally different group of antipsychotics is the *butyrophenones*, the most popular of which remains haloperidol (Haldol). This group of medications resulted from the synthesis of well-known analgesics such as meperidine (Demerol). Atom substitutions of the butyrophenone nucleus led to the development of the *diphenylbutylpiperidine* group (e.g., pimozide, penfluridol, and fluspiriline) which, with the exception of the off-line use of pimozide (Orap), are not available in the United States. Of the *indolone* group, molindone (Moban) is the one most familiar to practitioners in the United States. Another alteration of the tricyclic molecule led to the development of the *dibenzodiazepines*, of which loxapine (Loxitane) is the most popular. A derivative of this class is the remarkable medication clozapine (Clozaril), an *atypical* antipsychotic that was the first new antipsychotic on the U.S. market in two decades. While it has its own risks, clozapine does not possess the typical neurological side effects (extrapyramidal symptoms) associated with conventional antipsychotics and no case of tardive dyskinesia has been reported with clozapine. Risperidone (Risperdal), a *benzisoxazole*; quetiapine (Seroquel), a *dibenzothiazepine*; olanzapine (Zyprexa), a *thienobenzodiazapine*; and ziprasidone (Geodon) are the remaining atypical antipsychotic drugs currently prescribed in the United States at the time of this writing and represent new chemical classes of drugs. It is worthwhile remembering that the initial discovery of the phenothiazines and butyrophenones was serendipitous, that is, accidentally found during a search for something else, while their therapeutic effect was the result of close clinical observation rather than "directed" research. The newer atypical antipsychotics, however, were specifically designed with the pathophysiology of schizophrenia in mind. The mapping of the human genome should lead to the development of safer and more effective medications that target the proteins of specific schizophrenia "candidate" genes.

In the early years following the introduction of chlorpromazine, the term "antipsychotics" was used interchangeably but incorrectly with the term "phenothiazines," since the latter is simply one of many groups of antipsychotics. Likewise, all antipsychotics were earlier referred to as being "neuroleptics" in that their side effects resembled those observed in neurological disease. However, the newer "atypical" antipsychotic drugs tend to have less and in some cases none of these extrapyramidal side effects at recommended doses, and hence the term has less meaning today. Clearly antipsychotics are not "tranquilizers" since they are as likely to energize as to selectively sedate a patient. This class of medication is referred to as the "antipsychotics" because of their specific effect on psychotic behaviors. Among responsive patients, the typical neuroleptics are essentially equivalent in their therapeutic effect and mode of action. Important differences in side effects, however, tend to distinguish the recently approved atypical antipsychotics, although comparative efficacy studies of these medications are still in their infancy.

All antipsychotic drugs (typical and atypical) can be further classified in terms of their potency: high, intermediate, or low. The more a drug "binds" to a specific group of neuron receptors in the brain (e.g., the receptors for the neurotransmitter dopamine), the greater is its potency. The more potent the drug, the *lower* the dose required for "binding" and hence for a therapeutic effect. Low-potency typical neuroleptics (such as chlorpromazine [Thorazine] and thioridazine [Mellaril]) require *higher* doses but tend to have somewhat fewer motor side effects (extrapyramidal symptoms) and have greater initial sedation, higher anticholinergic side effects (e.g., dry mouth, constipation, urinary retention, blurred vision), and a greater effect on blood pressure (orthostatic hypotension) than do high-potency antipsychotics such as fluphenazine (Prolixin) or haloperidol (Haldol). But the latter antipsychotics have a greater incidence of extrapyramidal side effects. Hence, the typical neuroleptics differ in their potency (the degree to which they relatively bind to different receptors) and side effects more than in their therapeutic effects. However, for reasons that are unclear, sometimes a patient who is nonresponsive to a drug from one group of typical neuroleptics (e.g., a phenothiazine) *will* respond to a drug from another group (e.g., a buterophenone). Between the mid-1970s and the mid-1990s, there had been a gradual change in the use of neuroleptics from low-potency to high-potency drugs. Unfortunately, the earlier low-dose advantage of these high-potency antipsychotics was often lost as doses and hence attendant side effects became unnecessarily increased over time. The dosage studies of the 1980s and '90s, however, have seemed to curb this excess among patients who continue to be maintained on traditional neuroleptics (see below).

Conventional antipsychotic drugs variously come in oral form (tablets and capsules), in liquid form for patients who might "cheek" their medication, as intravenous injections, sometimes but questionably used for the management of acute cases, and in the popular intramuscular (IM), long-acting (depot) injectable form. Two antipsychotic drugs, fluphenazine (Prolixin) and haloperidol (Haldol), have these widely used, long-acting, decanoate forms available, and in the case of fluphenazine, the less frequently used enanthate form. (Other decanoate preparations are not available in the United States, such as zuclopenthixal and flupenthixal.) These depot preparations are the fatty acid esters of the parent drugs that are mixed in oil and, after injection, are widely stored in fatty tissue and only slowly released into the blood stream. The half-life of these esterized medications in the body can be measured in days to weeks rather than hours for the oral (hydrochloride) forms. Active metabolites can often be found for months after a single injection.

Typical neuroleptics are not generally prescribed for persons who have a preschizophrenia history of serious blood disorders such as agranulocytosis (indicated by a low granulocyte count), nor for patients with severe pulmonary decompensation (obstructive pulmonary disease), and are used with caution in patients with a serious history of liver, kidney, heart, or intestinal disease. While few teratogenic effects (influences on the fetus) occur in pregnant women, the "benefit" of preventing psychotic episodes with low-dose antipsychotics often outweighs the "cost" of medication to the mother and unborn child. Breastfeeding, however, is usually avoided. Neuroleptics are generally ineffective in psychotic states that are secondary to seizure disorders where anticonvulsants are the drug class of choice. Neuroleptics, in fact, lower the seizure threshold even further, including the atypical antipsychotic clozapine (see below).

For the indicated conditions, antipsychotic drugs exert a special and direct influence on the core symptoms of psychosis. These include formal thought disorder (illogical thinking, loose associations, autistic preoccupation, thought insertion, thought withdrawal, thought broadcasting, neologisms, and word salad), sensory experiences without discernible external sources (hallucinations), and false beliefs (delusions). They may not "cure" delusions, but frequently the patient's investment in the strength of the false belief is modified. They tend to have little or no effect on such thought disorders as "concrete thinking." There is a clear effect on the hostility and uncooperativeness that is frequently associated with the psychotic process. However, it remains equivocal whether any antipsychotic drug (typical or atypical) has an effect on the impoverished thinking, amotivation, and blunted, flat, or reduced affect involved in the so-called negative symptoms, beyond the reduction of extrapyramidal symptoms (particularly akinesia) associated with the newer atypical agents. Studies indicate a gradual but slower improvement in negative symptoms during the treatment of the acute episode for most antipsychotic drugs (Breier et al., 1987). However, 15–20% of schizophrenia patients, for example, will have a persistence of these negative or "deficit" symptoms *after* the resolution of an acute episode, and higher maintenance doses of a neuroleptic appear to actually increase their severity. It remains unclear whether atypical antipsychotic drugs can relieve these primary negative symptoms. Sometimes psychotic patients might seem less anxious or agitated on antipsychotic medication, but these are "nonspecific" effects. Anxiety and agitation are not the sole or primary indications for antipsychotic drug use and are better managed by other medications (e.g., lorazepam [Ativan]).

Dosage of Typical Neuroleptics

In this brief overview of dosage, a discussion of drug dose "equivalencies," which has traditionally been part of psychopharmacology texts, will not be offered. Many problems exist, not the least of which is that so-called equivalencies were often determined in open practice studies during the early years of antipsychotic drug use, among somewhat different patients, and at a time of limited experience. Further, blood levels following a fixed dose of a given drug can vary 10- to 20-fold, patient to patient. As a general principle, a dose of 100 mg of chlorpromazine (a low-potency antipsychotic drug) is equal to about 2 mg of a higher-potency drug within the same group (e.g., fluphenazine hydrochloride), or 1 or 2 mg of a high-potency drug from a different group such as haloperidol hydrochloride, and is equal to 10–12 mg of a drug with intermediate potency (e.g., perphenazine [Trilafon]). These equivalencies, however, are only approximate.

For patients who remain on typical neuroleptics by choice, indication, or default, there is no support for the belief that "if little is good, a lot must be better." The minimum effective dose (MED) is one that confers all the therapeutic benefit that is possible while minimizing unwanted side effects. (With the exception of risperidone, MED strategies are less important for the newer atypical antipsychotics because the margin of safe dosing is greater and the risk of extrapyramidal symptoms and tardive dyskinesia is less or absent.) The concept of appropriate dosing is simple but difficult to implement. If the patient is one of the 75% likely to respond to a typical antipsychotic drug, careful studies have demonstrated that he or she *will* respond therapeutically during an acute episode (McEvoy et al., 1991) and prophylactically during maintenance treatment (Hogarty et al., 1988) to the MED. Neuroleptic MED is crucial to psychosocial practice and other rehabilitation strategies since it can often provide the optimal condition for the application of psychosocial interventions and the avoidance of treatment noncompliance. Side effects of antipsychotic drugs can often be lessened and the need for anticholinergic (antiparkinsonism) medications either circumvented or reduced, as mentioned earlier. The latter is important since these medications can interfere with short-term verbal memory and hence the learning upon which psychosocial treatments are based (McEvoy & Freter, 1989). In the past, practitioners observed that responsive patients did improve with high doses, and the subsequent relationship between dose and response was viewed as "causal," even though low doses ultimately proved to be equally effective. Side effects, it was thought, were simply the price one had to pay for symptomatic improvement. For reasons best attributed to decreasing lengths of inpatient stay, pressure from utilization review personnel to move patients out of hospitals as quickly as possible, and concern among family members who often needed to be reassured that "everything possible had been done," the neuroleptic dose was increasingly but unfortunately prescribed in the higher approved ranges, particularly for the high-potency drugs.

Regarding the dose needed for the acute episode, a number of studies have clearly documented that "more" antipsychotic drug does *not* lead to a faster or more complete therapeutic response (Kane, 1996)! "Rapid neuroleptization" had been a very popular practice prior to 1980 (and apparently remains so among some prescribers), when in fact the sedative effect of a high dose was often incorrectly believed to be synonymous with the antipsychotic effect. Many inpatient dosage studies have disproved the rapid neuroleptization hypothesis in that it takes approximately the same time for a therapeutic effect to emerge whether the effective dose is low, standard, or high. Increasingly it has been shown that the more appropriate MED is sufficient for a therapeutic response among those patients who will respond to neuroleptics and that agitation can be controlled by an "as-needed" (PRN) dose of an antianxiety drug, most often one of the benzodiazepines such as lorazepam (Ativan).

For example, a very basic hypothesis put forth many years ago by the German psychiatrist H. Haase has been subject to rigorous testing. This hypothesis stated that the dose at which very mild muscle rigidity first appeared (not gross extrapyramidal symptoms) represented the "neuroleptic threshold dose"—the MED at which patients would receive *maximum* therapeutic benefits and *minimum* side effects *if given the requisite time to respond*. Higher doses, according to this hypothesis, would not lead to greater therapeutic improvement but only to greater side effects. In a large inpatient study (McEvoy et al., 1991), over 70% of consecutively admitted and acutely psychotic, nonrefractory schizophrenia or schizoaffective disorder patients did respond to the neuroleptic threshold dose, which averaged about 4 mg a day of haloperidol (Haldol) and most often was in the range of 2–6 mg a day. Compared to the average daily dose of approximately 25 mg of Haldol used in the United States at the time, the neuroleptic threshold dose was indeed quite low. High doses did not lead to greater improvement among nonresponders to the neuroleptic threshold dose, except that high doses *did* seem to have a circumscribed therapeutic benefit among hostile and uncooperative patients. But side effects among these high-dose patients were also greater. About 15% of patients responded to the neuroleptic threshold dose between 10 and 14 days. An additional 40% of patients responded between 2 and 4 weeks, and the remaining responders did so by 6 weeks. Response to the neuroleptic threshold dose was greatest among patients with a "rapid" onset of symptoms (often their first exposure to antipsychotic medication) and lowest among those with a slow or "chronic" onset.

Thus, the clues to a therapeutic neuroleptic response during the acute episode are patient type, time, and the MED. The neuroleptic threshold dose is individually determined, and its effect is reminiscent of earlier animal studies which suggested that the underlying mechanism of therapeutic response might indeed be the "either/or" depolarization blockade. In the early years following the introduction of antipsychotic drugs, a discrete population of seemingly nonresponsive, younger (under age 40), and less chronically hospitalized (between 2 and 10 years) schizophrenia patients did respond differently to "high dose" treatment. However, no study in recent decades has endorsed the value of such treatment dose as a general strategy.

There is a clear parallel to the inpatient dosage studies reflected in the results of outpatient maintenance studies that randomly assigned patients to either a "standard" 25-mg dose of intramuscular fluphenazine (Prolixin) decanoate biweekly or to a "low" dose that represented only 20% of the prescribed dose—roughly 5 mg of fluphenazine decanoate every 2 weeks (Hogarty et al., 1988). About 77% of stabilized outpatients could be maintained on this biweekly low dose over 1 year. There were no significant differences in relapse rates between the two doses at 1 or 2 years, although low-dose patients did experience more "minor" but aborted episodes in the second year, particularly those who lived in highly stressful households, as described in Chapter 1. At least four other studies confirm these results (Kane, 1996). Side effects were less troublesome and more patients were vocationally active by 2 years if they received the low dose. In the PT studies, where dose was not experimentally controlled or manipulated, a majority of patients was successfully maintained on the MED of fluphenazine decanoate, as described in Chapter 2.

Another dosage strategy that has been studied is called "intermittent medication management," a variant of the "drug holiday." This approach has recently been well tested in five studies but found wanting (Kane, 1996). In this strategy, stabilized schizophrenia patients had their medication discontinued, but with the reappearance of prodromal signs of an episode, medication was again reinstated. Approximately the same number of patients needed to be reinstated each year as those in other studies who were observed to relapse following placebo substitution. While the total dose might be somewhat less over time, intermittent dosage was inferior to a modest but continuing maintenance dose on many criteria tested. The social cost of intermittent destabilization, particularly the burden on the patient's family, was noteworthy in one study. We do not recommend these intermittent strategies except in the rare case when a patient refuses medication but would consider restarting medication if prodromal signs reappeared.

The lesson from the dosing strategies of recent years is thus important: The PT therapist should assume that the patient will be one of the 75% who will respond to a low dose of conventional, neuroleptic medication, *until proven otherwise!* (Strategies for the management of the suboptimal responding patient are presented below and in Chapter 5.) For the acutely psychotic, nonrefractory patient, the neuroleptic threshold dose is the preferred dosing approach when typical neuroleptics are used. For the recovered and stable outpatient, the minimal effective maintenance dose is the preferred approach, namely, that dosage *below* which prodromal signs appear and *above* which more than minimal, cogwheel rigidity occurs.

The Depot Advantage

While an increasing number of patients appear to better tolerate and thus better comply with atypical antipsychotics, a minority of patients survive without relapse because of depot neuroleptics. Traditionally, intramuscular depot fluphenazine (Prolixin) or haloperidol (Haldol) decanoate had been recommended largely on the basis that the patient was or would be "drug noncompliant." While this justification is important, it remains incomplete. Depot preparations also avoid "first-pass" metabolism in the gut and intestinal tract, and hence facilitate the acquisition of therapeutic blood levels, thereby circumventing a problem that is sometimes encountered among patients who are "atypical metabolizers" (and so might appear to be nonresponders) or who are taking other substances that might interfere with the absorption of oral antipsychotic medications in the gastrointestinal tract. Most important, depot preparations permit the physician to deliver the least amount of medication needed for the maintenance of therapeutic gains. Costs of depot medications are also decreasing over time, and a single injection can last from 2–6 weeks (Carpenter, Buchanan, Kirkpatrick, & Breier, 1999), thus precluding the daily struggle that often arises with oral medications. On the downside are, of course, the risks of extrapyramidal side effects, including akathisia (internal restlessness) and tardive dyskinesia, which are lessened or avoided with the atypical antipsychotics.

Patients maintained on depot medication often present specific management concerns for the nonphysician who values "self-determination" around issues of medication taking. In practice, however, it is often easier to encourage patient independence in other areas of life once the issue of medication taking has been placed under control. A trade in "control" issues can often be made to the general benefit of the patient. For example, if the patient can be convinced that multiple and simultaneous changes in day-to-day living often contain the provocations of a new psychotic episode, then the need to ensure stable and protective plasma levels of the antipsychotic drug by way of intramuscular injection is often more understandable and acceptable. (In the face of extraordinary life concerns, medication taking and dosage become two issues that the patient, the family, and the therapist need not worry about on a daily basis.) When the patient is motivated and well enough to seek an independent residence, or establish a new relationship, or return to school or work, then he or she can be informed that *all* personal resources, skill, and independent judgment will be needed in order to successfully and autonomously negotiate these important life events. Such challenges need not be complicated by the rituals and forgetfulness that characterize daily dosing.

A compelling justification for depot neuroleptics among psychosocial therapists is that the "mystery" surrounding the reasons for a relapse can be better understood and managed. Were the patient prescribed an oral medication exclusively, the therapist would find it difficult, if not impossible, to accurately determine whether or not a subsequent relapse, should it occur, was due to stress itself or to covert medication noncompliance. *Destabilization while the patient is receiving a depot neuroleptic usually indicates the presence of an independent life stress or that the intensity of the psychosocial treatment plan was excessive!* Individual treatment planning becomes inherently more rational with depot preparations, since the clinician has a better appreciation of what steps in the rehabilitation process can and cannot be comfortably handled, information that is uncontaminated by the question of medication noncompliance. With no convincing evidence that any psychosocial intervention for schizophrenia has a positive effect in the absence of medication for the majority of patients, it can also be confidently said that weeks, months, or even years of successful psychosocial treatment will become undone when the patient noncomplies with oral medication. The ultimate condition for establishing psychosocial treatment effects will be realized once a depot preparation for an atypical antipsychotic medication becomes available, a likely possibility in the immediate future.

Atypical (Nonconventional) Antipsychotic Drugs

Much to the relief of schizophrenia patients, their families and those who care for them, the 1990s saw the first wave of atypical antipsychotic drugs introduced in the United States that at least spared most patients from the chemical restraint of extrapyramidal side effects, including the effects on willed behavior and spontaneity. Equally important, these new medications significantly lowered or effectively eliminated the risk of the much feared tardive dyskinesia (TD). The latter is a largely involuntary and often persistent drug-induced movement disorder that primarily involves the mouth and face but can also appear in the extremities, body trunk and breathing muscles. A pursing or smacking of the lips, jaw movements, tremor or "fly catcher" movements of the tongue, and facial grimaces are the signs most often observed. Most of the typical neuroleptics have a 5% per year cumulative incidence of TD. However, most of the atypicals tend to have few if any TD effects, and the granddaddy of the newer antipsychotics (clozapine [Clozaril]) is often a recommended treatment for those with persistent movements induced by earlier-prescribed neuroleptics. Risperidone (Risperdal), introduced in 1994; olanzapine (Zyprexa), marketed in 1996; quetiapine (Seroquel), approved in 1998; and ziprasidone (Geodon) introduced in 2001—all are now heralded as "first-line" antipsychotics to be used in place of the typical neuroleptics. In fact, a recent study of olanzapine proved superior to haloperidal among first episode schizophrenia patients (Sanger et al., 1999). Clozapine, introduced in 1990, is intended for those patients who are refractory to, intolerant of, or suboptimally responsive to at least two trials of other antipsychotic drugs.

This is not to say that these newer medications are without side effects. Rather, one often substitutes a new class of side effects for the old. These range from a troublesome weight gain to the rare but potentially life-threatening disorder of agranulocytosis observed with clozapine. We comment below on patient management with these newer medications based as much on our own experience as on the results of controlled and published studies, which characteristically represent industry-supported studies that did not extend much beyond 6 weeks during drug development. Our preferences of the moment might change with continuing experience. Clearly for the refractory patient, clozapine has been nothing short of an extraordinary gift, a claim that stands in some contrast to the relatively few patients (about 150,000) who have been prescribed clozapine in the United States, whereas a quarter to a half million patients are likely to be eligible (see Conley & Buchanan, 1997). Each drug has its advantages and disadvantages, which we highlight below. Before offering this overview, we should note that we are not impressed with occasional reports that cite first-line atypical antipsychotics as being significantly more effective for patients who were refractory to typical neuroleptics, although important studies are in progress. In our experience, if a patient had responded to a typical antipsychotic drug, he or she will likely respond to an atypical drug as well. But refractoriness also occurs with the first-line atypical antipsychotics, thus suggesting an abiding and important role for clozapine.

Indications

For the most part, the choice of a first-line atypical drug at this time is influenced more by its side-effect profile than by valid differences in efficacy among drugs. Only two nonindustry supported trials have been published at the time of this writing that compared two different atypicals directly, and these studies suffered problems in design and/or sample size. (Other reports that we have seen can be similarly characterized, although the National Institute of Mental Health [NIMH] has now initiated multisite studies that will include a wide range of severe mental illnesses and atypical drugs in their protocols.) If there is any selective indication used by us, it is one that includes a *supplemental* low dose of risperidone (e.g., 1–3 mg a day) for more symptomatically unstable patients when we seek some greater dopamine (D_2) antagonism while attempting to establish a maintenance drug regimen. We view risperidone as something of a medication that lies midway between the typical and atypical antipsychotic drugs in effects, pharmacokinetics, and side effects.

There are, however, quite different side-effect profiles between the atypical and the conventional antipsychotic drugs that serve to indicate the advantage of atypicals. The atypicals not only have a reduction or avoidance of extrapyramidal symptoms, akathisia, and tardive dyskinesia, as mentioned earlier, but also a suggestion of improved therapeutic effects. The latter include patient reports that they do not feel as mentally "dull" taking an atypical, an effect that might speak more to a reduction in subtle behavioral akinesia as it does to the amelioration of negative symptoms. Also, in our experience, the atypicals seem to have better mood stabilizing properties regarding the management of concurrent anxiety and/or depression. It remains unclear whether this is a reflection of the same phenomenon that often occurs among patients who are successfully treated with conventional antipsychotics during the acute episode or whether the effect differentially extends to those with persistent impairments of affect following the resolution of positive symptoms (see Chapter 5).

The indications for clozapine were identified earlier, that is, a second-line antipsychotic medication for those patients who fail to show improvement with, had a suboptimal response to or appeared intolerant of conventional and/or first-line antipsychotic drugs. However, there is also growing evidence of clozapine's selective efficacy that extends to a reduction in suicide and an improved engagement with and response to psychosocial treatments, as well as greater maintenance of quality of life (e.g., Rosenheck et al., 1998). (We clearly subscribe to these observations in that nearly half of patients participating in an ongoing study of cognitive-enhancement therapy [CET] are being maintained with clozapine, patients that would not have likely been able to utilize such rehabilitation approaches as recently as 1990.) Clinical evidence further suggests a reduced craving for illicit drugs and a decrease in smoking among some clozapine-treated patients (e.g., Drake, Yie, McHugo, & Green, 2000).

Side Effects

With the exception of risperidone, a transient but often bothersome *sedation* characterizes the initiation of treatment with the other atypical antipsychotic drugs, including clozapine. (We attempt to manage sedation through a conservative dosing strategy to be described below.) *Weight gain* might be the most frequently encountered obstacle when one is using olanzapine, a problem that deters some patients from accepting clozapine as well (Henderson et al., 2000). Weight gain is an important issue for schizophrenia patients, given the increased risk of diabetes and other life-compromising conditions that accompany obesity (Devlin, Yanovski, & Wilson 2000). Fortunately, in our experience, obesity is not an inevitable consequence of olanzapine or clozapine therapy. (We approach the issue of weight gain with a comprehensive discussion of the advantages and disadvantages of these medications, including the risk of weight gain. A plan is then offered that includes referral and alliance with our medical center's skilled nutrition and weight management program, coupled with an integrated program of feasible and enjoyable exercise.) Otherwise, at doses of 4 mg or more, risperidone opens the door to mild *extrapyramidal symptoms* and an occasional and troublesome akathisia for some patients. Extrapyramidal symptoms seem less with olanzapine (although a recent study suggests otherwise [Conley & Mahmoud, 2001]), and for all practical purposes are rare or nonexistent with quetiapine and clozapine. However, *anticholinergic side effects* of olanzapine are common (as is hypersalivation and constipation with clozapine). Transient *hypotension* (low blood pressure) is also problematic among risperidone-, quetiapine-, and clozapine-treated patients.

Sexual dysfunction (likely associated with increased prolactin release) has been a frequent side effect among conventional neuroleptics, but the problem differs widely among the atypicals: at one extreme risperidone tends to increase and sustain prolactin levels in a manner that is similar to the traditional neuroleptics, but at the other extreme quetiapine has no important persistence of prolactin elevation. Olanzapine has a relatively low incidence of sexual dysfunction side effects. The characteristics of quetiapine can make it a good alternative for young women who face long-term maintenance treatment. Associated with a lower sustained prolactin level, for example, is a reduced risk of drug-induced osteoporosis, which when coupled with a lower incidence of weight gain makes quetiapine a particularly attractive choice for many women. However, we do not have an extensive clinical experience with quetiapine at this time and must reserve judgment on its differential therapeutic efficacy, particularly its long-term efficacy in maintenance treatment. Finally, there are selective and often serious side effects associated with clozapine that were mentioned earlier. The first is agranulocytosis, which occurs among 1–2% of patients, as well as the risk of seizure at higher doses. The risk of agranulocytosis requires monitoring through routine blood tests. Such patients cannot be restarted on clozapine. Patients who develop a sore throat or fever should be immediately referred to the prescribing physician. While all antipsychotic medications lower the seizure threshold such that approximately 1% of treated patients in general experience a drug-induced seizure, the risk rises to about 3% among clozapine-treated patients that are maintained at higher doses. Constipation, as mentioned above, is also a life-compromising side effect that occasionally occurs among clozapine-treated patients. Since constipation often tends to be overlooked, the clinician needs to query the patient about constipation on a regular basis and to initiate the appropriate dietary and medical interventions when indicated. Overall, an analysis of our current research caseload indicates that the most frequently prescribed (second-line) antipsychotic is clozapine, followed by olanzapine and risperidone as the first-line choices. Our choice of a first-line atypical antipsychotic will likely change as new medications come onto the market in the coming years. As mentioned earlier, development of a long-acting intramuscular atypical antipsychotic is eagerly awaited.

Dosage of Atypical Antipsychotic Medication

Among patients that have been maintained on a conventional neuroleptic but are judged to be candidates for an atypical drug, we will not abruptly stop the former and initiate the latter. More often we will "cross-titrate" these medications (lowering one while increasing the other). However, there are exceptions. For patients with an established history of intermittent relapse and/or behavioral acting out, we will first overlap the two medications in question before tapering, that is, maintain the conventional drug dose until the atypical medication is near the assumed therapeutic dose, then taper the conventional drug. For medications that have short half-life and are excreted rapidly (e.g., clozapine and quetiapine), we routinely divide the dose. We have seen a number of suboptimal responders to these medications improve when their single daily dose is divided.

Otherwise, our approach to dosing with the atypicals, including clozapine, represents a strong adherence to the guiding maxim: *Start low and go slow!* In this regard our starting dose tends to be lower than that recommended in the Expert Consensus Guidelines (McEvoy et al., 1999). For example, we will typically initiate risperidone at 1 mg a day and increase the dose to 2 or 4 mg over a period of 2 weeks. For olanzapine, it is not uncommon to begin treatment with as little as 2.5 mg a day and to reach the desired maintenance dose of 10–15 mg a day in 2–3 weeks for female patients. (Doses for male patients are often higher in our experience, reaching the 15–25 mg a day range.) Treatment with quetiapine typically begins at 25 mg twice daily with the goal of at least 300 mg reached by 3–4 weeks. (Many patients will require a dose of 600 mg a day or more.) So too with clozapine: a starting dose of 12.5 mg a day for 2 or 3 days, followed by 25-mg increments every 3 or 4 days until a maintenance dose of at least 350 mg a day is reached, or more precisely a blood level that is at least 350 ng/ml. (Some patients require higher doses in order to reach this plasma level.) Again, the frequency of a dose increase depends on how well the patient tolerates the current dose. For medication with a short half-life, even intermittent drug noncompliance can confound the issue of therapeutic efficacy. The strategy of divided doses for these drugs is again important. Should a patient need to be discontinued from clozapine, it is critically important to "cover" the patient with another medication at the beginning of discontinuation if possible. (This would not be a strategy for the patient suffering from agranulocytosis, who would need to have clozapine discontinued abruptly.) The maintenance dose of an atypical drug will likely vary among patients, being somewhat lower for well-stabilized and infrequently relapsing patients, and somewhat higher for those with an unstable history of intermittent psychosis. The guiding strategy for dosing and the rapidity of dose increases is greatly influenced by the patient's own report. We cannot emphasize enough the need to remain in frequent contact with and to carefully listen to the patient's own account of his or her mental state and side effects during the initiation and subsequent adjustment of medication doses. Blood level is a useful guide for determining therapeutic efficacy with clozapine, but not for the other atypicals at the moment.

Given our caution in both initiating and increasing doses, we do not always subscribe to the recommendations that an adequate trial of a typical antipsychotic is only 6 weeks. Given that it might take 3–4 weeks for the atypicals and 3 months for clozapine before a maintenance dose is established, we are more likely to continue treatment for 12 weeks with the first-line antipsychotics and for as long as 6 months with clozapine, increasing dose to the maximum maintenance level tolerated in the face of an incomplete response before "switching" to another drug. The 6-week recommendation can be a useful rule of thumb once the optimal maintenance dose is achieved. In Chapter 5 we describe the fine-tuning medication procedures that we use when attempting to achieve an optimal level of stabilization, including the use of augmentation strategies and the pharmacological management of comorbid impairments such as anxiety, depression, and negative symptoms.

Other Medication Issues

Duration

For chronic psychotic disorders, particularly schizophrenia and schizoaffective disorders that are characterized by *two or more episodes*, indefinite maintenance on an appropriate dose of an antipsychotic drug is indicated, at least over the age when the patient remains at risk. While some poorly characterized patients might appear to fully recover and no longer need medication in later life, most adults with recurrent illnesses require a judicious maintenance dose of antipsychotic drug, at least through the age of 70.

A problem does exist, however, for first-episode schizophrenia or "schizophreniform" disorder, first episodes of schizoaffective disorder, as well as atypical psychotic states where the diagnosis is often uncertain and only time can lead to a final diagnostic decision. In these cases, it is wise to continue maintenance chemotherapy for at least 1 year following the resolution of the index psychotic episode. Together with the physician, the patient, family, and other concerned mental health professionals, the PT therapist should develop a treatment plan that contains a clear description of the patient's prodromal signs (see Chapter 4), should the patient insist on a trial off medication. Medication can then be gradually discontinued.

Based on the treatment contract, should prodromal signs reappear, medication should be quickly reinstated. Knowledge of the patient is the best source of individual prodromal signs and is a primary focus of PT. Again, it is worthwhile stressing that these early indications of a new episode are often not psychotic signs per se. Rather, they frequently include anxiety, depression, excitement, frustration, sleep or appetite disturbances, and somatic complaints, as much as a mild increase in thought disorder or suspiciousness. A recent and sobering study of first-episode schizophrenia patients provides a very strong argument against drug discontinuation in this population at any time (Robinson et al., 1999). About 82% of first-episode patients experienced a relapse within 5 years! The hazard ratio (risk of relapse) was nearly *five times greater* for patients who discontinued medication than for those who remained on medication.

Unfortunately, controlled maintenance studies of multiepisode psychotic conditions have rarely equaled 3 years and none have exceeded 5 years. In these studies, the 1-year risk of a new psychotic episode following drug discontinuation appeared to be about 65% whenever medication was discontinued. The average is misleading, however, since risk can equal 95% in patients with five or more episodes, as described earlier (Hogarty & Ulrich, 1998).

Drug Interactions

Frequently the most troublesome management problem for the nonphysician (and an abiding concern for the family), surrounds the issue of what can and cannot be taken safely by the patient who has been prescribed antipsychotic medication. Often the most successful management plan can become effectively undone by the inappropriate use of "street drugs" and/or over-the-counter medications.

Illicit Drugs. Drugs with hallucinogenic properties such as amphetamine, LSD (lysergic acid diethylamide), PCP (1-[1-phenylcyclohexyl]piperdine, or phencyclidine), cocaine, and marijuana, for example, can exacerbate the positive symptoms of psychosis since they facilitate the release or synthesis of important neurotransmitters believed to underlie these symptoms. Numerous studies, for example, have concluded that marijuana abuse will often lead to a new episode of schizophrenia among patients with a history of schizophrenia. A very restricted use of *d*-amphetamine among negative-symptom schizophrenia patients (but not those with positive symptoms) has been shown to have some circumscribed value, but the limited effect, potential neurobiological consequences, and the legal complications in prescribing amphetamine render this strategy impractical if not unwarranted.

Alcohol. Alcohol is a potent central nervous system depressant and hence can intensify certain side effects of antipsychotic drugs, particularly sedation or the motor difficulties associated with extrapyramidal symptoms. Patients that are receiving antipsychotic medication should definitely not "drink and drive"! Alcohol significantly influences the mood of the patient as well as critical judgment, thought processing, and reaction time, all of which have been demonstrated to be important in the pathophysiology of psychotic disorders. As it does in the presence of all anesthetics, an antipsychotic drug will also enhance the effects of alcohol. Recent evidence suggests a relationship between alcohol abuse and cerebellar deficits in males with schizophrenia (Sullivan et al., 2000). Alcohol can also increase metabolism and hence might lower therapeutic plasma levels over time and hence the wanted effect of the antipsychotic drug. Often a management dilemma exists as to whether the therapist should take on the issue of "a beer or two a day" when other pressing problems need negotiation. In these instances, both the patient and the family should at least be clearly informed regarding the potential problems that follow alcohol consumption while a patient is receiving antipsychotic medication.

Tobacco. Smoking increases metabolism and hence could lower antipsychotic blood levels and therapeutic effects, including the atypical antipsychotics clozapine and olanzapine. Nicotine, however, does appear to facilitate attention and neuronal functioning. This combination of circumstances might well explain the propensity of many chronic patients to smoke heavily, perhaps as a form of "self-medication" or as a circuitous way to lower extrapyramidal side effects. A recent report indicates that smoking reduces monoamine oxidase activity in schizophrenia patients (Simpson et al., 1999), thus likely increasing available neurotransmitters. Aside from the known health hazards associated with smoking, patients with impaired judgment, sedation, or compromised motor skills are at a particular risk for setting accidental fires that follow indiscriminate smoking.

Caffeine. Tea, coffee, and colas often contain significant levels of caffeine, and "caffeinism" can complicate the differential diagnosis of akathisia or concurrent anxiety. Coffee and tea also appear to precipitate many conventional antipsychotic drugs (causing them to settle down in more solid form), which are then more rapidly eliminated from the body, thereby decreasing therapeutic effects.

Over-the-Counter Drugs. Antacids such as milk of magnesia and kaopectate all interfere with the absorption and hence the blood levels of orally taken antipsychotic medications. Thus, they can decrease the wanted therapeutic effects. Decongestants, particularly those containing epinephrine and phenylephrine, can increase hypertension, sedation, and depression. Antihistamines also increase sedation and can enhance anticholinergic side effects. Among patients suffering from high blood pressure, antipsychotic drugs can decrease the effects of antihypertensives but increase postural hypotension among patients taking (thiazide) diuretics.

Antidepressants. Most antidepressants (both tricyclics and the newer selective serotonin reuptake inhibitors) can cause the blood levels of the antipsychotic drug and/or the antidepressant to rise when combined.

Medication Noncompliance and Advocacy

Sometimes a psychotic patient will refuse either treatment, in general, or an antipsychotic drug, in particular, a cause that even today might be endorsed by the therapist or legal advocate. A critical analysis of the issue is needed, however, in order to ensure that such a decision is appropriate and informed. (It rarely is, in our opinion.)

In general, laws exist throughout the country that permit the civil commitment of psychotic patients who have been certified to be a danger to themselves or others. Nonetheless, following involuntary inpatient treatment, such patients can and do "vote with their feet" when it comes to accepting a long-term maintenance program. (Few states currently provide involuntary outpatient commitment that, at best, is difficult to enforce.) More often than not, a patient's refusal of antipsychotic drug treatment has a clear foundation in personal experience, as described in Chapter 4. Many such patients have been inappropriately medicated in the past and are well aware of the "bad results," most often unwanted (and sometimes unnecessary) side effects. At other times, denial of illness (see Chapter 5), memory loss of the consequences that followed prior episodes, and stigma underlie the issue of treatment rejection. Sensitivity, psychoeducation, and patience are the best approaches to the issue of medication refusal.

In many cases, the therapist can listen to the nature of patient concerns and together with the physician should offer a different treatment plan, designed to avoid past negative experiences, if these are important obstacles to compliance. A lower dose is often an effective option. Compromises on dose, route of administration, and antipsychotic drug choice are also possible and often necessary. Patients and/or family members who continue to resist medication need to be calmly and competently informed about the risks for relapse that apply, the possible adverse consequences of prolonged or recurrent psychosis, and the limitations of psychosocial strategies when used in the absence of medication. Before this "psychoeducation" process is attempted, the clinician must come to a personal decision as to whether a patient has a "right to psychosis" or the "right to grow" through a psychotic experience. If the answer is affirmative, in fairness to the patient and the family, another professional opinion is *absolutely* necessary. Patients noncomply with medication for reasons that have been documented through careful studies (see Table 3.1). Examining these factors in a "health belief model" (Fenton, Blyler, & Heinssen, 1997) could lead to an individualized understanding of and response to medication noncompliance, that is, a review of the reasons why a patient refuses to take medication, such as fears of physical harm, side effects, a reminder of illness, moral failure, and the like.

Information offered to family members concerning the need for antipsychotic medication, its mechanisms of action, therapeutic effects, and the nature and control of side effects has also contributed greatly to the

---

TABLE 3.1. Empirical Correlates of Noncompliance in Schizophrenia

Patient-related factors
    Greater illness symptom severity, grandiosity, or both
    Lack of insight
    Substance abuse comorbidity

Medication-related factors
    Dysphoric medication side effects
    Subtherapeutic or excessively high dosages

Environmental factors
    Inadequate support or supervision
    Practical barriers, such as lack of money or transportation

Clinician-related factors
    Poor therapeutic alliance

Note. From Fenton et al. (1997, p. 645).

therapeutic alliance. In our program, patients have rarely discontinued treatment once family members have been provided information regarding the illness and its treatment along with the package of practical survival skills. Clear evidence is available demonstrating that medication noncompliance is significantly reduced among patients whose families have participated in psychoeducational programs (Hogarty et al., 1991). Further, other investigators have shown that the maintenance dose of medication is frequently lower in these family programs, possibly because of reduced familial stress that follows a cognitive mastery of psychosis and its treatment (Falloon et al., 1985). Information related to the psychobiology of psychotic conditions, the influence of medication on these processes, and the positive and negative effects of environmental factors on treatment response and course have all represented an important metacommunication to patients and families that they could not possibly have "caused" a brain disorder in their loved one (see Chapter 4). Rather they, as well as clinicians and other concerned friends, relatives, and employers, have a potentially strong influence on subsequent outcome by supporting medication decisions.

The opportunity for legitimate advocacy can present itself in the face of wrong diagnostic indications for psychotropic drugs, misinformation, or no information provided by the prescriber regarding side effects, and clearly inappropriate drug or dosing strategies. The format for exercising advocacy in these circumstances is, however, difficult. A very sensitive and all-too-frequent problem can occur, for example, when the nonphysician therapist has concern about medication management but feels unable to "reach" the prescribing physician or otherwise comfortably share observations that on the surface might appear to question prescribing practice. However, it must be noted that the overwhelming majority of physicians in our experience are open to and actively solicit the observations of other clinicians, family members, and patients themselves. Also, studies related to medication management, particularly regarding the newer medications, are always appearing in the literature, and many reports might have understandably escaped the attention of the physician, given the unprecedented number of mental health publications available, as well as their variable quality. Most physicians today labor under the constraints of managed care that limit available time per patient yet increase caseloads. While clinical psychopharmacology has an important empirical knowledge base, the practice, much like psychotherapy itself, remains an "art form."

However, should communication regarding legitimate concerns not be possible following sincere attempts to do so, the recommended approach is the same as one would follow with a nonphysician colleague who is not open to peer suggestions. In such cases, it is acceptable practice to suggest to the patient and family that it might be worthwhile to seek a second opinion. Should any practitioner, physician or otherwise, object to a second opinion, there is a clear basis established for simply seeking a new responsible clinician. Such decisions should not be made lightly, since an *inappropriate* referral could seriously disrupt continuity of care. Consultation with a competent supervisor or senior colleague should occur before such a recommendation is made. In facilities where absolutely no option is available to the patient or nonphysician therapist (e.g., in rural areas), the provision of relevant reading lists, case presentations, guest lecturers, or journal clubs can often provide the opportunity to discuss patient management and to acquire pertinent information as well.

Integrated Treatment

Finally, we close our discussion of medication management with some principles of integrated treatment that have come from our many studies of medication and psychosocial therapies, including PT:

1. Antipsychotic medications are central to the regulation of attention and arousal that underlies the psychotic process. But psychosocial interventions are equally important for the control of stress that frequently exploits this process, stressors that arise in the context of an overstimulating home, work, recreation, clinic, or school setting.

2. When psychotic patients who were definitely receiving medication have a relapse, most often than not a severe and independent life event occurred that might have been addressed by the clinician. Loss of Social Security or welfare benefits, a close relationship, or a permanent residence are but a few examples of disruptions that can lead to relapse and that are the proper object of psychosocial intervention.

3. Similarly, patients who remain disorganized, hyperaroused, withdrawn, aloof, or have little insight while receiving antipsychotic medication might be particularly susceptible to the stress of aggressive problem-solving efforts, rehabilitation initiatives, or therapeutic attempts to develop insight. Destabilization among patients who were faithfully taking medication can thus suggest a psychosocial treatment plan that needs to be changed, rather than the medication.

4. Minor exacerbations of psychotic symptoms can often be traced to environmental stressors that can be negotiated by the therapist, rather than retreat to a permanent increase in the dose of an antipsychotic drug

or the prescription of additional medications. Some evidence exists that the effective dose of medication might be less in the context of appropriate psychosocial interventions. Often a short-term supplemental (oral) dose of medication is useful for the patient that has been maintained on a low dose of fluphenazine or haloperidol decanoate while attempts at environmental manipulation are being made.

5. Rehabilitation and problem-solving strategies need to be slowly introduced after a stable dose of medication is achieved. The resolution of residual psychotic symptoms through the use of maintenance chemotherapy takes time, and patients frequently pass through months of inactivity, increased sleep, and lack of motivation before they are ready to take on the challenge of a fuller life.

6. Once initiated, rehabilitation tasks need to be simple "single steps at a time" for many recovering psychotic patients, with medication being closely monitored during each new initiative.

7. One change at a time is also essential. If a patient is beginning a rehabilitation program or obtaining a new residence, initiating work, or resuming a close interpersonal relationship, it is not the time to also negotiate a change in the type or dose of medication. This is particularly true today as new medications are increasingly being introduced.

8. The therapist must not be misled by the seeming improvement that frequently follows drug noncompliance. Side-effect reduction is largely responsible for the apparent improvement in such cases, and the continuation of depolarization block by medication stored throughout the body will often keep the patient free of psychosis for weeks or even months. Given time, however, a relapse will most often occur and the relationship to earlier drug discontinuation will often not be made in the mind of the patient or therapist.

9. Low dose does not mean "no dose." If a patient is responding well to psychosocial treatment while receiving a low maintenance dose of medication, this is not an indication that medication is no longer needed.

10. For many chronically psychotic patients, the failure to sustain treatment effects associated with psychosocial interventions can often be traced to the same reason that the maintenance of medication effects does not endure. The reason is that once the treatment ends, often the effect does as well Over time, reasonably recovered patients might need fewer psychosocial treatment contacts, but they still profit from the "safety net" assured by the continued availability of the clinician and periodic "booster" and review sessions.

11. Since the nonphysician therapist usually has more ongoing con-

tact with the patient (much like family), he or she needs to remain attuned to medication issues, even though his or her therapeutic interests and priorities might remain elsewhere. One of our most experienced and skillful clinicians recently remarked that even after years of practice, "it is still easy to become passive about medication issues and to narrowly focus on PT or supportive therapy. It is always important to think about what can be affected by medication and what is likely to be influenced by therapy or other support systems."

12. Beware of one's covert *false* assumptions! These can often include the presumption that—

    a. Residual or persistent psychotic symptoms (or anxiety or depression) will be refractory to more aggressive medication management (i.e., such symptoms are an "inevitable" part of schizophrenia).

    b. Supplemental medication strategies will not work, so why bother?

    c. Psychotic symptoms are really nonpsychotic symptoms that do not need to be aggressively managed.

    d. A more useful medication (e.g., clozapine) will not be effective because the clinician can predict how the patient will respond (e.g., with weight gain or other side effects).

    e. The diagnosis of early schizophrenia should be avoided for fear of "labeling" (but at the price of mistreatment).

    f. Comorbid substance misuse, mental insufficiency, brain damage, learning disabilities, or hyperactivity do not require specific diagnosis and selected interventions.

    g. A prolonged use of anxiolytics rather than a more appropriate use of antipsychotics (or supplemental mood stabilizers or antidepressants) can better manage the primary or associated symptoms of schizophrenia.

    h. One's knowledge is correct and complete without seeking further information from the patient, family, community agencies, or other providers.

In summary, a careful regulation of neurobiological factors by an antipsychotic drug and skilled negotiation of internal and external environmental factors by psychosocial intervention will continue to offer the best foundation for achieving and sustaining recovery of function for the patient with schizophrenia.

CHAPTER FOUR

The Basic Phase

As we begin the formal description of PT, it is worthwhile to recall the fundamental goals that we wish to accomplish: *the achievement and maintenance of clinical stability*. These objectives are intended to keep patients as free from disabling psychotic symptoms as possible and in better control of their illness. Without such mastery, even minor exacerbations can be demoralizing and disruptive of social and vocational achievements. Aside from avoiding the potential neurobiological, psychological, and social consequences of an unwanted symptom exacerbation, it is well known that the probability of a future exacerbation is reduced dramatically the longer a patient can survive without a psychotic episode (Hogarty & Ulrich, 1977). Thus, we need to be persistent and aggressive in attempts to achieve and maintain symptom stabilization. The following basic phase principles should help both clinician and patient to gain confident control of the processes that perpetuate or exacerbate the positive symptoms of psychosis.

This chapter describes the components that characterize the first—or basic phase of PT. These include the following:

- Getting ready for PT
- Joining with the patient
- Establishing a treatment plan

- Providing the rudimentary elements of psychoeducation regarding schizophrenia and its treatment
- Creating a plan for the resumption of tasks and responsibilities
- Describing the initial relationship between "stress as a trigger" and important psychotic prodromes (the beginning of "internal coping")
- Learning the basics of social skills training that facilitate appropriate avoidance of stressful situations as well as the proactive use of positive remarks

The chapter concludes with a discussion of the criteria that a patient would need to satisfy before proceeding to the more cognitively demanding intermediate phase of PT.

From the preceding outline, the experienced clinician will quickly recognize that there will be little that is novel to the basic phase of therapy, which is precisely the frame of mind that we wish to establish at the outset. The initiation of internal coping, elementary psychoeducation, and basic social skills training are the components that might extend beyond the core procedures of routine care outlined in Chapter 3, but that depend on these fundamentals for their efficacy. Good care, as we have emphasized, is knowing and doing the basics very well. PT strategies, whether innovative or progressive, build upon but never supersede the basics. The tried-and-true practice principles of the basic phase have come from three sources. First, the principles of joining, case management, and psychoeducation (along with support and medication management) also constituted the supportive therapy control condition during the studies of PT and, as described in Chapter 2, yielded positive results on relapse and adjustment that few experimental psychosocial treatments have approximated. Most contemporary outpatient programs, for example, would be delighted to have scarcely a third of their schizophrenia patients experience a psychotic relapse in the 3 years following an index hospitalization, even though gains in personal and social adjustment might have been modest. But such were the outcomes among our supportive therapy recipients in the recent studies. Second, from a study described earlier (Hogarty et al., 1986), we recall that only 19% of very-high-risk patients relapsed in a skills training condition during the first postdischarge year (and 0% relapsed in the combined skills training/family psychoeducation condition), a rate that stood in some contrast to the 38% of control subjects who relapsed in that study. It seemed difficult for us to improve on the first-year relapse results of skills training, support, and medication, and it was precisely the gains from this patient-centered therapy that we wished to preserve by integrating the strategies that had proven especially useful in establishing clinical stabilization. In treatment, as in life, one can profit most by building on existing strengths and prior successes. Closely associated with the premise of "doing the basics well" is our desire not to reinvent the therapeutic wheel. Most of the practice principles contained in the basic phase of PT have been described by us and many others elsewhere (e.g., see Anderson et al., 1986), including the broad guidelines of an early (unpublished) working manual that influenced our initial efforts at PT.

Thus, the goals of basic phase PT are similar to those followed by us for many years—namely, to (1) achieve stabilization of symptoms and the living condition of the patient; (2) acquire entitlements, housing, medical care, and subsistence for the patient as indicated; (3) facilitate patient cooperation with medication taking and clinic appointments; (4) assist in developing a fundamental knowledge of the illness and its treatment; (5) encourage resumption of the patient's customary responsibilities in the household beginning with self-care and personal hygiene; (6) introduce the concepts of stress, reactivity, and prodromes; and (7) provide a few basic coping strategies appropriate to the early stage of recovery. The following basic phase principles will each hopefully contribute to the attainment of these goals. The components constitute a process more than a prescription, and flexibility in order and emphasis should be determined by individual patient needs, rather than by fidelity to a seeming recipe. In many ways the process of "blending" these treatment components will be among the most challenging PT tasks that the clinician will encounter. Many therapists might typically approach the treatment process using techniques in a serial fashion. Such an approach would render a disservice to PT and, we suspect, to the patient as well. Rather, the clinician will want to keep in mind at least four facets of blending: (1) the integration of PT techniques with the patient's own autoprotective strategies; (2) the blending of PT techniques *within* a phase, such as stressor identification and the rudimentary social skills components of the basic phase; (3) the blending of PT techniques *across* phases, such as deep breathing (intermediate phase) and criticism management (advanced phase) with the cues of distress; and (4) the application of selective techniques to the realities of the patient's current life circumstances. Blending serves to individualize the patient's treatment and provides the basis for acquiring an increasingly relevant repertoire of adaptive strategies that is appropriate to the stage of clinical recovery and the patient's abilities and immediate needs.

PT CREDENTIALS

We have no precise credentialing that would be appropriate for identifying a prospective PT clinician. In our own program, PhD clinical psychologists who had a strong behavioral training background and experience with schizophrenia patients were the largest in number, followed by master's-level psychiatric nurse clinical specialists. The nurses found PT particularly compatible with their training insofar as knowledge of body systems and clinical psychopharmacology made the psychosocial and biological treatment of PT a seamless and easily integrated process for the patient. By intent, the practice of PT is best reserved for a potential therapist who has achieved at least a master's-level competency in psychosocial treatment, including social work practitioners as well as those in counseling education and rehabilitation. The task will be more difficult for the nonphysician, however, in the absence of knowledge regarding maintenance chemotherapy, particularly the absence of experience in collaboratively working with a prescribing physician. Knowledge of schizophrenia, including the contemporary findings on neurodevelopment and pathophysiology, as well as a relevant work experience with schizophrenia patients are highly desirable.

A good candidate for the practice of PT would be an empathic, noncynical, and above all hopeful person who maintains professional boundaries and is ever mindful of conditions that precipitate a countertransference. Such an individual would also be sensitive to the pathophysiological vulnerabilities of schizophrenia patients, to the slow curve of recovery, and to the value system and culture of the patient. Those who view schizophrenia as the result of faulty parenting, dysfunctional family systems, or other nurturing calamities, rather than as a developmentally based brain disorder, would not likely warm to PT. We encourage PT for therapists who realize the potential for an enhanced quality of life for even the most impaired patients. Clinicians that are curious, resourceful, flexible, respectful (of patient autonomy, opinions, and boundaries), open, directive, active, and comfortable with positive and negative symptoms are prime PT candidates. Therapeutic optimism, however, is not synonymous with naïveté. Rather, it is an attitude tempered by the reality that achieving modest yet very attainable goals is an important objective. Symptom stabilization, relapse prevention, and fostering the capacity needed to form, maintain, and enjoy interpersonal relationships and vocational pursuits constitute these core objectives.

Today, the available forms of psychotherapy number in the hundreds. Providers of service to the schizophrenia patient might want to think of limiting their interventions to those practice principles that arise from relevant data regarding the psychosocial and biological bases of schizophrenia, and for which empirical evidence of efficacy can be found, evidence that extends beyond the anecdotes of the therapy's originator or the testimonial of followers. As we attempted to describe earlier, even the most carefully considered, disorder-relevant intervention for schizophrenia patients holds the potential of doing harm as well as good. In this regard, a modicum of PT supervision is desirable. Facilities that adopt PT have a special opportunity to implement the *peer supervision* approach to treatment fidelity, one that we used successfully during the studies of PT. In this setting, the relevance of selected strategies can be collaboratively determined for the difficult-to-manage patient, the integrative process can be periodically reviewed, and the experiences of advanced practitioners can be shared. Weekly sessions are most useful in the first 6–9 months of PT implementation. Once comfort and confidence increase, biweekly sessions are generally sufficient. Peer supervision also provides a needed continuity to the culture and process of PT, as either new clinicians join the facility or others depart.

PT SESSIONS

At first, it was believed that weekly PT sessions of approximately 45 minutes each would be indicated. In practice, however, patients attended clinic for approximately three sessions per month during the first year of treatment, and somewhat fewer (though typically biweekly) sessions in subsequent years as described earlier. For patients who suffered prominent difficulties in attention and information processing, hyperarousal and impaired problem-solving abilities, sessions would often not exceed 30 minutes, especially when additional time for fine-tuning medication was needed. The length and frequency of sessions were thus found to vary according to patient needs, strengths, and liabilities, as well as the presence or absence of interim crises. In short, the trajectories of sessions were typically a function of patient needs and desire, tolerance for therapy, the rate of learning as constrained by neuropsychological problems, and hence the level of recovery, each of which differed within and between patients at any given time. If we have learned anything in the past 30 years, it is that time is needed for the schizophrenia patient to heal and seal over, a precious commodity in the era of managed care. Premature, aggressive attempts to speed the recovery process will typically set it back to the beginning, as we have described in earlier chapters and repeatedly experienced. As shown elsewhere (Hogarty et al., 1988), it most often takes 6 months and for some patients 10–12 months to simply achieve a reasonable remission of psychotic symptoms following an acute episode and, for many of these patients, to experience the return of physical stamina appropriate to the resumption of life roles. In times past, most of this initial period of recovery occurred in the context of a hospital (asylum), but today it falls to the outpatient therapist to create a "holding environment" in what is often a stressful and unaccommodating world (Winnicott, 1965). With ever-decreasing lengths of hospitalization available for the acutely psychotic patient, the challenge of outpatient stabilization becomes a formidable task.

The format for an individual session might appear intimidating, given the multiple phases and the multiple components within a phase. But, in practice, the process can quickly become predictable to both patient and therapist, once the therapeutic alliance and the treatment contract are established. A typical session will begin with a status check of clinical stability, including persistent positive or negative symptoms, mood disturbance, possible medication side effects, and concurrent use of alcohol, illicit drugs, or over-the-counter medications. Such inquiries are fundamental to the successful management of medication. Similarly, a status check of environmental stability can alert the clinician to continuing or potential problems that need to be addressed in the areas of housing, finances, conflicted relationships, or other individual sources of perceived stress. Clinical and/or environmental instability provide the blueprint for selecting PT strategies as well as the associated homework assignments. For example, were paranoid ideas to increase in a volunteer job setting, the clinician could evaluate possible stressors associated with the position, assess the patient's cues of distress, provide a brief educational review, and begin to work on, let us say, a basic social skills technique that could be practiced at home. Otherwise, the session would move to a review of progress on a specific PT component, particularly one represented in a recent homework assignment. According to the patient's phase of PT, the review might focus on the component at hand or it might represent the integration of components already worked on, including (1) an element of acquired and applied psychoeducation; (2) the resumption of a specific task in, or later out of, the home; (3) the use of an internal coping strategy; or (4) a specific social skill technique. Finally, the next step designed to further develop competency in one of the preceding areas (1–4) can be introduced, discussed, and—when appropriate—enhanced with a relevant homework assignment. The introduction of any new material is supported with a rationale for how this component fits into the overall treatment plan. Enlisting the patient as an ally in the process of identifying and implementing progressive tasks requires that the therapist act as an expert regarding the steps needed for recovery, while offering the patient distinct choices at each step as a way to ensure that the process remains collaborative. Reference to the long-term treatment plan tends to appropriately move patients away from the "crisis of the day" mentality that often characterizes outpatient maintenance treatment.

GETTING READY

Preparation for PT begins with the selection of an individual patient at a specific juncture in the course of illness, most often during a period of destabilization. For us, the first application of PT began with the identification of a hospitalized patient shortly before discharge who had experienced an acute psychotic episode, either the first or, more often, the most recent in a series of episodes. For some readers of this volume, PT candidates might be drawn from an existing caseload of patients who are at least partially stable. For others, patients will be at various levels of stabilization such as a postdischarge referral from an inpatient unit, a referral from another community provider or family member, or a self-referral. Prior knowledge of the patient, the degree of symptom remission, and the level of current functioning will make the basic phase more or less difficult to complete.

For the patient who might be new to a therapist or a treatment program (but is otherwise characterized by an extensive psychiatric history), nothing can be more disheartening than an initial encounter that appears to treat the patient as though this was his or her first contact with the mental health system. We have often wondered whether a patient's so-called resistance to a new treatment opportunity simply reflects a frustration with new requests for historical information that has been repeatedly provided on prior occasions. A newly hospitalized patient, for example, that had been treated in an established aftercare program carries an anthology of important information related to personal history and prior treatment, including outpatient care. Because the patient has recently relapsed is rarely an indication that existing information is irrelevant and that the current treatment regimen, particularly medication, is ineffective and in need of immediate change. Patients relapse for many reasons, not the least of which follows an independent life event that almost always can be identified among medication compliant patients who were otherwise appropriately medicated (McEvoy, Howe, & Hogarty, 1984). Existing medical records typically contain a wealth of information regarding past history, the patient's environment, and his or her treatment response. If the identified candidate comes from the PT clinician's own health care system, the observations, insights, and treatment strategies (successful and otherwise) of the previous primary clinician are simply invaluable and should be immediately sought.

Once a successful engagement with the patient has been made, permission to obtain release of the medical history, including contact with the previous therapist, if appropriate, should be tactfully sought. Similarly, the observations and reports of significant others who maintain an abiding interest and concern for the welfare of the patient should be solicited. As we have described elsewhere (Anderson et al., 1986), schizophrenia is not a "private event" that can be concealed from loved ones. Excluding family input into the treatment plan under the guise of preserving confidentiality is often an exercise in misplaced altruism and a deterrent to the patient's best hope for recovery of function. Such exercises in confidentiality are generally absent in non-Western cultures, an absence that might explain the relatively better outcome of these patients in developing countries (Leff, 2001). Certainly the *content* of therapy sessions should remain within the boundaries of confidentiality and respect for the patient's privacy. But schizophrenia remains a very "public event" to those most concerned about the patient, and their observations and efforts are crucial to treatment planning and outcome. Some states do not allow information to be shared with the family if the adult patient objects. In these instances we follow the National Alliance for the Mentally Ill guideline that obligates clinicians to assure patients that neither they nor the family are responsible for the illness and that outcome is far more likely to be better if "all interested parties work together."*

In constructing the needs assessment to which PT will be targeted, the types of information that the clinician will want to seek from existing sources prior to initiating therapy include the following:

1. Past episodes of schizophrenia, including the identification of possible precipitants and a potential pattern of reactivity that might precede symptom exacerbation.

---

*See *www.nami.org/update/platform/htm* [# 3.0].

2. Identification of the patient's individual prodromal signs and symptoms to the extent possible.
3. Past medication regimens and the patient's subjective experience, including a positive response as well as unwanted side effects.
4. Problems in medication compliance, including contributing factors such as obvious or subtle side effects, false beliefs, issues of control and autonomy, denial of illness, or the patient's own plan of recovery that might preclude medication.
5. The existence of family or significant other support and, conversely, conflicted relationships or the absence of needed resources related to stable housing, financial benefits, medical care, food, clothing, and transportation (significant mental illness in close family members or friends, as well as conflicts with community care providers, also should be noted).
6. Comorbidity in the form of drug or alcohol use, abuse, or dependence, affective disorder, personality disorder, medical illness, and limited intellectual capacity.
7. Patient strengths, including "premorbid" and recent social and vocational competencies, as well as past difficulties in establishing and maintaining instrumental or expressive roles.
8. Residual cognitive difficulties in maintaining attention, working memory, problem solving, or abstract reasoning.
9. Prior successes or lack thereof in response to other psychosocial interventions, whether supportive, behavioral, family, educational, or vocational in nature.

Prior knowledge can go a long way toward facilitating the process of joining with the patient, forming the treatment contract, and allowing the principles of supportive therapy and medication management to be implemented. It is often helpful to maintain a simple checklist of this essential information before and during PT.

Finally, "getting ready" often means *not* introducing many basic phase components (e.g., internal coping or role resumption) until residential stability is ensured. As described in Chapter 2, patients who lived independent of family, were unsettled in their place of residence, and/or who lacked access to such fundamental necessities as financial assistance, food, clothing, and medical care often relapsed prematurely when faced with the challenges of the basic phase. In retrospect, it is not difficult to appreciate the negative consequences of PT's cognitive demands among patients who lived independent of family and were preoccupied with whether they might be "on the street" the following day or without food and clothing in the immediate future. Therefore, the need for basic case management strategies, including material support, should be dealt with first, as described in Chapter 3. *For residentially unstable patients who struggle with the challenge of meeting basic needs, PT should be reserved to the principles of joining, support, medication, and case management until safe and predictable housing and other basic necessities are secured!* Again, the task of the clinician is one that resembles the psychoanalytic concept of the "holding environment" (Winnicott, 1965), an empathic understanding of the patient's turmoil in the face of overwhelming life events and the communication that a safe, dependable environment constitutes the immediate therapeutic agenda to be pursued by the clinician.

When beginning PT, the clinician will often be more narrowly focused on the tasks of achieving symptom stabilization and reducing the risk of relapse, especially in the first year following a recent episode. (Once stabilization is achieved, the risk of relapse should significantly decline over time, to 15% or less per year [Hogarty & Ulrich 1977].) Depending on the pretreatment clinical state, the typical risk of relapse in the first and subsequent years should be significantly reduced with the addition of PT, as demonstrated by the results of the PT study among patients who resided with family. Basic phase goals will likely take up to 8 months for most patients to achieve, again depending on their clinical state.

JOINING

More often than not, a candidate for PT will present at a time of crisis as perceived by the family, patient, or another mental health provider. Sometimes the crisis will have been the first occurrence, or more likely the recurrence of acute psychotic symptoms. Should the new episode have required hospitalization or a change in provider status, the patient could be described as now being "out of the therapeutic container" in terms of an interrupted treatment plan. As difficult as this disruption might have been for the patient, there is at least the opportunity to introduce the concept that PT goals and strategies can represent a hopeful new beginning. The fear, anxiety, blame, denial, and confusion that accompany a first episode of schizophrenia are often equaled only by the demoralization and despair associated with a recurrence of symptoms. Slowly, the reality dawns that this is an illness that will not be easily managed, readily denied, or wishfully attributed to transient events. Nor is it an illness for which "warm medication" will be the exclusive prescription for the resumption of social and vocational roles and the acquisition of a meaningful quality of life.

No matter what form psychotherapy has taken throughout its history, each approach has emphasized the essential need for a therapeutic relationship, or "alliance," and each has acknowledged the difficulty in establishing one. The latter is especially true regarding the patient who is suspicious, angry about the consequences of illness, in denial of the illness or the need for treatment, is extraordinarily ambivalent, thought disordered, projecting, blaming, or simply indifferent to any change in the status quo. In such situations, Fenton and McGlashan (1999) recommend flexibility, creativity and patience, a prescription that we readily endorse.

Commentators on the obstacles to joining have uniformly cited an alleged patient "distrust" of human relationships, historically interpreted as originating in early dependent relationships with an inept, cold, uncaring adult (principally a parent) who was unwilling or unable to meet basic needs for emotional support, understanding, and nurturance. We gratefully note that much of this etiological speculation on the source of mistrust (and on the nature of schizophrenia itself) has now been tempered by the absence of empirical support for such beliefs (see Hirsch & Leff, 1975). The strength of other explanatory models, including developmental neurobiology and human genetics, are welcomed alternatives. In our own experience, an initial mistrust of the therapeutic relationship has frequently had a legitimate foundation in reality, best understood using the established psychotherapeutic principles of empathic listening, validation of the patient's feelings, initiating the search for information surrounding the details of these experiences, and a willingness to become the likely object of criticism from the patient (McGlashan, 1983). Prior to the introduction of the newer atypical antipsychotic medications, for example, a primary source of mistrust was often an unpleasant experience with typical neuroleptics. Our success in enrolling and maintaining patients in treatment over the years can largely be attributed to an acknowledgment of these unfortunate medication experiences and a simple pledge to the patient that chemical restraint in the form of extrapyramidal side effects, akathisia, and the assault on affective life and willed behavior is *not* the price that one has to pay for recovery. (See the disussions of *medication management* in Chapters 3 and 5.) The patient can clearly and confidently be told that options are now available regarding patient input into medication decisions, including the use of minimum effective dosing (MED) strategies for those maintained on typical neuroleptics, the route of administration, and the choice of an appropriate atypical antipsychotic drug. Patient distrust of the therapeutic relationship in recent years has also followed upon having "serial service providers" that have appeared and disappeared in the patient's life. As experienced and credentialed clinicians have been "downsized" because of cost, or forced to seek employment outside the patient's provider network because of an inequitable reimbursement for service, or asked to serve more patients per hour, the dependable and available therapeutic relationship has become a rare commodity. It is most comforting to patients when assurances can be offered that a clinician will likely remain in place during the PT experience. Potential disruptions in the continuity and predictability of the therapeutic relationship is unfortunately a major obstacle to the implementation and maintenance of psychotherapy today.

Otherwise, many patients lack awareness or understanding of the nature and severity of their illness and some see no need for ongoing treatment. In such cases, it is often unproductive to either argue about the presence or absence of symptoms or to be overly confrontational about symptom-driven behavior. Encouragement can sometimes move patients to accept treatment, if not for themselves then for loved ones who are greatly distressed by the illness. Often the fear that dependable day-to-day services provided by their family might become jeopardized can also be motivating. Proposing that medication might simply contribute to the patient's "feeling better" (or get providers and family "off the patient's back") are sometimes more successful strategies for compliance than describing the specific antipsychotic effects of a drug. For some, a compromise that the patient will "try treatment for awhile" at least buys time to establish a therapeutic relationship and to initiate the recovery process. For patients who live with their family and/or depend on the family for support, there is often the inclination to pronounce "ultimatums" (e.g., eviction, involuntary commitment, withdrawal of support) if the patient refuses treatment. We typically discourage such ultimatums unless the family is prepared to follow through on them. There are, of course, exceptions should the patient terrorize the family or become a source of danger to him- or herself or others.

The tasks of joining include a communication that the clinician understands something of the distress associated with an episode or hospitalization and the associated feelings of hopelessness, sadness, grief, mourning, anger, or apprehension. Hopefulness about recovery and the means to achieve it are gradually introduced in the form of PT. For the acutely psychotic patient, brief but regular visits to the patient (most often on the inpatient unit) will serve to ensure his or her familiarity with the clinician and to begin the process of establishing rapport. Even for the patient who denies illness, is involuntarily hospitalized, or who initially rejects the need for treatment or at best is ambivalent, these brief contacts often serve to reinforce the reality that a caring clinician and a potentially useful outpatient treatment do exist. Often these visits represent little more than socializing contacts with a reassuring clinician. Empathic or "active" listening is employed as the medium for obtaining the details of the patient's life experience from his or her perspective and for identifying and labeling the strong associated affects. Lengthy discussions regarding the content of psychotic symptoms should be avoided, but the associated feelings can be acknowledged. ("It must be upsetting to feel that your neighbor had been poisoning your food.") Dwelling on psychotic material tends to socialize the patient to the unhelpful expectation that "therapy" is essentially an opportunity to discuss symptoms. Less attention is paid to displays of emotional dysregulation and more to the fact that these affects are understood by the clinician. Communication should be simple and uncomplicated. Clinicians should also be prepared for a negative response or resistance to the need for treatment. But even such resistance can be viewed as a "rudimentarily healthy kernel of willful autonomy" (McGlashan, 1983, p. 913), one that holds the potential for being channeled into health-promoting behavior.

As acute symptoms remit with medication, gentle confrontations might be used with the persistently resistant patient in terms of identifying apparent discrepancies between the reality of psychotic episodes, social and vocational dysfunctioning, and family distress, for example, and the patient's belief that continuing treatment is not indicated or desired. On the other hand, acknowledging the validity of patient concerns that personal life goals have been compromised or family life disrupted by the illness can serve to reinforce the potential of a realistic treatment plan. More often than not, the real "treatment resistance" experienced by PT therapists has come in the form of unrealistic patient goals such as wanting an immediate return to academic classes that would exceed the patient's level of cognitive organization or hoping for a full-time job that would not accommodate his or her limited capacity for information processing. By not colluding with such short-term unrealistic goals, the joining process might be extended somewhat, but nevertheless sends the message that the treatment strategies being suggested are attainable forms of self control and autonomy. A helpful message might be something like this: "PT is first a way to reduce and control stress in your life and avoid hospitalization. Over time it will help you to gain confidence in managing important relationships and job opportunities in the community."

Again, as the more florid symptoms abate, strategies to be used, such as medication management, psychoeducation, as well as the choices available for prodromal management and coping, can be simply described without great elaboration. For the more stable outpatient candidate, these PT goals and strategies can be introduced earlier. More problematic for the new outpatient is the logistic issue associated with regular clinic attendance. Obstacles to transportation should be reviewed and, until they are resolved, irregular clinic visits can be supplemented with telephone calls. Public or private support that can help to defray transportation costs is among the most cost-effective of strategies for avoiding "no shows." Our transportation costs during the PT studies averaged about $65.00 per patient year (paid by the program) and led to an extraordinary rate of treatment compliance. We suspect that this compliance often contributed to the low rate of relapse across all treatment conditions.

Finally, a key element in joining is once again the successful connection with family for patients who either live with their family or maintain regular contact. While PT was designed as a patient-centered treatment for reasons described earlier, even the informal inclusion of the family can contribute to a more comfortable household, more satisfying relationships, and the provision of information and support that are crucial to the treatment plan. The therapist should strive to open and maintain lines of communication with family members, and to share with them the nature of and reasonable expectations for PT. Basic education about the illness and its management should be offered when discernible gaps in knowledge are apparent. Long term, the family should feel comfortable in calling the clinician in order to obtain answers to their questions, to offer their own suggestions and observations, and to develop confidence in the treatment approach. Family members should ultimately feel that their loved one is receiving high-quality care and that they have a central role in ensuring a good treatment outcome. For those less familiar with the concerns of family members and the approaches to family engagement when schizophrenia affects a loved one, we again refer the reader to our earlier text (Anderson et al., 1986).

THE TREATMENT PLAN

The foundation of the treatment plan is the clinician's assessment of individual needs, strengths, goals, personal coping strategies, as well as environmental supports and constraints. The latter include family and personal resources related to stable shelter, financial assistance, food, clothing, transportation, medical care, and any current disruption in these relationships and support systems. Careful inquiry and attentiveness to patient concerns can often reveal a possible pattern of events that typically lead to symptom exacerbation, views toward and fidelity in taking prescribed medication, and recurrent or persistent sources of stressful life events. These dialogues will typically reveal the patient's own perceptions of "what went wrong," their acknowledged vulnerabilities, expectations for recovery of role function, and plans for achieving these goals. It is during these discussions that one or more of the PT strategies can be introduced as the means of facilitating the patient's own perceived goals. It is important to stress that PT is not something that the clinician will do to the patient, but rather it is a process to be shared with the patient, since patient recovery also depends on individual resiliency, strengths, and health-promoting initiatives. The patient's notions of "causality," the level of preserved insight, and the degree of hopefulness or pessimism about the future can also be identified. (The pretreatment assessment derived from existing records, prior therapist reports, past treatment response, and the premorbid competencies are most crucial sources of information at this point in establishing the treatment contract.) Systematically identified as targets of the treatment plan should be *individual prodromal signs* such as the following: neurovegative features that include changes in sleep, appetite, and energy; affective symptoms such as anxiety, agitation, irritability, anger, or depression; behavioral changes that include avoidance or arguing; and cognitive changes that appear as rumination, decreased concentration, and impaired comprehension, as well as ambivalence and residual thought disorder. Such information can also serve to prioritize the content of the treatment plan around three broad classifications or symptom typologies: (1) the affectively unstable patient, (2) the negative symptom patient, or (3) the persistently psychotic patient. Throughout these assessment sessions, patients can be offered reassurances that their symptoms will become better controlled and their level of functioning will gradually improve through systematic collaboration. For patients who find it difficult to conceptualize or verbalize past history, cognitive and emotional states, or future goals, the clinician can restate the patient's thoughts, feelings, expressed needs, and plans in a nonthreatening manner that often increases trust and personal comfort. Such reframing should be clearly and repeatedly stated for patients who suffer obvious impairments in attention, information processing, and recall.

The content of the treatment plan as it relates to achieving the patient's individualized goals will include a rational medication regimen and its careful management, so designed as to reduce unwanted side effects and achieve symptomatic relief. Further, patients can be told that formal education regarding the essential features of schizophrenia, including sensitivity to environmental stress, will be provided. Patients should be assured that new coping strategies, which will further develop and expand upon their own existing skills, can be learned and that the eventual resumption of work and relationship roles will be pursued. Each of these treatment plan components should be integrated with the patient's own perceived goals and defined as being either short term (e.g., symptom stabilization) or long term (e.g., resumption of work) in nature. "Therapy" is described for the patient as a series of steps needed to—

1. Maintain survival without psychosis.
2. Gradually resume roles and responsibilities.
3. Develop awareness and foresight regarding the relationship between relapse and the cues of distress arising from internal or external events.
4. Acquire strategies designed to reduce stress and avoid psychotic or affective decompensation.

In order to help patients understand and accept the treatment plan, it is often useful to discuss the following elements: (1) how and in what situations therapy will work to achieve the patients goals (e.g., coping with a perceived source of stress, (2) the time frame to be used for achieving these goals, and (3) the number of sessions and types of PT schedules to be followed. The patient should be informed that sessions will begin on a weekly basis and the length of a session will range between 15 and 45 minutes depending on the patient's ability to concentrate and tolerate discussions. Once the patient achieves a reasonable degree of stability, sessions will likely be reduced to biweekly visits.

The treatment plan emphasizes the importance of regular patient attendance, fidelity in taking the prescribed medication, and the negative consequence of alcohol and drug abuse. The patient is encouraged to discuss any obstacles to attending regular sessions and to share information about what he or she perceives to be sources of stress and support. Information sharing about persistent or recurrent symptoms, beliefs about medication and side effects, and any other concerns that might influence a willingness to participate should become an agreed-upon component of the plan. An effort should be made to elicit an explicit assurance that the patient will call the clinician whenever thoughts arise of harming oneself or another. (The issues of depression and suicidality are addressed in Chapter 5.) Finally, the plan includes an agreement between the patient and the clinician to work together on the set of established goals. The clinician agrees to help the patient reach the objectives that are consistent with promoting stabilization, preventing relapse, and recovering function. As the patient comes to better appreciate what PT can provide, the clinician details what the patient's own role will be in achieving a successful outcome, including regular attendance, medication adherence, and the application of learned strategies to stressful encounters outside the clinic.

PSYCHOEDUCATION

Whether stimulated by the success of family psychoeducation or because of its own intrinsic value, the provision of information regarding the nature and treatment of schizophrenia has become an increasingly important component of direct patient care itself (Sullwold & Herrlich, 1992). For patients whose understanding of schizophrenia had been little more than a chaotic, frightening, and inexplicable alteration of perceptions, beliefs, and emotions (and an alienation from family and friends), education has provided a sense of cognitive mastery. With correct information, schizophrenia can be readily understood as a "no-fault" brain disorder that has an increasingly clear origin, a well-described pathophysiology, and an array of effective treatments that can positively influence course and outcome. Further, not only does psychoeducation reduce anxiety, guilt, hopelessness, and blame, but it can also free patients to develop and use their own coping resources in order to better negotiate stress, avoid a relapse, and resume functioning. Knowledge about the illness provides an explicit rationale for the treatment plan, including the need for a gradual, stepwise resumption of functions, an appreciation of the vulnerabilities imposed by the illness and the subsequent need for realistic short- and long-term goals. With education, patients tend not to attach idiosyncratic meaning to their symptoms and most often come to appreciate how their own individualized treatment plan offers the real possibility for a better future.

In PT, education is an integral part of most treatment sessions, the content of which varies in quantity and depth depending on the patient's level of symptomatic recovery and the capacity to process and understand information. It is often possible for the therapist to provide a formal psychoeducational workshop as well, where 8–10 patients can be collaboratively introduced to the core information regarding schizophrenia and its treatment. This is especially true in programs where multiple therapists practice PT. Not only are such workshops economically feasible, but they tend to legitimize the expert knowledge of the PT therapist, provide an opportunity for peer support and generate comfort among patients who are learning that others share similar experiences. In our program, a formal workshop typically occurred following symptom stabilization (usually 4–6 months after hospital discharge).

Numerous textbooks, journal articles (particularly those to be found in the *Schizophrenia Bulletin*), and pamphlets from the NIMH or the pharmaceutical industry are now available that describe schizophrenia and its treatment in an easily understood, comprehensive, and accurate format. We continue to rely on the basic psychoeducation principles that we previously published for family members (see Anderson et al., 1986, Ch. 3), although the content has clearly changed with time. For example, over the 16 years that we tested and developed family psychoeducation, no two workshops were ever identical in content. Information on the nature and treatment of schizophrenia was modified as new insights from the basic and clinical neurosciences and treatment research evolved. In the present volume we attempt to update this information, but it is not intended to replace basic information regarding the nature of schizophrenia (Anderson et al., 1986). While this evolution carries with it the responsibility to remain familiar with current literature, the metacommunications of psychoeducation remain constant: (1) schizophrenia is not a volitional or learned disorder; (2) schizophrenia leaves the brain exquisitely sensitive to life experiences that need to be wisely negotiated; (3) schizophrenia has a clear pathophysiology, as shown from scientific studies; and (4) increasingly definitive and effective therapeutic interventions are available that respond to this pathophysiology. The therapist can simply complete these messages with current information. We tend to rely on reviews that are periodically updated in the *Schizophrenia Bulletin*, an inexpensive, comprehensive, and authoritative NIMH publication available from the U.S. Government Printing Office.

In the following pages, we might at times emphasize the biological substrate of schizophrenia disorders, even though our primary interest is on the psychological and social components associated with recovery. We do this because many of the nonphysician clinicians who work with the severely mentally ill might not have been exposed to recent thinking about the origins of schizophrenia, if one recent study is any indication: Rubin, Cardenas, Warren, Pike, and Wambach (1998), reported that in spite of extraordinary research advances in the past two decades, nearly half of the experienced clinicians they surveyed continued to believe that parenting behavior was etiologically significant in severe mental illness and "getting them [the parents] to recognize their own culpability should be an aim of therapy" (p. 420). While most clinicians known to us recognize the importance of biological factors (as was found in the above Rubin et al. survey), we suspect that a bit of confusion might continue to exist between a "cause" and a psychosocial "risk factor" for schizophrenia symptoms. Developmental experiences, such as the attitude embodied in "expressed emotion" that characterizes the behavior of parents, other family members, therapists, landlords, friends, and bartenders, is one of many potential risk factors in schizophrenia. (Loss, expectations that exceed cognitive competencies, isolation, and substance abuse are a few others.) "High" expressed emotion (EE) can precipitate an episode of schizophrenia (and other medical and psychiatric disorders), and "low" EE can influence a good outcome in already affected patients, that is, in the presence of other causes. But risk factors do not "cause" the disorder themselves. One analogy that comes to mind is the "risk" for a diabetic patient that is represented by the candy counter at a neighborhood grocery store, but the local grocer is clearly not the cause of a diabetic crisis for the affected patient who overindulges.

During the basic phase, the components of psychoeducation that are offered include the following: (1) information on the origins of schizophrenia; (2) its clinical presentation as experienced from the subjective and objective points of view; and (3) how treatments work, including their modification of vulnerability and stress. While we shall attempt to remain true to the science that supports these themes, the PT therapist will want to reframe and translate the content according to the patient's needs, clinical state, and ability to process information. Over time, various aspects of psychoeducation content are *reintroduced* when they bear upon a specific PT component such as discussion of a vulnerability, a prodromal sign, a source of stress, a medication side effect, or the acquisition of a coping strategy. Whenever new concepts are introduced in the education process, patients should be strongly encouraged to take notes in a readily accessible notebook.

Origins of Schizophrenia

Until recently, we avoided speculation on the "cause" of schizophrenia and preferred to limit our comments to a reasonably well-described pathophysiology or brain dysfunction that often characterized individuals who were already affected by this illness. But with the substantial research contributions from the "Decade of the Brain," the modern neurosciences have now provided a more extensive database regarding the possible origins of many schizophrenia disorders, such that we have been moved to attempt an integration of relevant work (Keshavan & Hogarty, 1999) that we briefly summarize in the following paragraphs.

Clearly a genetic basis can be established for some cases of schizophrenia, although critics cite the limitation of genetics for purposes of prevention in that only 10% of patients have a clear family history of schizophrenia. However, neuropsychological, psychophysiological, and neuroanatomic markers of these disorders may occur in as many as 50% of first-degree family members, particularly offspring, who might never manifest the phenotype or clinical presentation of schizophrenia itself. Hereditability has been estimated to account for 60–70% of schizophrenia cases with environment accounting for the remaining 30–40%. The failure to express this genetic vulnerability implicates the important role of poorly understood environmental influences as well as developmental experiences that confer protection or resiliency. But well-known genetic studies do indicate an important biological substrate to the origin of manifest schizophrenia, with rates of 1% in the general population rising to approximately 3% among the nephews and nieces of an affected individual (25% genetic relatedness), and from 10% to 14% among siblings and offspring (50% relatedness), to 35% or 40% when both parents have suffered schizophrenia and up to 50% among identical twins when one is affected (100% genetic relatedness).

In recent years, more attention has been paid to the neurodevelopmental hypothesis of schizophrenia, which implicates brain anomalies that might follow upon genetically mediated environmental insults and/or developmental failures. A broad literature implicates two important developmental periods that might impact on the origin of schizophrenia: the early intrauterine and perinatal period, and the later developmental epochs of adolescence and early adult life. Early cerebral insults that might underline schizophrenia have been referred to as the "first hit," and later problems as the "second hit." In the early developmental model (Weinberger, 1987), a brain insult that occurred during gestation might likely have remained symptomatically "silent" until provoked by the developmental challenges of adolescence or young adult life, a hypothesis supported by the study of neonatally lesioned young animals. Evidence of early insult in schizophrenia has been drawn from studies of the following: viral infection associated with season of birth, including retrovirus in recent studies; perinatal anoxia; DNA mutations associated with advanced paternal age;

nutritional deprivation; and indirectly by studies of neurological "soft signs" and childhood asociality. Perhaps more compelling is the evidence from autopsy studies that describe the cortical cytoarchitecture anomalies of many schizophrenia patients. Errors in neurogenesis and migration (typically those that occurred in the second trimester of pregnancy) have been found in various studies such that an inappropriate decrease in neural connectivity in superficial cortical layers is accompanied by an equally suspect increase in neural density in deeper, subcortical, white matter layers. These early insults might likely have influenced various structural and functional brain anomalies that include enlarged ventricles, a smaller hippocampus and amygdyla, and impaired neuronal viability in the anterior cingulate that have been observed among adult schizophrenia patients as well as the high-risk offspring of parents with schizophrenia. Such anomalies can also account for the ubiquitous alterations in neuropsychology, electrophysiology, and neurochemistry that characterize adult schizophrenia. It remains a matter of debate, however, whether these apparent anomalies are specific for schizophrenia, or are nonspecific indicators of severe mental disorders overall.

Later in normal adolescence, neurodevelopment continues with a surge in synaptic "pruning" as well as reductions in delta sleep, membrane synthesis, gray matter volume and prefrontal metabolism. In schizophrenia, these various reductions in structure and function seem to represent an exaggeration of normal developmental processes, perhaps an indirect indicator of excessive synaptic pruning, particularly in the prefrontal cortex. The absence of normal cerebral asymmetry in many schizophrenia conditions (i.e., a failure to lateralize brain function and structure) might also be a consequence. It is not that neurons themselves die off, but rather that synaptic or axonal pruning might have become accelerated, as evidenced by reduced synapse-rich neuropil, synaptophysin, and the density of dendritic spines. Further, the myelination of important pathways between the frontal and limbic regions of the brain that normally continues through middle age might also have been compromised in schizophrenia, particularly among early-onset males. Lieberman et al. (1997) have suggested a three-stage neurochemical model that integrates these neurodevelopmental epochs in an attempt to explain both the origin and the onset of schizophrenia as well as its residuals. These authors focus on developmental deficits in neurochemical regulation and plasticity that could influence neuromodulation perinatally, neurochemical sensitization during adolescence and young adult life, and perhaps neurotoxicity during the postonset phase of illness that might account for the residuals of this disorder. "Sensitization" is a key concept in this unifying hypothesis, a concept that reflects a "progressive and enduring enhancement of behavioral response" to noxious stimuli (Lieberman et al., 1997, p. 208), rather than an adaptation to, or "tolerance of," such adversity. Patient psychoeducation could profitably include a description of this neurochemical sensitization deficit as a likely basis of vulnerability to stress.

The "environment" that represents one's personal developmental experience also clearly influences brain function. The synaptic and neural proliferation observed during perinatal brain development provides the playing field upon which a profound diversity of individual life experiences will ultimately shape and preserve selected neural circuits, as the growing child adapts and interacts within its own "socioecological niche" (Eisenberg 1995). The interactive process of selective pruning, reinforcement, and the continued strengthening of surviving neural circuits through learning influences most individual differences and has been described as "experience-dependent synaptogenesis" (Greenough & Black, 1992). As surmised from animal studies at least, many adverse early developmental experiences (such as those that include disruptions in important attachments or social isolation) are also capable of altering the structural and functional integrity of the brain, alterations that ultimately might be uncovered behaviorally by the challenges of young adult life. (A recent study raises the possibility that such vulnerability might be genetically influenced [Ellenbroek & Cools, 2000]). We have recently suggested (Keshavan & Hogarty, 1999) that the neurodevelopmental anomalies of at-risk individuals might lead to a delay in the acquisition of important social cognitive milestones that subsequently predispose the vulnerable individual to an interpersonal discomfort or social naïveté prior to the onset of schizophrenia symptoms. Even a mild disadvantage in social cognition might lead other, better socialized children or adults to avoid or greatly limit interaction with the vulnerable child, a well-known phenomenon that can lead to the process of desocialization (Cameron & Margaret, 1951). Social dysfunction and withdrawal (which typically follow desocialization) have been shown to characterize the adjustment of schizophrenia patients for more than 2 years prior to onset (Hafner et al., 1998). Social isolation effectively precludes the opportunity for the continued development of social cognitive abilities (e.g., perspective taking and context appraisal) that are necessary in order to successfully manage the challenges of young adult life such as academic achievement, emancipation from one's family of origin, the acquisition of a mate, and pursuit of a career. (An important goal of treatment would therefore include the systematic resocialization of the patient.) Thus, the interaction among the vulnerabilities that are represented by the anomalies of heritability, neurodevelopment, and cognition might likely account for schizophrenia risk, onset, and residual disability, particularly during the stressful transitional periods of late adolescence as well as early adult life. Whatever manner the PT clinician chooses to convey this information, the metacommunication should be absolutely clear: schizophrenia is without doubt a no-fault brain disorder.

What Is Schizophrenia?

The PT clinician has a broad selection of materials from which to choose when describing and defining schizophrenia for the patient. These materials might include the scholarly contributions of the neurosciences, to the formal characteristics of the disorder presented in DSM-IV, a vast array of clinical descriptions, and vivid first-person accounts contained in each issue of the *Schizophrenia Bulletin*. We continue to use the personal (subjective) and public (objective) perspectives of behavior that are associated with schizophrenia as we described them some years ago (Anderson, Reiss, & Hogarty, 1986, Ch. 3), and refer the reader to this source for a more complete description.

One can begin the patient's education by correcting misinformation. Many schizophrenia patients seem to be in denial of their illness, but what we have often observed being denied is the popular misconception of schizophrenia as "split personality" or as someone who is "crazy," that is, someone whose behavior is unpredictable or violent, or a person without moral character. (When dramatic cases do make the headlines, patients often need to be assured that violence is not inevitably associated with schizophrenia. To the contrary, violence is less common among those who have schizophrenia than in the general population; see Stuart & Arboleda-Florez [2001].) The clinician needs to regularly probe for the patients' understanding of their problems and how the illness has affected their ability to work and relate to other people. We review for patients the history of arbitrary classification and labeling of these behaviors and define precisely what we mean when we use the term "schizophrenia." We comment on the subjective experience of schizophrenia, emphasizing components that might have characterized the patient's own reality, such as problems with distraction and attention, sensory overload, and sensitivity to stimuli, as well as misperceptions. (These "disabilities" of schizophrenia are more fully elaborated in Chapter 5 in the sections headed *Psy-*

choeducation and Adjustment to Disability.) Davidson et al. (1998) provide a very moving and comprehensive account of these subjective experiences, including the barriers to relationships and the fears that surround social interaction. The public presentation of this subjective terror often includes thought disorder (such as a loose association among ideas, or illogical or incoherent speech), delusions, hallucinations, and an associated reduction in feeling and social withdrawal. Negative symptoms, such as amotivation, loss of interest, and poverty of speech or thought content, often accompany positive symptoms and continue in a number of patients long after positive symptoms abate; these negative symptoms are often associated with frontal lobe anomalies. In a substantial minority of cases, clinical depression will accompany or follow a psychotic episode. It is often reassuring for the patient to learn that these terribly distressing thoughts and feelings are in fact the common signs and symptoms of this widespread illness. Patients are often surprised to learn that more than 2.5 million people in the United States alone have experienced schizophrenia, a disorder that is three times more frequent than such well-known illnesses as multiple sclerosis or muscular dystrophy, and about as prevalent as diabetes mellitus.

How Do Treatments Work?

We underscore the importance of both medication and psychosocial treatment, the former being indispensable to symptomatic relief and the latter being entirely necessary for achieving clinical stability and recovery of function.

Perhaps the most difficult area of psychoeducation for the nonphysician to understand is the possible mechanism(s) by which medications actually operate on brain systems in order to influence the thinking and feeling of a patient that has become obviously impaired. A basic understanding is not only central to the educational needs of patients but is often important to the content of practice itself in that theoretical notions concerning the nature of mental disorders are likely to be altered as the clinician's understanding increases concerning the brain, behavior, and the effects of medication. Hence, in keeping with our intent to better elaborate the less familiar aspects of practice, we offer a fuller description of this process.

First and foremost, we stress that psychotropic medications are not "symptom covers" that keep patients from "facing their problems," as aspirin might alleviate a fever that is symptomatic of an underlying infection. Nor are they "curative" of an illness, as antibiotics are for many bacterial infections. Rather, psychotropic medications influence the underlying process (pathophysiology) of the disorder, much like the antihypertensive effect that other drugs have on high blood pressure or the way that insulin compensates for defects in glucose metabolism among diabetics. They stabilize behavior and thus prepare patients and clinicians for the difficult task of addressing the interpersonal and social problems that often influence the manifestation, recurrence, and course of the disorder. Today, fortunately, the newer antipsychotic medications can facilitate this focus on recovery by avoiding the side effects of earlier medications that often dulled affect and cognition. While an understanding of the precise mechanisms of drug action is still evolving through modern neuroimaging techniques, all psychotropic medications variously affect the underlying neurochemical processes of neurons that are presumed to influence affective and cognitive states. A very basic if not crude description of these processes follows.

The brain contains literally billions of nerve cells, or neurons. Not all contain the chemical messengers (neurotransmitters) that are central to human cognition and emotion. The messages involving thoughts and feeling travel electrically from a nerve cell (neuron) along its single long branch (axon) and its many short branches (dendrites) to the end of each of these nerve fibers. There the electrical message encounters a space, or *synapse,* that exists at the end of a neurofiber between the pre- and postsynaptic neurons. Each neuron and its axon and dendrites contains hundreds of these synapses which are selectively responsive to particular neurotransmitters. It is at these synapses that the neurons "communicate" with each other, either dendrite to dendrite or axon to axon or dendrite to axon. Some neurons and their transmitters serve to "inhibit" the message, whereas others serve to "excite" or intensify the message. When they coordinate their activity, or "fire" together (Shatz, 1992), the ensuing effect is to regulate a type of behavior. When grouped together as a "family," these effects account for such behaviors as movement, sight, touch, decision making, and emotions. More than 40 of these neurotransmitters have been identified. While neurotransmitters are only contained within the neuron and the synaptic space, they interact with neurohormones, produced by such important glands as the pineal, pituitary, adrenal, and thyroid. These hormones are excreted directly into the bloodstream and eventually pass the blood–brain barrier.

When the electrical message reaches the presynaptic nerve ending, a process occurs (exocytosis) that releases the chemical messenger from the presynaptic neuron into the interneuronal space, or "synaptic cleft." The neurotransmitter then crosses the space and finds its special harbor at the postsynaptic receptor, much as a key fits a lock. There, a secondary messenger system converts the neurochemical message back to an electrical message that continues along through the next neuron (called its "action potential"). If "too much" of a neurotransmitter is released into the synaptic space, then various neurochemical "Pacmen" of sorts (e.g., monoamine oxidase [MAO] or catechol-3-O-methyltransferase [COMT]) are available to oxidize or otherwise neutralize the neurotransmitter. Some years ago, a popular theory claimed that chronic psychosis was due to "too little" MAO.

In general, different classes of psychotropic drugs attempt to correct the problem of either too little or too much of the selected neurotransmitters that are presumed to influence a specific mental disorder. These problems in neurotransmission are likely to be secondary to developmentally altered neural circuitry and neurochemical deficits referred to above. The action of psychotropic drugs has given rise to the popular notion of correcting a "chemical imbalance" in the brain, often the metacommunication that has the most potent effect on patient understanding. While these mechanisms of action have only been studied directly in lower animals, the complexity of the human brain and the ability of researchers to only indirectly assess their action (via urine, blood, or cerebrospinal fluid) had made extrapolations to human brain chemistry difficult in the past. However, modern imaging techniques such as functional magnetic resonance imaging (fMRI) and its spectroscopy, as well as positron emission tomography (PET scan), increasingly provide visual images of drug action at specific brain sites.

Psychotropic drugs variably exert their influence in one or more ways: (1) by blocking (antagonizing) the postsynaptic neuron; (2) by blocking the reuptake of the neurotransmitter into the presynaptic neuron following its release; (3) by stimulating the release (agonism) or emptying the neuron of its neurotransmitter contents; (4) by initial sensitization (stimulation) of the presynaptic neuron through small or intermittent doses; (5) through a complex feedback system involving depolarization of the electrical potential of the presynaptic neuron, similar to discharging a battery, an action that serves to place the neuron in a resting state and hence limits the amount of neurotransmitter released; (6) by inhibiting or weakening the action of a given "Pacman" such as MAO; or (7) through autoreceptor sensitivity, a mechanism that would also lower the firing rate of the presynaptic neuron. Drugs also appear to act by increasing the forerunners (precursors) of important neurotransmitters, such as lithium's ability to increase tryptophan, the precursor of the neurotransmitter serotonin. All drugs variously influence intracellular and cell membrane functions by their effects on such crucial ions as potassium, calcium, sodium, and phosphate. Often the nature of a receptor's neighbor will influence its particular action as well (the "firing together" phenomenon referred to above). Given the numbers of cells, synapses, neurotransmitters, brain areas, and hormones involved, including the dynamics of cell physics, electrical polarity, and the extraordinary but minimally understood intrabrain connections, much of our understanding of drug mechanisms is incomplete at this time.

In general, the two neurochemical mechanisms most frequently studied among antipsychotic drugs include (1) *postsynaptic blockade* and (2) the associated feedback to the presynaptic neuron called *depolarization blockade*, an action that effectively "turns down" the release of a neurotransmitter. Most information covering these actions have come from the study of the neurotransmitter dopamine, a chemical messenger (one of the biogenic monoamines or catecholamines) believed to be important for many human behaviors such as the processing of information from the external world, maintenance of a sense of self and memory, initiation of action, and emotional investment. (Arvid Carlsson, Paul Greengard, and Eric Kandel, the Nobel laureates in physiology and medicine for 2000, received the award for their pioneering work on this neurotransmitter and its mechanism of action in normal and disease states.) Other neurotransmitters are also involved in psychosis, principally norepinephrine, glutamic acid, and serotonin—one of serotonin's receptors being selectively antagonized by the atypical antipsychotic medications. The study of dopamine in schizophrenia was stimulated by the very early observation that the dopamine agonist amphetamine (which increases the release or synthesis of dopamine and other neurotransmitters) can in high doses produce a clinical state in "normal" individuals that is similar to paranoid schizophrenia itself. Such agonists can also evoke psychotic symptoms in already affected patients.

Dopamine-containing neurons can be found in discrete but interconnected areas (or "tracks") of the brain. The foremost area, and one believed to be important to an understanding of therapeutic effects, is called the mesolimbic dopaminergic tract. This mesolimbic area encompasses the circular border (cortex) of the oldest part of the human brain. Best visualized as a "fist and wrist," the wrist represents the brain stem and the fist represents the important midsection of the brain (e.g., the hippocampus, amygdala, and basal ganglia) that contains connections to the hypothalamus and the pituitary gland as well as projections to and from the cortex of the frontal and temporal lobes, areas that are central to attention, memory, cognitive organization, perception, and abstraction—or, in clinical terms, to "executive functions." All information from the senses passes through this limbic system, where bits and pieces of data are attended to or ignored, evaluated, and charged with feeling if deemed important. The basic needs of hunger, thirst, and sex, as well as scanning the external world and a readiness to respond to it (arousal), are all represented by one or more interacting parts of the limbic system. Studies of the mesolimbic system in nonhuman primates have revealed that antipsychotic drugs block the action of dopamine (and other neurotransmitters) in postsynaptic neurons contained there. To put it simply, antipsychotic drugs (because of their somewhat similar molecular structure) can selectively take the place of molecules of real neurotransmitters at the postsynaptic receptor, but act rather like "phoney" transmitters since they do not pass the message along through the neuronal chain in quite the same way as true neurotransmitters do. Following their competitive battle with the true neurotransmitter molecules, postsynaptic blockade is achieved by the phoney molecules and feedback occurs, over a period of days or weeks, that results in depolarization, a process that might explain the therapeutic response. From animal studies of the typical neuroleptics, this action seems to be an "either/or" phenomenon: once it is achieved at a given dose, higher doses do not seem to result in more depolarization. Recent neuroimaging studies in patients have shown that once a certain percentage of dopamine (D_2) receptors are occupied (about 65%), clinical improvement will follow. Greater occupancy will lead to side effects, but not necessarily to greater improvement, even when atypical antipsychotics are used (Kapur & Seeman, 2001). The delay in achieving depolarization might also explain the fact that therapeutic effects are not observed immediately after the first dose of an antipsychotic drug. Nor does recurrence of symptoms occur in the days or weeks or even months following the discontinuation of medication, a reality that often obscures the relationship between medication noncompliance and relapse.

Whatever the individual antipsychotic drug might be, many studies in neuropsychology indicate that the primary behavioral mechanism of action for all antipsychotic drugs includes the normalization of arousal and the ability of the patient to correctly redeploy attention. Following a half century of study, these disorders of information processing (selective attention, distraction, vigilance) and arousal (very high or low) have been shown to be at the heart of psychosis and many of its residual deficits.

While less so with the newer atypical antipsychotics, particularly quetiapine, clozapine, and olanzapine, traditional neuroleptics exert a major blockade on other dopamine receptors located in an important area of the brain known as the nigro-neostriatal dopaminergic tract. This area regulates motor behavior of the extrapyramidal nervous system, a regulation that extends from leg and arm movements to facial and tongue movements, as well as posture and muscle tone. Blockade of these receptors can lead to side effects that include acute dystonia, akinesia (or pseudo-parkinsonism), akathisia, and tardive dyskinesia. In the tuberoinfundibular dopaminergic tract, antipsychotic drugs, including some of the newer ones, also block dopamine-containing neurons in the hypothalamus that regulate the release of prolactin (in women and men) by the pituitary gland, a hormone responsible for milk production in women following childbirth. Galactorrhea, amenorrhea, sexual dysfunction, and weight gain are other side effects that follow this blockade. These are the two tracks, then, that appear to account for many unwanted effects of antipsychotic drugs, but less likely account for their therapeutic effects. (For detailed information on the side effects of antipsychotic medications and their management, the reader should consult the useful recent reviews by Hansen, Casey, & Hoffman, 1997, and Egan, Apud, & Wyatt, 1997.)

Once clinicians understand the biological vulnerabilities that are common in schizophrenia, they are better able to integrate the concept of psychosocial stress within this biological diathesis when explaining to patients just how stressful life experiences can either provoke or sustain the illness. More importantly, the mechanism by which psychosocial treatment such as PT can serve to modify stress and its noxious effect on biological vulnerabilities can also be illustrated. (Again, the biological markers of vulnerability are not specific to schizophrenia per se, but are often shared among many mental disorders.) Further, if stress itself were sufficient to "cause" schizophrenia, then the world would obviously find schizophrenia patients in the majority. In the extreme, either catastrophic stressors or extraordinary biological vulnerability could theoretically be sufficient for psychotic symptoms in one model (Zubin & Spring, 1977), but for most patients the presence of stress and vulnerability can vary over time, even within the same subject. For example, a good responder to and faithful complier with antipsychotic medication appears to require a quantum increase in stressful life events in order to experience a reemergence of psychotic symptoms (McEvoy et al., 1984; Leff, 1981). In the absence of antipsychotic medication, the same patient might succumb to even the mild stress of everyday life (e.g., Leff, 1981). The ability of patients to variably achieve a remission of positive symptoms as well as to recover and maintain functioning is viewed as convincing evidence of the validity of the "stress vulnerability" model (Nuechterlein & Dawson, 1984). These authors also provide a rich "heuristic schema" of how vulnerability factors, personal and environmental protective factors, as well as external stressors interactively impact on genetically influenced information-processing capabilities and arousal to produce either the prodromes or episodes of schizophrenia or the recovery and maintenance of function. Factors that tend to insulate patients from the effects of stress include the action of maintenance antipsychotic medication on their neurobiological vulnerabilities, the protection of a safe, predictable, and supportive environment, and the effectiveness of improved coping strategies that can abort the prodromes often leading to a reemergence of symptoms. As described in Chapter 1, psychosocial treatments for schizophrenia seem to have succeeded either by directly modifying the environment that the vulnerable patient needs to negotiate or by increasing the patient's own capacity to manage the environment itself. We feel that PT further addresses the destabilizing *subjective* effects of stress that might persist despite successful environmental manipulation. Explaining how medication and PT work together to achieve clinical stabilization, avoid relapse and increase functioning is a message of hope and empowerment.

Aside from the formal education workshops of the basic and intermediate phases, information on schizophrenia and its treatment is individualized in most every PT session. Patients can be assured that over time they will come to learn about (1) their personal vulnerabilities, including sensitivity to specific sources of interpersonal stress, interference from information-processing and working memory difficulties, or the adverse effects of alcohol or illicit drug use; (2) how their particular symptoms come to unfold and remit; and (3) how the symptoms can be managed with medication and PT strategies. Without subjecting patients to a host of frightening statistics, they should at least be informed about the relapse risk that can be expected if medication is refused or discontinued (see Chapter 1), or the constraints on recovery that can be anticipated if medication is accepted but a definitive psychosocial treatment is not used (see Chapter 2). Although such risks are particularly difficult to discuss with first-episode patients, given the often equivocal nature of diagnosis, variability of the course of the illness, and the likelihood of denial, it is of paramount importance to address these risks, as they apply to the majority of first-episode patients. In the initial weeks and months following an acute episode, less emphasis should be placed on the complex issues of etiopathophysiology and a stronger message should be communicated regarding the real possibility of a recovery. As symptoms abate and attention improves, the clinician can move to a fuller discussion of brain function and schizophrenia, how information-processing deficits and hyperarousal can effect mood and behavior, and the role of medication and PT in managing the illness.

Repetition is a characteristic of psychoeducation in the basic phase, particularly while positive symptoms persist and executive functions remain impaired. Eliciting feedback is a way to determine the degree of patient comprehension, since it is often unwise to assume that even basic information on schizophrenia and its treatment can be correctly understood during the early months following an episode. Reference to the patient's notebook should be made routinely. Finally, rudimentary education provides the vehicle for most patients, particularly first-episode patients, to begin the process of "making sense" about their psychotic experience and the need for a plan of recovery. If successful, the basic phase of psychoeducation should equip the patient with a general notion of schizophrenia, how symptoms tend to arise and remit, the necessity for monitoring prodromal signs and the provocative sources of stress, and how a treatment plan that includes medication and PT can serve to manage vulnerability and prevent recurrence. It is a fundamental principle of PT that the more patients learn about their illness and its course, the more personal responsibility they can assume in its management.

RESUMPTION OF DAILY TASKS

Task assignment proved to be a most useful strategy in the earlier family psychoeducation approach and was thus incorporated into the initial phase of PT. It represents a less abstract and practical strategy that can provide a thread of continuity from session to session, an important consideration during the early months of PT. As the patient recovers, more demanding PT assignments related to the acquisition of coping skills will ultimately replace these basic tasks and the associated homework assignments.

A psychotic episode frequently leads to the suspension of instrumental role performance, even such fundamental tasks as maintaining *personal hygiene* and *nutrition*. Not infrequently, this disruption in daily routine has been a source of frustration and despair, if not resentment, among family members and friends. Since positive psychotic symptoms might continue as private experiences for the patient and not be fully appreciated by significant others, impairments in self-care might often seem willful, extreme, or without justification, and this critical response itself could become an enduring source of stress for the patient. PT does not emphasize a resumption of responsibilities until there are signs that clinical recovery has indeed started. These signs include the following: a decrease in affect lability, including depression; a decrease or modification of hallucinatory experiences; a normalization of sleep, energy, and/or appetite; an increase in concentration and recall; and a reduced investment in or preoccupation with delusional beliefs, or a renewed interest in the external world, including the interests and concerns of significant others. Our lengthy experience has repeatedly reinforced the finding that if expectations exceed clinical state, the consequence to the patient will often represent a continuation or recurrence of symptoms.

When initiating a plan for the resumption of responsibilities, the clinician should review what the patient had typically undertaken in the past, not only those activities that were routinely mastered but those that conveyed a sense of fulfillment and satisfaction as well. This appraisal not only helps to attain instrumental success but also ensures that expectations are reasonable and tasks are graduated in difficulty. The presence of an explicit plan once again deemphasizes the recurrent "crisis of the day" mentality to which patients and often clinicians have become accustomed. Success in the achievement of small steps very often reenforces the patient's own active role in the recovery plan. Even though tasks might appear simple and mundane, they achieve a special meaning when associated with the larger and often long-term goals related to the resumption of work, school, or household management responsibilities. The value in establishing a routine, building stamina and energy, and tolerating the ordinary if not boring activities of daily living becomes the rationale for achieving long-term career and life goals. This association between immediate tasks and long-term goals needs to be emphasized, repeatedly if necessary.

The initial tasks assigned often represent the most pressing (yet easiest to achieve) and most often center on self-care activities. In extreme cases, the tasks might begin with the negotiation of a shower twice a week or attendance to neglected grooming. Otherwise, the progression can include the performance of household tasks typically performed premorbidly, including cleaning, meal preparation, shopping, laundry, or household maintenance. (Over time the tasks will become social and recreational, first with other household members and eventually with people outside the home as described in Chapter 5.) For many patients, the challenge is to temper the inappropriate resumption of major role obligations that exceed cognitive ability and stamina. The PT session will most often include a homework review of the earlier assigned task and, when indicated, assignment of a new task. Setbacks in performance can be seen as an indication of poorly timed expectations by the therapist and an opportunity to return to tasks that were effectively mastered. Offering task choices to the patient not only makes the process less authoritarian but is likely to further reaffirm the notion that the patient is indeed an active participant in his or her own treatment.

Finally, a note on the context of household task assignment might aid the therapist when dealing with patients who had been ill for a lengthy period of time and had effectively given up, or perhaps never assumed, expected household responsibilities. In the patient's absence, the family would inevitably have established its own routine for meeting household responsibilities and tending to the welfare of other family members. The therapist needs to respect this order and not be quick to disrupt established routines. Often we have found that the plans of other family members related to the pursuit of interests and activities might have been suspended following the patient's illness (Anderson et al., 1986). Encouraging these activities often results in the opportunity for patients to assume a role or two that might free the family to pursue their own neglected interests. Otherwise, when informed of the treatment plan, most families will see some value in the patient's participation in household routines that might have historically fallen to other family members (even if the latter feel that they can continue to perform these tasks more easily and with greater success than the patient). There is rarely a family that is unwilling at least to allow a "trial-and-error" approach to the assignment of household responsibilities. The family can be reassured that the treatment plan is not necessarily attempting to re-create past successes or rekindle interest in prior activities, but rather is designed to initiate a plan of recovery that might just as likely lead to new roles and new interests that remain within the patient's ability to pursue and enjoy.

INTERNAL COPING

Internal coping is a technique that clearly elevates PT beyond the realm of supportive therapy. If the neurochemical sensitization theory described earlier is at all relevant, then many schizophrenia patients will likely respond to ordinary life events, let alone personal conflicts and catastrophes, with increased *reactivity*. Clearly patients cannot be trained to the specific negotiation of each and every noxious stimulus they might encounter. Nor is the response to a given stimulus likely to be constant across individuals. Rather, it is essential that PT provide a way to identify not only the clear prodromal signs that have preceded prior psychotic episodes but eventually (in subsequent phases) the *earliest* cues or indicators of self perceived stress that often precede prodromes and symptoms. While the need to recognize early signs and symptoms has a long clinical history, the challenge remains formidable. The disorganized and affectively labile patient, for example, often needs a method for conceptually organizing his or her subjective response to stress; the persistently symptomatic patient might require assistance in segregating prodromes and individual cues of distress from abiding symptoms; and the negative symptom patient often needs help in simply articulating his or her subjective state. Not infrequently, distressed patients will answer "fine" or "OK" to any inquiry about personal discomfort, or at best be unaware that their familiar and automatic responses to stress might at times be the harbinger of a new episode. We share with patients our working definition of stress borrowed from Schafer (1983, p. 47), namely, that "stress is arousal of mind and body in response to the demands made upon it," a definition which acknowledges that stress is part of everyday life and can originate with "good" as well as "bad" events.

When PT was first conceived, it was felt that the principles of internal coping should be reserved for the intermediate and advanced phases, or—if introduced earlier—they should not extend much beyond the association between life events and potential relapse. But it quickly became apparent that the patient's response to external or internal sources of stress in the form of more apparent and easily identified possible prodromal signs was essential to the task of achieving clinical stabilization as quickly as possible, as well as maintaining it. Internal coping in the basic phase thus includes four tasks:

1. The definition of what a patient means by "distress," using the patient's own language.
2. An identification of the interpersonal context or life events that the patient associates with this distress.
3. Identification of the manifest prodromal signs that have preceded the onset of psychotic symptoms in past episodes.
4. Identification of the patient's existing "autoprotective" strategies for coping with stress, including helpful and unhelpful techniques.

The theme of early internal coping is to encourage patients to become more aware of the feelings and behaviors associated with self-perceived stress and to evaluate the options that are immediately available to reduce this distress, thus gaining a beginning sense of control and mastery.

During a session, internal coping can follow the review of a homework assignment since it is in the discussion of obstacles and difficulties in completing tasks that contexts often become identified which might be particularly stressful to the patient. Key relationships with family and friends are discussed, including recurrent and episodic conflicts identified by the patient. (Prior psychiatric history obtained during the formation of the treatment contract is particularly useful for the assessment of stressful situations and the potential prodromal signs that are provoked.) Often input from the family regarding current functioning can also help to identify the challenges and the strengths that characterize the patient's life at the moment.

Personal Definition of Stress

First, it is important to learn what the patient means by the term "stress." Definitions offered by patients have ranged from "upset" to "bad vibes," "dumped on," "blown away," or even more idiosyncratic responses. As simple as the inquiry may appear, nonetheless a modicum of skill and tact is required when attempting to understand the personal meaning of stress. Probing contexts and events to such a degree that the stress itself would be reactivated is not useful. A general discussion of the patient's social environment, economic and physical well-being, as well as key relationships is a useful entry (e.g., "How have things been going regarding . . . ?"). Inquiry about the patient's typical response ("So when that happened, how did you feel?"), serves to repeatedly focus the patient on the broad relationship between stressors and the arousal of mind and body.

Identification of Major Prodromal Signs

Identification of the most obvious and typical prodromal signs for the individual patient should begin as soon as possible following the initiation of PT since this information is crucial to establishing and maintaining clinical stability. The assessment of prodromal signs that need to be monitored should be obtained from the medical record as well as from the current reports of the patient and the family. Table 4.1 lists the more frequent and important prodromal signs identified by our own PT therapists

TABLE 4.1. Frequent Prodromal Signs of Psychosis

Anxiety
  *Tense or nervous
  *Restless, agitated, or hyperactive
  *Feeling overwhelmed
  "Something terrible" will happen
  *Hypochondriacal concerns
  Anger, belligerence, or negativism
    (*about little things)
  Ruminative preoccupation (*with
    one or two ideas)

Depression
  *Depressed mood (sad, worthless,
    inadequate, hopeless, guilty,
    pessimistic)
  *Social withdrawal, isolation, or
    emotional distance
  *Loss of usual interest

Sleep disturbances
  *Sleeping too much or too little
  Sleep reversal

Behavior and functioning
  *Eating much less or much more
  Recent difficulty performing as a
    wage earner, student, or
    homemaker
  Recent conflicts with others
    (*spouse or mate)
  Recent impaired social judgment
  Recent increase in dependency
  Clear changes in daily routine
  Deterioration of hygiene or
    appearance
  *Increase or start of alcohol/drug use

Thought disorder increases:
  *Difficulty concentrating or
    remembering
  *Suspicion/ideas of reference
  Conviction concerning delusions
  *Quantity or quality of hallucinations
  Odd or unusual thinking
  Distractibility
  *Religiosity
  *Not making sense

Note. Signs preceded by an asterisk (*) are included in Herz (1985).

and also contained in earlier studies (Herz, 1985; Herz, Glazer, Mirza, Mostert, & Hafez, 1989). While later PT phases will probe deeper into the earliest and highly individual affective, cognitive, physical, and behavioral cues of distress, at this stage of treatment the emphasis is on clear and less ambiguous prodromal signs that have led to previous episodes. This review of historical prodromal signs is steeped in the long-standing psychotherapeutic tradition of reconstructing the patient's "path to breakdown" (McGlashan, 1983).

Unfortunately, not every patient shows an immediate reactivity to adverse experience, although positive symptoms of schizophrenia seem more easily precipitated by stress than negative symptoms (Doherty, 1996). Typically 45% of patients might have experienced a rapid onset of schizophrenia symptoms in less than 1 month (and another 34% within 1–6 months [see Hogarty & Goldberg, 1973]), thus suggesting reactivity to life events (Leff, 1981) as well as highlighting the importance and relevance of monitoring the specific prodromal signs listed in Table 4.1. However, for the minority of patients whose episode unfolds insidiously over a longer period of time, the emphasis will often shift to behavior changes that in and of themselves might not appear "pathological" but nonetheless represent a behavioral change that is clearly out of character for the individual patient. For example, an otherwise punctual patient might begin to arrive at the clinic an hour or more prior to a scheduled appointment; another mild-mannered patient might begin to complain about family, friends, or neighbors; and yet another usually nonreflective individual might initiate a discussion of vague existential issues such as the "meaning of life" or "never having been understood." Careful listening can often reveal whether these changes in usual behavior patterns are associated with other (subjective) prodromal signs of an episode or whether they are, in fact, a part of the recovery process. Once prodromal signs are clearly identified by the patient and therapist, the primary coping strategy is fairly simple: *call the PT therapist!* In the initial weeks or months of recovery from a psychotic episode, for example, medication is frequently in need of adjustment and very often a dosage increase or the addition/adjustment of a mood-stabilizing medication can abort what might otherwise be an important prodromal indicator of decompensation (e.g., restlessness, depression, or an increase in thought disorder). With less serious prodromal signs (e.g., everyday worries), support and reassurance can be offered together with the hope that PT will lessen these general concerns over time.

Autoprotective Strategies

Independent of prodromal severity, the initial coping repertoire should also include an appraisal of the patient's own traditional way of adapting to symptoms, and support should be given to those health-promoting strategies that the patient claims are helpful. These techniques have been identified over many decades as *autoprotective strategies* (Brenner, Boker, & Muller, 1987). Arieti (1974), for example, described cognitive states that served as precursors to hallucinations and paranoid delusions, thus allowing patients to employ coping strategies in anticipation of these troubling symptoms. Breier and Strauss (1983) emphasized three phases of symptom self-control: awareness of prepsychotic symptoms through the self-monitoring of "targeted" behaviors; an appreciation of their potential implications; and the application of self-control techniques, principally self-instruction and a reduction in or increase of activity, such as distraction. Meichenbaum and Cameron (1973, 1974) had earlier developed an effective behavioral approach in the form of self-instruction.

In the more definitive study of Carr (1988), no less than 350 individual coping strategies were identified. In this study, as in others, anxiety and depression more than psychotic signs were the symptoms more likely to be targeted for management by patients. Behavioral control strategies were used by 83% of patients, the most frequent of which included passive distraction (e.g., listening to the radio or watching television) or active distraction (e.g., reading, writing in a diary, or performing personal hobbies). Others sought to change their environment by going for a walk or a ride, or attending church or a movie. Inactive forms of behavioral control were also common, such as resting or relaxation, as were active forms of physical activity, such as running, swimming, or vigorous exercise. Still other patients indulged themselves when dealing with thought disorder (but not hallucinations) by eating, drinking (both alcohol and nonalcoholic beverages), smoking, and at times using illicit drugs. Others sought supportive contact by phoning or visiting with family or friends, particularly to relieve symptoms of depression and delusions. Forms of cognitive control directed at managing hallucinations and delusions included "suppression" (attempts to deliberately exclude symptoms from consciousness) and a shifting of attention. Strategies that actually *increased* symptoms were used by 29% of patients, particularly those with delusions (e.g., sleeping with a weapon). These results, as noted by Carr (1988), were similar to those reported by Cohen and Berk (1985), a survey which showed that in response to schizophrenia symptoms, patients most often tended to "fight back" (with types of self-instruction) or to "pray." Similar to a substantial number of our own patients, however, about one-third of patients in the Cohen and Berk study could not identify a specific coping strategy. An early study by Falloon and Talbot (1980) showed that auditory hallucinations were responded to by patients in the form of passive or active behaviors, increased social contacts, or attempts at regulating attention and arousal.

In our experience, patients can often identify valuable coping strategies but tend to apply them inconsistently, such as various forms of exercise. It thus becomes important to support and reinforce techniques that the patient had found to be helpful in the past. For many, increased sleep is a frequent form of stimuli control, particularly in the early stages of recovery. A majority of patients are inclined to use "distraction" or self-perceived forms of "relaxation" (which PT builds upon in later phases) as useful coping mechanisms. Unfortunately, symptom-provoking coping strategies are also common, particularly the use of alcohol, drugs, caffeinated beverages, and overeating. Helping patients to review these latter behaviors as unhelpful coping mechanisms while emphasizing their own health-promoting techniques often proves useful. Autoprotective strategies that were helpful for other patients with similar symptoms can also be shared and discussed. Beyond "calling the therapist," the process of identifying and activating autoprotective strategies is within the first line of coping with prodromal signs, a method that serves to reinforce the association among stressors, symptoms, and self-control.

BASIC SOCIAL SKILLS TRAINING

The second line of coping with prodromal signs relies on previously tested, effective, and easy-to-master social skills taught during the initial period of recovery from a psychotic episode, a time when patients often remain symptomatic and neurocognitively challenged. These strategies are once again blended into the discussion of prodromes and are described as well-documented techniques that the patients can add to their own repertoire of autoprotective coping mechanisms. In the early stages of recovery, the patient will most often continue to experience symptoms that significantly impair social perception and the sophisticated responses that are useful in managing exchanges with others. The therapist should assist the patient in deciding what can be done to promote or reinforce relationships in the immediate household as well as to reduce conflict and stress. Social skills strategies promoted in the basic phase include the following: (1) the structuring of role obligations; (2) teaching of successful conflict-avoidance techniques that direct the patient to absent him- or herself from such exchanges in a direct yet dignified manner; and (3) teaching simple positive exchanges designed to facilitate relationships in the household by identifying when and to whom praise and appreciation can be given. The patient is asked to describe daily interactions that provide the therapist with contexts in which to target praise statements or conflict-avoidance strategies.

Role Restructuring

In the basic phase, patients are typically discouraged from taking on new social challenges such as school or work until symptoms are stable. If, in spite of this counsel, patients return to school or work, they are encouraged to reduce their "social load" while they are symptomatic. They may be asked to consider reducing the total number of classes they are taking or the hours worked or time spent on extracurricular activities, for example. Patients are also encouraged to decrease the amount of social stimulation when they feel particularly stressed. (See Chapter 5 for a fuller discussion of these techniques.)

Conflict Avoidance

As the therapist and the patient review the contexts and impact of social stress, they will begin to identify specific hot spots. The therapist instructs the patient to avoid both real and potential conflict situations. While there are many conflict resolution skills a person might use, social skills training emphasizes two basic methods. In the first, patients are advised not to use behaviors that evoke negative reactions from others, such as speaking loudly, swearing, complaining about symptoms (e.g., delusional beliefs), blasting the television or stereo, maintaining poor self-care (hygiene), or displaying annoying mannerisms. The therapist assists the patient in viewing these negative behaviors from the other person's perspective and understanding others' feelings as well as his or her own. The patient is encouraged to see that controlling a negatively perceived behavior should improve the relationship and make the patient feel less stressed. The second conflict avoidance strategy simply encourages patients to physically leave stressful situations, rather than remain in a situation that has the potential to escalate or increase stress to the point where it might overwhelm their coping capacity. Although this is not what is commonly thought of as "conflict resolution," it is felt that more sophisticated methods of social skills training may actually increase stress and conflict in the early months of treatment, before patients have clinically stabilized. Also, many patients may not have the expressive skills needed to effectively resolve conflicts. Even if they are successfully able to make their point, the aftermath of an intense interaction may result in added stress and arousal.

However, it is often difficult for patients to perceive when and where conflicts might arise. For this reason, the therapist should give specific advice and direction. Based on the earlier assessment of the patient's relationships, the therapist identifies the people and the situations that are best avoided. Patients are educated about common behavioral signs of anger in themselves and others that could serve as cues for leaving a difficult situation. When conflict is escalating, the patient is instructed to withdraw in a nonrejecting manner. Leaving the situation allows the patient to feel a greater sense of control. Patients are instructed to express their feelings, if possible, and to request a time out (e.g., "I'm feeling a bit overwhelmed—

I need some time by myself"). Patients are encouraged to go to their room, take a walk, and otherwise try to quiet their strong feelings, using effective autoprotective strategies, if available At these times, it is also useful to limit the amount of social stimulation in order to lower arousal.

Specific conflict situations are identified for practice with the patient. (Skills training procedures have been described in detail elsewhere [Liberman, DeRisi, & Mueser, 1989].) In very "hot" and potentially destabilizing situations, the patient must withdraw, make some appropriate comment on their feelings, and do so without escalating the situation further. Initially, patient responses are clear one-statement comments such as "I need to take a break" or "I would like to be alone right now." The patient is coached about what to say and how to deliver the message. After the therapist has modeled the appropriate behavior, the two rehearse and the patient performs the appropriate response with the therapist offering corrective feedback. Feedback rewards effective elements of patient response and identifies areas that need improvement. Feedback is offered both on content as well as paralinguistic and nonverbal aspects of social performance such as voice tone and volume, eye contact, gestures, and facial expressions. Typically, each role-play situation is rehearsed several times. As patients show improving capability, they are asked to perform more extended role-play interactions where the antagonist role is assumed by the therapist, who attempts to escalate the conflict. In these role-play scenes, the patient is asked to imagine being angry and upset yet still able to avoid further conflict and to leave the situation gracefully.

After successful role-play practice, patients are given a specific homework assignment focused on conflict avoidance. They are asked to record their performance on a homework sheet. At the next session, the homework is reviewed. The patient is reinforced for completing the assignment despite the results achieved. Problems that arise are used for further role-play practice and future homework practice. These assignments can be interspersed with the resumption of tasks.

Positive Assertion

In addition to learning conflict-avoidance skills, patients are encouraged to interact more positively in their relationships with significant others. During the acute stage of illness, many patients are rarely rewarding to others. Even if they have not been irritable or hostile, they are commonly self-absorbed and preoccupied with symptoms, a behavior that can impact negativity on friends and family. Being able to be more positive with significant others is likely to decrease stress in relationships and promote a more stable and predictable social environment. For this reason, basic social skills training focuses on increasing the patient's expression of positive feelings toward others.

Key relationships in which positive messages will be introduced are identified and types of positive messages are described by the therapist, such as giving compliments, showing concern or interest in another, and expressing appreciation. The therapist informs the patient about the importance of rewarding others through positive comments and gives a rationale for building relationships through positive assertion. Most patients have the capacity for expressing positive comments, but many will not use this ability optimally during the early recovery period unless encouraged.

As part of teaching the expression of positive messages, the therapist again uses the traditional social skills procedures of instruction, modeling, role-play, feedback, and homework assignment. The content of positive assertion scenes is guided by common situations in the patient's life and by the behavior of significant others. Patients living with family members usually have different (and obviously more frequent) opportunities for positive assertion than patients living alone. For example, a patient living with his or her family might compliment their mother on dinner or thank her for driving to the store or clinic. A patient living alone could be encouraged to initiate positive comments with a landlord, other tenants, or shopkeepers.

Initial situations selected for role-play are brief responses that later progress to more complex positive messages. Through collaborative discussion, the therapist and patient identify a specific social situation for role-play practice. The patient is instructed on what to say and the therapist often models the response. Then, the patient role plays the response. The therapist provides positive reinforcement after each role play and identifies areas for further practice (e.g., "That was a good first try. I really liked what you said. Next time, you might want to speak a bit louder"). Again, the response is practiced several times, and the patient is given specific feedback on the content of the message and nonverbal elements as well as paralinguistic elements of the message.

After mastery in the session, the patient is again given a written homework assignment to give a positive message to an identified person and record the interaction. The therapist will often select a homework task that has a high probability of meeting with success, especially in the beginning of treatment. Individuals are targeted for positive messages that are generally receptive to the patient and likely to react in a positive way.

At the subsequent session, the homework assignment is reviewed. Independent of the outcome, the therapist supports the patient for expressing the positive message and uses information about performance for planning further opportunities for positive assertion. Often, patients receive positive remarks from others that increases their motivation to continue to develop skills in making positive comments.

In summary, the basic social skills component of PT is highly reflective of the individual patient's level of stability as well as the types of social situations that most often occur. Although all patients learn avoidance skills and the expression of positive messages, the pace is variable. The amount of role-play practice differs from case to case depending on need, and the content of role-play practice is always uniquely tailored to the patient's life circumstances. Not all basic phase PT sessions contain social skills training, but every patient learns skills in conflict avoidance and positive assertion.

We hope the reader can now appreciate the flow of basic phase sessions, particularly the active treatment components of alliance formation, task assignment, identification of stressors that are associated with episode prodromes, education, and skills training. Once prodromes are identified, initial coping strategies can be activated: (1) contact the therapist, (2) use self-generated techniques that are deemed to have been useful in the past, and (3) utilize the basic social skills strategies of avoidance and positive assertion.

TRANSITION FROM THE BASIC PHASE TO THE INTERMEDIATE PHASE

What was stated at the outset of this chapter should now be apparent, namely, that the basic phase of PT (including support and medication management) is itself a comprehensive treatment that few schizophrenia patients would likely encounter in the public-care sector today. The neglect is unfortunate because most patients (93%) are clearly able to master these basic phase skills within the early months that follow an index psychotic episode. (The few who struggled with basic phase components were patients who experienced severe and persistent positive symptoms that remained refractory to medication and who might profit from exposure to cognitive-behavioral therapy [Garety et al., 2000].) The therapist should be comforted by the realization that basic phase PT could stand alone as an effective, relevant, and comprehensive approach to the competent management of schizophrenia. Later phases will simply expand on these principles. Even though a patient (or a beginning therapist) might not advance to or master the elements of intermediate and advanced phase insights and techniques, neither should feel discouraged. Clinicians can confidentially return to the basic phase components assured that their efforts are appropriate and effective. For example, an ongoing study of ours that relies on Basic Phase components as an "enriched supportive therapy" control condition is showing within-group incremental advances over time in personal and social adjustment, as well as cognitive competencies. Elsewhere, Herz et al. (2000) have shown impressive effects on relapse using a *prodromal management program* that is similar to many basic phase components.

Since a principal goal of PT is to maintain the clinical stability achieved, assurances are needed that incremental therapeutic demands (much like other sources of stress) do not exceed the patient's cognitive capacity. Thus, PT includes criteria for the subsequent application of incremental therapeutic components that we feel offer protection to the patient and guidance to the therapist as well. The criteria that should be met prior to proceeding to the intermediate phase are next described, although some flexibility in judgment is obviously needed on the individual case basis. For example, minor exacerbations of symptoms for 1 or 2 weeks (a miniepisode) might necessitate a medication adjustment in an otherwise stable patient who satisfies remaining criteria. The criteria are offered as guidelines rather than rigidly enforced rules. Before advancing to the intermediate phase—

1. Positive symptoms should be in remission, or if present should be relatively stable. The patient's behavior should not, for example, be greatly influenced by persistent hallucinations or delusions. Further, symptoms should not be of such intensity that they interfere with regular clinic attendance.
2. A maintenance dose of antipsychotic medication should have been achieved, with a relatively consistent dose established.
3. The patient should keep appointments for PT sessions at least 75% of the time so that the requisite ongoing assessment of clinical state and role performance can be made.
4. The patient's place of residence should be relatively stable, safe, and predictable so as to ensure the opportunity to focus on im-

portant and abiding relationships in the patient's life. (As mentioned earlier, this condition should be satisfied prior to initiating the basic phase of PT.)

5. It is important that the patient be able to maintain an attention span sufficient for a discussion of symptoms, medication issues, and basic social skills for at least half an hour at a time.

6. The patient should have a basic understanding that schizophrenia is an illness for which treatment is necessary or that treatment may be beneficial in achieving the patient's goals (i.e., there should be some agreement regarding the content of the treatment plan).

7. There should be some evidence that the patient is making appropriate use of positive comments to significant others or is showing some ability to effectively reduce stress by appropriately avoiding conflict situations.

For tracking purposes, we include in Appendix B our Process Rating Scale, which includes micromeasures of these various criteria, as well as the opportunity to scale their degree of attainment. Twenty-four items are provided for basic phase performance, and ratings of "almost never" should alert the clinician that caution needs to be exercised in moving beyond the basic phase.

CHAPTER FIVE

The Intermediate Phase

The intent of the intermediate phase of PT is to capitalize on the gains realized during the basic phase. A popular poster found in many clinics says it best: "Staying well is the hardest part of getting well." Among those who are recovering from a recent episode, the beginnings of clinical stabilization will become the foundation upon which to build self-initiated coping strategies that will be tailored to the subjective cues of distress. The relatively greater consolidation of information regarding schizophrenia, its treatment and the influence of stress on subsequent course and outcome will serve a similar purpose for those whose entry into PT was further removed from an episode of psychosis. The dominant theme will be to preserve and build upon the clinical stability thus far acquired with the primary goals of maintaining oneself in the community, free of positive symptoms and with a growing sense of mastery and personal comfort.

Since the intermediate phase will primarily build on the methods and procedures of the basic phase, the description of this extension will often make reference to Basic Phase components. The clinician should again be reassured that 93% of schizophrenia patients have been able to enter and clearly respond to intermediate phase techniques. More than half of these patients, for example, successfully graduated to the advanced phase of PT following 6–9 months of intermediate phase participation. While this proportion of patients falls short of 100%, it needs to be emphasized once again that the majority of schizophrenia patients do engage and profit from the information and associated adaptive skills contained in the intermediate phase, interventions that might not be routinely offered to patients because of therapist (or program) reservations concerning "lack of insight," insufficient cognitive capacity among schizophrenia patients, or alleged "cost."

To appreciate the process needed to achieve these seemingly straightforward but nonetheless challenging objectives, this chapter describes the following key components of the intermediate phase:

- The maintenance and enhancement of *clinical stability*
- The personalized crafting of *psychoeducation*
- The continuing resumption of *responsibilities within the home*
- Initial efforts to facilitate *adjustment to disability*
- Most important, the extension of *internal coping* to the interface between the highly individualized cues of distress and their management
- As the management strategies of choice, the introduction of *relaxation* and *social skills* techniques that extend beyond avoidance and prosocial statements

In this chapter, the integration of intermediate and basic phase PT should become more apparent. The goals of psychoeducation, the identification of gross prodromes of a new psychotic episode, the beginning plan to resume self-care responsibilities, and the elementary skills of avoidance and positive assertion that were characteristic of the basic phase all clearly bear a close resemblance to the objectives of the intermediate phase identified above. The second phase of PT will differ essentially in the level of sophistication and complexity needed to (1) sustain clinical stability; (2) actively engage the patient in his or her own treatment plan; (3) stimulate the patient to initiate "quality of life" enhancing interactions with those in the immediate environment; and (4) enable the patient to engage in lower levels of stressful encounters without exacerbating cognitive, affective, and behavioral symptoms.

ENHANCEMENT OF CLINICAL STABILITY

Medication Management and Stability

While a modicum of stabilization needed to graduate from the basic phase is crucial to survival in the community, clearly the level of persistent positive, negative, or affective symptoms will vary from patient to patient and thus affect stabilization to a greater or lesser degree. In the service of reserving psychosocial approaches to those aspects of personal and social adjustment that remain independent of or unresponsive to appropriate and judiciously used chemotherapy, the initial approach to enhancing clinical stability involves fine-tuning the patient's medication regimen. As mentioned earlier, it is important not to accept residual symptoms (psychotic or affective) as being inevitably "untreatable."

The first medication consideration is directed to those patients whose *positive* symptoms have persisted, albeit at a lower or less incapacitating level. Foremost is the need to revisit the patient's feelings about medication taking in general, including side effects and any lingering reservations that might contribute to covert noncompliance. (In the intermediate phase, compliance issues often involve the patient's taking medication at a lower dose or less frequently than prescribed.) Otherwise, the familiar inquiry regarding the use of alcohol, caffeinated beverages, illicit drugs, medications prescribed by a physician other than the responsible psychiatrist, or over-the-counter medications can often reveal the presence of substances that provoke or sustain positive symptoms directly or by way of interaction with prescribed medication. If a patient had been maintained on a conventional antipsychotic drug at a therapeutic dose *without* apparent noncompliance, this often becomes the occasion to introduce the need for a change to one of the atypical antipsychotics, particularly if the response to conventional neuroleptics during prior episodes had been less than optimal. If the patient, however, is being maintained on one of the newer atypical antipsychotics and noncompliance does not appear to be an issue, then the dose should be increased, if tolerated. When neither noncompliance, substance use or abuse, or medication changes can explain persistent positive symptoms, then an indication for clozapine clearly presents itself. In general, when it comes to changing medications, we tend to subscribe to the principles endorsed in the Expert Consensus Guidelines (McEvoy et al., 1999) for medication management, but not always. For example, we will not inevitably include a trial of an atypical antipsychotic if the patient had been a suboptimal responder to a number of previous trials with traditional neuroleptics or had experienced a serious tardive dyskinesia. We will often consider clozapine immediately. Further, if the increase in an otherwise therapeutic dose of an atypical antipsychotic medication fails to achieve the desired remission and the patient had earlier failed a trial with a conventional neuroleptic, we will likely consider clozapine without initiating what usually becomes an unsuccessful trial with yet another atypical antipsychotic drug.

In the less frequent instances where positive symptoms persist despite an adequate trial of clozapine, we will initiate augmentation strategies. These include adding an atypical or conventional neuroleptic or lithium and, if this is unsuccessful, an anticonvulsant such as divalproex sodium (Depakote), gabapentin (Neurontin), or more recently topiramate (Topamax) or lamotrigine (Lamictal). If all else fails, we will turn to a course of electroconvulsive therapy (ECT), which has often proven to be efficacious in the most seriously refractory cases. Sometimes we have been able to trace the suboptimal response to antipsychotic medications that have a short half-life (e.g., clozapine and quetiapine) to a failure to have divided the dose.

Persistent *negative* symptoms represent another challenge, particularly the difficulty in differentiating among negative symptoms, behavioral akinesia for patients who are maintained on a conventional neuroleptic, and clinical depression. It is very important to remember that negative symptoms will frequently coexist with positive symptoms during the acute episode and that many negative symptoms will also remit as the positive symptoms subside, albeit more slowly (Breier et al., 1987). Thus, the primary focus should be on achieving the best possible resolution of positive symptoms *before* one begins to fire away pharmacologically at negative symptoms. Negative symptoms are best characterized as deficit or nondeficit in nature (Carpenter, Heinricks, & Wagman, 1988), the former being a more enduring state that appears to have a strong neurobiological basis (e.g., frontal lobe impairment) and the latter being secondary to other phenomena such as medication side effects, an understimulating and isolating environment, or the transient effects of an acute episode.

If positive symptoms had been well managed with a conventional neuroleptic but negative symptoms persist, one would want to consider subtle behavioral akinesia as a contributing factor (e.g., by examining for minimal cog-wheel rigidity, a loss of spontaneity or usual interests that followed the introduction of the neuroleptic, as well as motoric slowing). Sometimes an intramuscular challenge with a centrally acting anticholinergic drug (e.g., 2 mg benztropine mesylate [Cogentin]) can confirm subtle akinesia if the patient feels better immediately. Otherwise, lowering the dose of the conventional neuroleptic to the MED has been the most useful strategy for us in the past (see Chapter 3; also Hogarty et al., 1988, and Hogarty, McEvoy, et al., 1995).

If positive symptoms are well maintained with an atypical antipsychotic drug but negative symptoms persist, we see no real value in switching to yet another atypical antipsychotic drug—with one exception. Given the possibility of extrapyramidal symptoms (e.g., akinesia) among patients treated with risperidone, particularly at doses of 4 mg or higher, we would support a change to a different atypical antipsychotic. (A recent study attributes a similar rate of extrapyramidal symptoms to olanzapine [Conley & Mahmoud, 2001].) It is worthwhile remembering that significant improvement in persistent negative symptoms was observed following receipt of PT (see Chapter 2). It is a matter of debate whether or not this improvement occurred among primary deficit symptoms, but clearly psychosocial treatment has had an effect among secondary negative symptoms that arise from social isolation and perhaps the residuals of the acute episode. At the moment, we remain unconvinced that any atypical antipsychotic drug, including clozapine, has an unequivocal effect on primary deficit states beyond relief from subtle akinesia. The inclination among some practitioners to chronic dosing with *d*-amphetamine appears to be largely an ineffective treatment of negative symptoms and might open the possibility for adverse long-term consequences. Our own (unpublished) study of intermittent dosing with amphetamine revealed no important effects among negative symptom patients. Based on available clinical evidence, we consider that the addition of a psychosocial intervention likely represents as good a chance for the amelioration of secondary negative symptoms as any treatment at the moment.

Beyond persistent positive and negative symptoms, the comorbid impairments of mood, primarily *anxiety* and *depression*, remain the most significant clinical obstacles to stabilization and recovery and have characterized as many as 42% of patients in our prior surveys. Not only have these impairments been cited as prominent contributors to adjustment handicaps, but they are often the heralds of treatment noncompliance, psychotic decompensation, and a heightened risk of suicide. (Suicide remains a likely cause of premature death for as many as 10% of schizophrenia patients [Caldwell & Gottesman, 1990].) In fact, treatment of depression has been cited as one of three interventions most likely to positively influence the quality of life for schizophrenia patients (the others being family psychoeducation and the control of medication side effects, as shown by Sullivan, Wells, & Leake, 1992). Since an important goal of PT is to better manage affective dysregulation psychotherapeutically, we would enlist a rational pharmacological approach as the needed prerequisite whenever possible.

Having said that, we note that the evidence for supplemental thymoleptic efficacy in treating the comorbid affect impairment of schizophrenia is very much a case of mixed findings. Using evidence from controlled studies as the basis for the pharmacological management of comorbid anxiety and depression, we shall turn briefly to our own large sequential study regarding the pharmacotherapy of impaired affect in recovering schizophrenia (the PIAS study), one of the two better-designed outpatient studies, in our opinion. Both Siris, Bermanzohn, Mason, and Shuwall (1994) and our own group (Hogarty, McEvoy, et al., 1995) studied the effects of desipramine on depressed or mixed anxious/depressed schizophrenia outpatients, the former for 9 weeks and the latter for 12 weeks. We also included a trial of lithium for nonmanic patients that presented with persistent anxiety (the only outpatient study of its kind) or with mixed anxiety and depression. All patients in our study were maintained with an MED of fluphenazine decanoate and were randomly assigned to a supplemental thymoleptic or its placebo and maintained under double-blind treatment conditions, that is, neither the patient nor the clinicians knew whether a thymoleptic or its placebo had been prescribed. All patients met criteria for clinical depression and/or anxiety by obtaining a score 7 at baseline on the Raskin Depression Scale or Covi Anxiety Scale, criteria similar to those used in the study of primary affective disorders.

Before identifying the highly selective effects of these medications, we should note that the nature of affective impairment in schizophrenia stands in some contrast to what conventional wisdom holds. First, while various studies report that a majority of schizophrenia patients present acutely with comorbid anxiety and/or depression, a substantial number will respond to antipsychotic medication alone during the acute episode (again more slowly than the resolution of positive psychotic symptoms). Supplemental thymoleptics appear to convey very little additional benefit during the acute schizophrenia episode. Antidepressants used in the *absence* of antipsychotic medication are clearly *contraindicated* (Kramer et al., 1989). Following recovery from the acute episode, studies further suggest that about 25% of patients, on average, will be characterized as having experienced a "postpsychotic depression." In our opinion, this description can be misleading. Rather than a distinct "episode" of depression, many of those with comorbid impairments of affect seem to have experienced a *persistence* of depressed mood that becomes revealed as positive symptoms abate (Knights & Hirsch, 1981). In the PIAS study, of 92 patients with depression and/or anxiety, approximately 75% had suffered this form of distress for as long as clinical records existed or that referring clinicians could recall. For the 25% with a more discreet episode, the median length of comorbid impairment was 1 year. (S. G. Siris also indicated [oral communication, November 1992] that depression was often of long duration in his sample as well.) Unfortunately, in our experience such persistent depression (or chronic dysthymia) can often lead clinicians to conclude that these impairments of affect are primarily characterological in nature. Patients are sometimes viewed as having a depressed "personality" and thus are not the proper recipients of chemotherapy (another false assumption, as described in Chapter 3). Others feel that the impairments are understandable reactions to stressful life events to which nondrug therapy had been directed "for years" (obviously unsuccessfully). While we subscribe to the latter explanation as a rationale for PT, often these comorbidities can be modified with appropriate pharmacotherapy used in combination with psychotherapy. But once again effects have been clearly circumscribed.

For example, in our trial of desipramine (an older, conventional tricyclic antidepressant), patients were maintained on an average dose of 150 mg a day. Specific measures of depressed mood improved significantly, but *only among female patients!* There was no evidence of a central antidepressant effect among males; rather, only the improvement of anxiety and residual psychoticism characterized the response of men (and also women). However, and this was one of the more important observations from the study, intermittent symptom "flurries," or miniaffective episodes, were significantly fewer in number in patients maintained on desipramine (12.5%) compared to those maintained on placebo (41.2%). This observation applied to patients of both sexes. Depression in male schizophrenia patients has remained something of an enigma, with some speculating that schizophrenia and its associated impairments of mood might be more of a neurological disorder in men and more of an affective disorder in women. Depression seems more enduring in males and at times could represent a variant of flat affect (negative symptoms) more than depressed mood. Females, on the other hand, tend to have a better preservation of affect overall. Thus, they might remain more disposed to associated mood impairments, but reassuringly to pharmacological management as well. Clearly the available evidence supports a better medication response among schizoaffective females than males (Coryell, Grove, vanEerdwigh, Keller, & Endicott, 1987).

In our studies of impaired affect, it also took time for antidepressant medication effects to emerge, perhaps an understandable phenomenon among schizophrenia patients who had been ill for many years and who had been treated with antipsychotic medication for a lengthy period of time. In our study, the effects of desipramine were not detectable until 12 weeks. Siris et al. (1994) also reported stronger effects at 9 weeks than at 6 weeks, and Johnson (1981) observed no effects from a supplemental antidepressant in a 5-week trial. Today, the newer selective serotonin reuptake inhibitors (the SSRIs), such as fluoxetine (Prozac), sertraline (Zoloft), paroxetine (Paxil), venlafaxine (Effexor), and citalopram (Celexa) seem to be widely prescribed for schizophrenia patients who suffer an apparent depression of mood. While we often use these new SSRIs for comorbid depression (Celexa and Prozac being more frequently prescribed, and buproprion [Wellbutrin] being used for anergically depressed males), we have also found some benefit in the control of phobia and obsessions with these medications. Unfortunately, research-based evidence of supplemental SSRI efficacy in schizophrenia is very limited and remains a public health concern given the magnitude of the comorbidity problem (Siris, 2000). Clearly this is a clinical issue that is in great need of comprehensive efficacy data obtained through appropriately controlled clinical trials of the SSRIs among schizophrenia patients with concurrent affective disorder.

Regarding comorbid anxiety, our trials of lithium among anxious or anxious/depressed patients attempted to maintain patients at lithium plasma levels between 0.4 and 0.8 mmol/liter, a modest range that was designed to avoid neurotoxicity given that patients were also being maintained on a conventional neuroleptic. While we will typically use a PRN dose of a benzodiazapine (e.g., Ativan) for discreet episodes of agitation or situational anxiety, patients in this trial suffered persistent anxiety that was variously described as feelings of torment, anguish, or drivenness. Once again, the positive effects of lithium treatment in this sample did not appear until 12 weeks. According to clinical raters, the anxiolytic effects were again reserved primarily to female patients; however, both male and female patients self-reported improvement in their anxiety/depression. Effects were particularly prominent among patients with a good premorbid history (but who did not necessarily have a good interepisodic adjustment). Those with a poor premorbid history seemed to suffer the side effects of lithium without enjoying any therapeutic benefits. As such, there are selected but nonetheless important aspects of comorbid anxiety and/or depression that can at least be partially managed with supplemental thymoleptics. But for the affective impairments that persist in spite of appropriate medication, PT adopts its own strategy during the intermediate phase.

PT and Stability

Each PT session begins with a brief scan of the intersession situations that appeared to be stressful for the patient, as well as an appraisal of the accompanying subjective signs (or cues) of distress, a familiar procedure in the stress management literature (Charlesworth & Nathan, 1984). By now, the patient should have been able to articulate, at least in broad strokes, the personal goals that he or she will seek through the treatment plan. The therapist will therefore want to focus initially on the most easily identifiable, customary, and predictable cognitive, affective, and behavioral indicators of stress that the patient encounters in the pursuit of personal goals. In the intermediate phase, a relative emphasis is placed on the labeling of these cues, more than negotiating the stressors per se (see the section *Internal Coping*, below). Over time, a certain continuity in the review of stressful situations will emerge. Even in the absence of current stressors, the therapist will want to revisit the status of an earlier situation that appeared moderately or markedly stressful for the patient. (At that time the consequences of a conflict, a loss, or even a positive event might not have been immediately apparent.) However, the process of scanning and recall is not designed to become a source of stress itself! If the patient's anxiety or arousal appear to escalate in the context of this review, the focus should immediately turn to reassurance and support even though this might mean that the agenda for the session is placed on hold. While an interim level of arousal is needed to maintain attention and active learning, patients tend not to process and retain important information when they are at the extremes of arousal. In this regard, it is well to keep in mind the classic Hebbian inverted U as a schematic representation of the relationship between learning and arousal (i.e., at either extreme of arousal, attention and thus learning become impaired).

Typically, the brief scan can occur around issues that have already been part of previous treatment sessions, such as during the review of a homework assignment, a discussion of recent instances of drug/alcohol use, the appraisal of continuing environmental supports or their absence (including current interpersonal conflicts), and abiding concerns regarding medication management. In PT, it is not at all useful (and in fact is contraindicated) to focus narrowly on early developmental conflicts that no longer directly impact on the patient's current life as a way to elicit characteristic cues of distress. In the face of persistent anxiety and or depression, the principles of basic phase psychological support should be utilized (see Chapter 3) as well as useful autoprotective strategies, with assurances offered that a medication adjustment, if indicated, as well as the imminent introduction of increasingly effective coping strategies, should prove useful in achieving greater personal comfort.

For depressed patients, inquiry regarding the possibility of suicidal ideation or preoccupation is clearly warranted. Depressed mood often becomes more apparent when positive symptoms have subsided. Should the patient reveal intent and/or a plan, appropriate action should be initiated, including rehospitalization if necessary. At the least, increased contact should be pursued. Invariably, the therapist will want to review the previously agreed-upon "contract" that obligated the patient to call upon the therapist before implementing any intent to harm him- or herself. Suicidality is an important source of persistent instability for some patients. Unfortunately, most risk indicators are nonspecific predictors of actual suicide (i.e., they have low specificity). While these indicators might have high "sensitivity" (broad and overly inclusive descriptions), they are often minimally useful to clinical management. For example, that males with schizophrenia might be at greater risk of suicide than females does not easily lend itself to a routine policy of "high surveillance" among all male patients. In our experience, the patients who seem most preoccupied with suicidal thoughts are younger males (under the age of 40) who are earlier in their illness, such as first-episode patients for whom recovery has been slow and tortuous, those who have resolved the initial stages of denial, or those who have had a decent recovery but have then experienced another episode. Comorbidity in the form of substance abuse or mood disorder can increase the risk. While PT is not a definitive psychotherapy of suicidality, in the review of depressed mood or sources of subjective distress the clinician will want to reappraise the patient's understanding of the illness, the often painful discrepancy between past and present performance, the mourning associated with lost or seriously altered personal aspirations, and the often increasing discrepancy between current status and the accomplishments of peers or siblings. Many of these issues are addressed in the *Adjustment to Disability* section, below, and again the principles of supportive therapy and autoprotection can be applied in the context of a hopeful message regarding recovery of function and illness management.

Alcohol and Drug Misuse

As described in Chapter 2, the studies of PT screened out the more obvious cases of substance use disorder. In fact, PT was not designed as an intervention that would be directly relevant to these comorbidities. Nevertheless, we should recall that 13% of patients were using alcohol at least at a moderately severe level, and 11% were using cannabis. Unexpectedly, these patients were among the better responders to PT as indicated in Chapter 2, suggesting that perhaps PT might also aid in the stabilization of this subgroup of substance use disorders. Further guidelines to managing substance misuse are offered in Chapter 6, which considers patients who are more likely to engage in community initiatives.

A review of the more successful treatment programs for comorbid substance abuse and severe mental illness (Drake & Mueser, 2000) reveals a number of similarities to PT that might account for the good outcome of our substance-misusing patients. First, patients allegedly use alcohol and/or illicit drugs for many reasons, not the least of which is to reduce social anxiety or to accommodate social expectations, behaviors that PT addresses through internal coping, relaxation, and social skills strategies. Moreover, PT focuses on illness management (such as prodromes) and the provision of associated adaptive strategies that are also characteristic of successful substance abuse programs for comorbid disorders. The attainment of *personal goals*, both social and vocational; *psychoeducation* about the illness and its consequences; *case management* services related to attaining material resources such as housing and entitlements, a *close monitoring* of clinical state and medication; and utilization of the fact that recovery from substance abuse disorder is also a *staged process*—all represent shared characteristics of successful programs for comorbid disorders and PT. Future modifications of PT that include the practice principles of harm reduction, motivational interviewing, and urine monitoring could elevate PT to a more relevant and effective intervention for comorbid substance abuse disorder. We doubt, however, that PT could easily accommodate more coercive techniques such as involuntary outpatient commitment or the use of a representative payee to manage patients' fiscal resources. Those clinicians who do not have an integrated mental health and substance abuse program readily available might at least feel comforted knowing that many PT strategies have found success in the treatment of cannabis- and alcohol-using schizophrenia patients.

In summary, the maintenance of stabilization includes a thoughtful and sensitive inquiry at the start of each session aimed at answering the following questions: how clinically stable is the patient today; how does the patient's present clinical state compare to that in earlier sessions; are the basic elements of safety, shelter, material needs, and emotional support secure; is the patient's comprehension of PT themes constrained by attention or memory deficits; and is the patient now able to attend to the next level of information and skill acquisition? An understanding of the material presented in the current session and previous sessions should be ensured through periodic inquiry. At the end of each session, it is helpful to have the patient briefly summarize what was discussed in the preceding hour.

PSYCHOEDUCATION

By now, patients should have a fundamental grasp of schizophrenia at both the symptomatic and psychobiological levels, including the concept of vulnerability to stress and how treatment might serve to lower the risk of decompensation. The intermediate phase of psychoeducation raises these basic themes to a more practical and highly personalized level.

As soon as stability ensures the requisite tolerance for new information and its appropriate processing, the formal introduction of intermediate phase psychoeducation should begin. Essentially, the curriculum is nothing more than an overview of the remaining components of PT that the patient will encounter, with emphasis placed on those that will occur in the coming months. While patients could be offered this information during individual sessions, once again there is much to be said for its presentation in a small-group workshop format (as was the custom during the PT studies). In agencies where other therapists utilize PT, patients will have a better opportunity to participate in a common workshop. As described in Chapter 4, the group approach tends to legitimize the central importance of the PT coping strategies that will be offered and serves to demystify if not destigmatize the issues involved in managing one's illness. Patients will typically share the obstacles that they have personally encountered in the process of resuming a social and vocational life, as well as how they have begun to come to terms with their illness. Often patients who might not spontaneously seek information or clarification are moved to further inquiry once a discussion of workshop themes has been initiated by peers.

If prescribed as a formal didactic, the psychoeducational content can be divided into three 20- to 30-minute presentations that include time for discussion and questions:

The first of these presentations includes a review of the initial *cues of distress,* including the more common physical, emotional, cognitive, and behavioral signs that will be initiated with internal coping (see below). It is emphasized that the acquisition of techniques that allow for easy detection provides the means for monitoring cues of distress *prior to* any visible behavioral effect and that such monitoring can often abort an escalation of symptoms. Even in the absence of symptom exacerbation, maintenance of an appropriate level of arousal will be essential to the ultimate resumption of social and vocational roles.

The second component of the psychoeducation session focuses on the types of *relaxation* that will be employed as a defense against the escalation of these cues of distress. The techniques will range from diaphragmatic breathing and the "relaxation response" of the intermediate phase to progressive muscle relaxation and guided imagery in the advanced phase. Further, the incremental skills that began earlier with avoidance and prosocial statements will expand during the intermediate phase to include aspects of verbal and nonverbal communication, taking the "emotional temperature" of another person, and ultimately the advanced phase essentials of conflict resolution and criticism management. Even though they were introduced in the basic phase, variations in voice tone and nonverbal expression (including gestures, eye contact, facial expressions, and posture) can again be modeled. *Social perception* is described as one of correctly timing and reading the emotional state of another person when initiating requests or dealing with anger and criticism. Patients themselves will frequently volunteer examples of the unwanted consequences that followed upon failing to make a correct social perception. The assertion of the patient's own concerns is illustrated by the utility of "I" statements (e.g., "I feel" or "I think") rather than "you-type" accusations. Handouts (described below) are provided that can be used to illustrate the contexts in which relaxation or social perception are to be applied and the results obtained. These handouts serves as a medium for eventually reporting homework assignments.

Finally, the third component introduces the concept of *adjustment to disability*, an often neglected component of care that can become a matter of some controversy if viewed as the "pathologizing" of common human responses to illness. We explore the pros and cons of this focus below in the section on *Adjustment to Disability*. However, even in the face of experience and prior education regarding the nature and treatment of schizophrenia, some patients might remain unconvinced of their own diagnosis or minimally appreciate how severe mental illness can affect their ability to work, play, and maintain important relationships. Others will not have come to terms with the disabilities and handicaps of their illness, in spite of prolonged illness and treatment. Fewer yet will understand the need for remediation if not compensation when confronted with persistent disabilities and handicaps. For some, the task can be as formidable as the forging of a new identity.

Before introducing the initial concepts of disability and its acceptance, the clinician should ascertain that the patients in the workshop will not be overwhelmed by an explicit description of the process that often begins with denial of disability, extends to the reality of disability, and (if all goes well) resolves as adjustment to disability. Knowledge of the patients' clinical state will influence the timing of disability discussions. Although patients might often maintain their "denial," they can use information that is relevant to their goals, even though an understanding of something called "schizophrenia" is incompetently formed or even absent. "Yes . . . but" is often the best accommodation a patient can make to disability information at this stage of recovery. The clinician can reinforce patient strengths and the belief that real achievements are possible, while gently suggesting that a slow, steady progression of practical compensations will likely get the patient to where he or she wants to be, safely and with a good chance of success.

The workshop provides the forum for drawing patients into sharing their past experiences and difficulties with work, school, or social interactions. The examples volunteered can represent the basis for illustrating how "disability" could have contributed to unsuccessful ventures. For example, a patient that shares how hard it was to "push myself to finish even small jobs" can be reminded of the price that an episode of mental illness can exert on stamina and mental energy. It can be emphasized that feeling "drained and tired" is not often thought of as one of the "disabilities" of schizophrenia during the recovery phase, but it is very real for most patients. Using analogies such as a heart attack, stroke, or other physical illnesses with which patients are familiar can begin to illustrate the relationship between a disorder that affects the brain and those that affect other organs, with often similar consequences and similar needs to adjust. Such examples provided by an individual patient can be followed with a question: "Did anyone else ever have a problem like that?" Attendees will often concur and share their own stories.

The point of the "adjustment to disability" component is to alert patients to some of the functional capacities that are affected by schizophrenia, to link these to the neurobiology of the illness, and to illustrate how PT will help them compensate for restrictions in functioning. Real-life examples will almost always provide an introduction to the disability "talking points" that are related to vocational difficulties, such as reduced stamina, amotivation, distractibility, and difficulties with supervisors or coworkers that might have followed upon impulsive or incorrect judgments.

The content of intermediate phase psychoeducation should become very clear to the PT therapist once all components of the intermediate phase have been reviewed. Following this review, the psychoeducational workshop will resolve to a summary of the essential intermediate phase components. Throughout the formal or informal educational presentation, it remains crucial that the therapist be attuned to how the patient is processing information both intellectually and emotionally. A simple inquiry can ensure the former, but the latter will often not be appreciated until a later series of exchanges reveals whether the patient is still engaged in the process of denial. Psychoeducation can be judged a success if patients indicate some increased awareness of their early warning signs as well as the strategies that will become available which might reduce a potential escalation of symptoms. Hopeful comments from the patient to the effect that self-management and improved functional status are possible in the future is another indicator of a successful psychoeducation. Patients who acknowledge that improvement is measured in contrast to their own prior status, rather than by way of comparison to the adjustment of unaffected peers or other family members, have clearly shown the beginnings of an adjustment to disability.

INCREASING RESPONSIBILITIES IN THE HOME

The assignment of incremental tasks that are directed toward the resumption of responsibilities within the home had been a core component of our earlier family psychoeducation approach (see Anderson et al., 1986, Chs. 4 and 5). While steps toward role resumption clearly remain important in PT, other homework assignments regarding cue identification and the associated coping strategies assume a more focal interest during the intermediate phase. Nevertheless, when it is critical to the very initiation of instrumental and expressive roles, the assignment of household tasks will continue to remain a technique of considerable importance for some patients. These circumstances are most likely to arise among patients whose behavior lies toward the extremes of role performance: those who are unmotivated to initiate behavior, and those who are motivated to resume responsibilities rapidly, as though an episode of severe illness had never occurred. Among these latter patients, there is often little or no appreciation of the restraints on capacity that exist in the form of residual vulnerabilities related to the regulation of arousal, attention, memory, and information processing.

The Undermotivated Patient

For unmotivated patients, it is important to review (with families as well) that a psychotic episode is something of a "catabolic catastrophe," with clear residual effects on stamina, energy, and motivation, effects not unlike the body's responses to any physical trauma. Such effects can often lead others to characterize the patient as being lazy, a shirker, or worse. Patients that are recovering from a recent episode can be easily overwhelmed by even the suggestion of increased household responsibilities or by fear that a lack of success might provoke the criticism of family members or friends. Among patients with little or no motivation, the necessity of contributing to the routine tasks that are essential to household functioning and to the well-being of other members can be nonjudgmentally described by the clinician, taking the perspective of the patient as well as the perspectives of other household members. A willingness to initiate even simple tasks can be seen not only as a way to achieve greater personal comfort in the home but as the means of incrementally building stamina and a routine that will inevitably be necessary for sustaining social and vocational roles outside the home. The benefits of a structured program for the incremental resumption of responsibilities can be presented as a method of avoiding the unreasonable expectations (and often the ensuing criticisms) that are frequently held by oneself or other members of the household. With the rationale discussed, the therapist can suggest a number of tasks that are both needed and appropriate to the patient's level of stability. At this juncture, an important opportunity arises that permits the patient's own choice of tasks and their sequencing. Sometimes this might be the first real chance that the patient has had to actively direct the agreed-upon treatment plan. Again, the sequencing of tasks should represent incremental steps in difficulty, with the absence of success representing a clear need to return to an earlier level of successful performance.

In the basic phase, patients with negative symptoms and reduced stamina would likely have been encouraged to focus on the tasks of self-care and personal hygiene, while those with greater stability and remission of symptoms would more often have been performing household tasks by choice or necessity. In the intermediate phase, the ultimate assignment of tasks is focused on those that can be *cooperatively* performed with another household member. (For those living alone, the task will focus on routine household maintenance and the paying of bills, for example, with the goal of ultimately ensuring competent performance of tasks outside the home related to shopping, health care, transportation, negotiation of needed services from social agencies, or effective collaboration with a case manager.) Sometimes the cooperative assignments will center on instrumental tasks such as tending to the yard or mechanical maintenance, preparation of food, and home cleaning. At other times, the focus will be on expressive roles such as the initiation of a conversation with another household member on a neutral subject (e.g., deciding what to watch on TV) or engaging in brief but appropriate exchanges with family guests who visit the home. The clinician should review these exchanges with the goal of ensuring clear and simple communications. For patients with little or no social life outside the home, these initiatives within the family (or with roommates or other supported-housing tenants) can often represent the first steps in resocializing the patient and thus provide the foundation for an eventual reentry into a wider social network. Otherwise, during the assumption of cooperative tasks, the therapist can review the *timing* of these tasks, that is, when it is most convenient to join other family members and when the patient's energy level is the highest during the day. When a homework assignment is reviewed during the subsequent PT session, it is often more important to reinforce the effort made in simply attempting the task than to analyze the extent of its completion or lack thereof. Even when task performance is successful, praise should be appropriately tempered. Most adults with a severe mental illness, for example, are quite aware that carrying out the trash twice a week is not a monumental achievement. Again, tasks should be relatively simple, relevant, compatible with clinical state, feasible with regard to completion, and graduated in difficulty.

The Overmotivated Patient

At the other extreme of motivation is the patient who by choice or necessity feels obligated to quickly resume the vocational or academic roles that were interrupted by the illness (a frequent concern among first-episode married or single-parent patients). As the PT results described in Chapter 2 revealed, some wage earner patients, particularly those who had household members that were dependent on their income, often successfully returned to work before symptoms had remitted or the underlying deficits had stabilized. But even in these cases, a task remained to temporarily limit the vocational or academic demands as much as possible, either through part-time employment, flexible hours, or a reduction in the number and/or complexity of academic credit hours. Even when such compromises cannot be negotiated, the opportunity to revisit the psychoeducational topic of "stress and vulnerability" should be utilized. In most cases, the patients will at least be willing to temporarily limit the amount of social stimulation outside the vocational role. For those with families, a review of customary patient responsibilities in the home can be made, and the willingness of other family members to temporarily assume one or more of these tasks can be determined for patients who feel the need to quickly return to work, school, or full-time homemaker roles.

ADJUSTMENT TO DISABILITY

The notion of "disability" following a severe mental illness can be difficult to accept (and therefore address), particularly if the clinician is negatively disposed toward the "medical model" or believes that the neurobiology of schizophrenia is nothing more than a collection of nonspecific observations that could just as likely support the effects of an adverse environment on brain function as the converse. But whether such a change in brain function is a cause or an effect, specific or nonspecific, decades of research now support the view that clear alterations occur in the structural, functional, and/or biochemical integrity of the brain during and following a schizophrenia episode (see Keshavan & Murray, 1997, and Chapters 3 and 4 for reviews). Further, this literature provides evidence for selected cerebral anomalies that predate the onset of schizophrenia in many cases, often arising perinatally (as described earlier). Whether clinicians subscribe to the "inside-out" or the "outside-in" hypothesis, most would agree that there are at least short-term functional behavioral consequences of compromised cerebral integrity.

Compared to the issue of adjustment to disability in mental illness, the concept of *psychological* adjustment to *physical* disability has received considerably more attention in the formal rehabilitation literature, but often with mixed findings (DeLoach & Greer, 1981). While there are obvious reactions and adaptive processes that the physically disabled must negotiate, it remains unclear whether the psychology of the physically disabled is significantly different overall than that of able-bodied individuals who face any number of life crises that also require adaptation. DeLoach and Greer (1981) have commented that getting an artificial leg on is no more upsetting than getting one's socks on. The relative neglect of psychological adjustment to *mental* disability in the psychiatric literature is therefore easy to understand. After all, the "strengths" model emphasizes *abilities* rather than disabilities, abhors the label of "abnormal" for what are often viewed as *normal* responses to adversity, and otherwise promotes patient *potential* rather than focusing on deficits. But unlike psychological adaptation in the physically disabled, the reality remains that the *brain* is the organ of impairment in patients with severe mental illness, and this acknowledgment carries with it important consequences, including the dilemma that the compromised organ is also the entity needed for disability awareness. Schizophrenia patients and their therapists can often be mistakenly led to believe that cognitive and affective disabilities are not "real" because they are less visible than other physical disabilities.

In our opinion, it is counterproductive to recovery when an *exclusive* strengths perspective precludes or seriously limits an acknowledgment and hence discussion of mental disabilities. Residual strengths will clearly be called into the service of adjustment during PT, but a failure to come to terms with the disabilities that follow a compromised neurobiological system can seriously jeopardize the goals of clinical stabilization and restoration of function. Without some appreciation of individual vulnerability and the associated psychological disabilities, patients might become unnecessarily exposed to risk factors that often precipitate recurrent psychotic episodes. Once disabilities become acknowledged and incorporated, self-worth, autonomy, and personal confidence will typically increase (DeLoach & Greer, 1981). In fact it is often difficult for clinicians to relate differently to the new patient identity that accompanies this adjustment to psychiatric disability. Following participation in our ongoing study of cognitive-enhancement therapy, for example, it has not been unusual for successfully treated patients to bemoan the need to adopt a former "patient" role (e.g., the recitation of symptoms litanies) once they return to a former mental health provider. At the opposite extreme are the therapeutic pessimists who also fail to address issues surrounding adjustment to disability, since it is implied in a wide literature that a majority of schizophrenia patients simply "have no insight" and thus the exercise of making such an adjustment would unlikely be successful. We have often encountered this form of nihilism, not only in clinical practice but in the scientific review process as well (e.g., disallowing promising treatment initiatives that "are not worth the cost"). The effect of such nihilism continues to manifest itself around the funding of psychosocial rehabilitation programs for the severely mentally ill, where the "deliberately disturbing" mentally ill routinely lose the competitive battle for financial resources to the "deserving victims" of physical disability (cited in DeLoach & Greer, 1981).

Among the stages of adjustment to (physical) disability that have been variously described in the literature (see DeLoach & Greer, 1981), the following have impressed us as being the more relevant experiences among patients with schizophrenia as well. When addressed, the subsequent growth in social and vocational effectiveness has been impressive, as the findings from the PT studies have clearly documented (see Chapter 2).

Denial

Once the shock, or even "emotional numbness," associated with a life-altering mental illness subsides, it is often followed by a period of denial. Such denial is not intrinsically maladaptive in the short run. In many instances it is a form of insulation against the overwhelming affects that PT attempts to control. Nor is strong denial the exclusive defense mechanism of the mentally ill. Think of the analogues in rehabilitation medicine: the paraplegic who believes that modern medicine will shortly solve the puzzle of connecting a severed spinal cord, or the recently diagnosed cancer patient who is convinced that diagnostic testing was erroneous or that a heroic medical procedure will reverse a broad metastatic process. Is it any wonder that schizophrenia patients might rely on similar *deus ex machina* solutions to the functional consequences of a covert impairment?

While denial often serves short-term goals, in the long run it is counterproductive to medication compliance and the demanding rituals of rehabilitation and recovery. Why bother with treatment if "nothing is really wrong" or if a temporary "problem" will take care of itself in time or with a few social services? In the absence of more obvious signs of disability that characterize physical disorders, those with severe psychological disabilities will often focus on the "shortcomings" of family members, peers, former coworkers or employers as the sources of their personal difficulty. "If only" analyses of the failure of others to have accommodated the patient are common, including a recitation of the alleged sins of omission and commission made by those who care most about the patient. This "search for a cause," while denying schizophrenia and its disabilities, can also extend to other explanations of the current problem: a misdiagnosed medical illness; the "wrong" psychiatric diagnosis; a rigid belief in an idiosyncratic cause; the result of another person's or society's failures; a questioning of the clinician's credentials; or at best an acknowledgment that some problem might exist but they are "not at all like the problems of people who are crazy." At times, the interaction between denial and delusions can represent a particularly difficult challenge for the clinician. For all the discussion of alternative causes, such patients often seem not to have a real appreciation of how their own symptoms present and affect others, let alone the functional consequences that might follow. Patients will often avoid the clinic and its "really sick people," as well as day treatment or resocialization programs that provide "activities for losers." Nonetheless, these very same patients will often lead lives of isolation, spending their days less personally groomed or less interpersonally connected than their "sicker" colleagues, often sipping coffee all day at one ubiquitous shop after another. Some patients, often less disabled, will muddle along unaware of the price that their unmanaged cognitive and affective disabilities exact on the patience, morale, and feelings of loved ones.

A most challenging twist on denial is the "flight to health." This preoccupation with being "normal" too often resolves to a dichotomous view of the human condition as either one of complete health or complete illness. Patients might acknowledge that they are ill now but insist that in a short time they will be entirely well. (In the meantime they will often prefer to do nothing until their health returns.) This stance effectively ignores the reality that recovery is often a long-term process that takes both personal effort and a relevant plan. At other times, patients might pressure the clinician to raise or lower a dosage, or add or delete a medication, as the likely action needed in order to get well "quickly." Sometimes the preoccupation with normalcy can take the form of unrealistic comparisons to peers. Since unaffected friends have often graduated college, some patients are anxious to return to school immediately following an episode, ignoring the fact that prior relapses often occurred in the face of untempered academic demands. So too with drinking. "All my friends drink beer," a patient might claim, "so having a six pack a day is normal for a guy like me," thus discounting the special health consequences to the patient and a likely sensitivity to alcohol (Drake & Mueser, 2000) that schizophrenia might impose. Medication taking, clinic appointments, the need to temporarily revise personal expectations, and a graduated approach to recovery are all reminders of "illness" and can serve as the antithesis to being "normal." Rarely is it acknowledged that "normal people" also have problems and that foresightful planning is the cornerstone of a successful life, one that carries with it a personal obligation to work at optimal functioning, independent of treatment. Disparagement of the therapist during these discussions of normalcy can also be difficult. It is not uncommon for patients to claim that the therapist is simply more "lucky" than they and therefore is insensitive to their current state. Some patients have argued that if therapists were in their place, they would be doing everything possible to get back on their feet "as quickly as possible."

The PT approach to denial is to adopt a sensitive listening posture, synthesize the details of the patient's account, and offer a reassurance that the underlying feelings are entirely understandable and upsetting. The therapist can acknowledge that anyone going through what the patient has experienced would likely feel the same way, but might also caution the patient to the effect that being constantly upset or overwrought by these issues has not and will not likely help in the long term. In contrast, PT will provide different ways to deal with strong feelings as well as a method to resume functioning as quickly as is prudent. The message communicated to the patient is that PT can help resolve the seeming dilemmas of health and illness, treatment or no treatment, by enabling the patient to increasingly recognize and control the strong affects and beliefs associated with these concerns and the associated symptoms as well. A treatment plan will allow the patient to safely move on with his or her life where the *patient* is in control, rather than the circumstances that led to the present or past crises.

Associated Affects

When denial begins to depart from the patient's repertoire of coping skills, all too often *grief* becomes the unwelcome visitor. The loss of one's ability to avoid or contain mental illness, the subsequent dependence on medication or a health system for support, the postponement of personal aspirations and goals, and the frustration of not being able to perform otherwise "automatic" activities can provoke affects that extend from demoralization to a profound mourning, and at times to clinical depression. *Shame* can also become the companion of grief. Many patients in recovery will eventually share the humiliation that was associated with acute symptoms, often embarrassing behaviors that now sustain a persistent guilt. At other times, patients will speak of the hurt that was inflicted on loved ones while acutely ill. In all but rare instances, the growing distance from an acute episode brings with it an awareness of how *stigmatizing* the illness can be in terms of both overt and covert messages received from friends, family, potential or actual employers, and the media (which are increasingly disposed to dramatize the sensational aspects of rare psychotic features or eccentric behaviors). Some patients become fearful that their illness might become a source of further public humiliation if revealed. Not surprising then, *anger* can become the natural response to shame, grief, and stigmatization. Again, this strong affect is unfortunately most often directed toward those loved ones or care providers whom patients feel have contributed most to their difficulties. Perceived slights, instances of alleged disrespect, failures to have appreciated the "uniqueness" of the patient's circumstances, or failures to have extended the desired support can spawn an irritability that becomes directed to either the employer that treated the patient "unfairly," the family member(s) that arranged for hospitalization, the clinician who insists on therapy, and even the agencies that appeared to withhold the support that the patient viewed as essential to recovery. Again, PT's response to the dilemma of being both "devil and deliverer" is to accept the legitimacy and understandable basis of these feelings, suggest how such strong affects can themselves be disabling, and offer the clear assurance that a way does exist to achieve both personal comfort and long-term goals.

Without an acknowledgment of the process of adjustment to disability, rehabilitation efforts can lead to the unhelpful prescription of vocational tasks at which patients have previously failed, or provoke an obsession with unrealistic career aspirations, especially when the less obvious cognitive and affective disabilities go unacknowledged. With a successful negotiation of denial and its associated affects, the stage can become set for an acceptance of disability. Such acceptance will serve to encourage patients to adopt a plan that is not only designed to capitalize on available strengths but that can also compensate for the more enduring disabilities or social handicaps. Acceptance is not the result of a bold confrontation, or one that requires patients to "confess" their illness and disabilities, but rather is a process that primarily leads to a different *understanding* by patients of their deeply held convictions and strongly felt emotions about schizophrenia and its consequences—a *metamorphosis*, in the words of DeLoach and Greer (1981), that seems as relevant to the mentally ill as it has been to the physically challenged.

Some Common Disabilities

The rehabilitation "point of entry" in adjusting to one's disability will likely have been established during the course of psychoeducation described earlier, particularly if the format included a more formal group presentation. Most often, patients will have experienced and be open to a discussion of common occurrences that few would have previously understood as "functional disabilities of schizophrenia." (Again, what is often being "denied" by patients is the medical or media characterizations of schizophrenia.) When disabilities are cognitively reframed in terms of the patient's personal experience, it is not unusual to see awareness and insight emerge.

The psychobiology of reduced *stamina* can often serve as the first example of a psychological disability. Reduced stamina can be conceptualized as the sequela of neurotransmitter depletion, catabolism and the neurobiological effects on executive functions. Or it can be cast in laymen's terms, such that the brain has experienced a profound "workout" during a psychotic episode, with the result that one needs considerably more mental effort in order to complete even the most mundane tasks. The patient can be told that many months are often needed in order to recover mental energy and that the exercises of PT are designed in a way that the patient can build "mental strength" just as the athlete will gradually build physical stamina following an injury. Further, since mental strength is such a valuable resource, the patient can be cautioned about expending or even wasting this energy by becoming overwrought about inconsequential matters. PT can be characterized as a series of strategies that will help to keep the mind from "overescalating" and thus preserve mental energy for really important tasks such as returning to work or school, maintaining a household, and enjoying friends, family, and social activities.

Closely associated with a reduced stamina that renders the effortful mental processing of information difficult is the common phenomenon of *amotivation*, which is both a (negative) symptom of schizophrenia as well as a residual disability for many patients. Again, with the assault that schizophrenia often makes on frontal-lobe executive functions, the patient can be assured that "getting motivated" is a frequent complaint of many patients during recovery—not that motivation is impossible, only that one needs to deliberately work at getting motivated since it will not always return magically on its own. The patient can be informed that success with PT exercises will become part of a wider "reward system" and that the satisfaction that comes from these successes, no matter how small, have been shown to be a consistent way to make motivation easier to sustain. Since a well-regulated dopaminergic system supports the mammalian reward system (Stellar & Stellar, 1985), both medication and skill accomplishments will work together to achieve and maintain this optimal neurochemical status.

In that PT prominently targets dysregulated affect, an important functional disability often presents itself in the form of *impulsivity*, a limbic-systemic-determined personal response (Taylor & Cadet, 1989) with which many patients can readily identify. The therapist can review recent instances where the patient might have become "worked up," anxious, angry, or even overly elated in the face of these strong, familiar, automatic, and often trusted feelings. Perhaps in the course of these feelings the patient might have said or did something that was later regretted. Some patients might have impulsively criticized those who were most involved in their care, whereas others were moved to quickly reestablish past relationships without providing time to repair interim damage. Even patients who resumed a prior role, such as a job, might have impulsively quit the first time a supervisor or coworker implied a criticism of performance. PT, it can be stated, will provide many ways to identify the earliest feelings that might lead to becoming "upset." Once the patient is able to anticipate these feelings, as well as the circumstances where they tend to "get out of hand," he or she can be assured that the calming self-control strategies of PT will often prevent the types of impulsive behavior that might have exacted a heavy price in the past.

Finally, there is a fundamental disability that is nearly omnipresent in schizophrenia, both acutely and during remission, and that is rarely conceptualized as a disability by patients or their providers. It is represented by the profound difficulty that many patients experience in maintaining attention, concentration, and working memory. (Working memory is the ability to cognitively hold information "on-line," which is essential to completing an instrumental task or a communication.) Best summarized as *distractibility*, this disability is associated with stimuli overload and/or the intrusion of irrelevant stimuli such that a substantial effort is subsequently required just to maintain vigilance. The process is often readily endorsed by patients who can no longer read, attend classes, pursue hobbies, or engage in tasks that require more than a moment or two of concentration. The clear effects of medication on arousal and information processing can again be reviewed. The manner is which PT will help the patient to gain control over environmental stimuli as well as the subjective effects of distress can serve as examples that will foster improved concentration, memory, and the pursuit of a personally satisfying life.

INTERNAL COPING

When PT was conceived in the mid-1980s, the field was awash in the techniques of "stress management," from simple avoidance to relaxation, desensitization, positive assertion, self-instruction, and cognitive reframing. Since we desired a systemic approach that fairly captured the elements of stress management that had proven to be successful with schizophrenia patients, our choices were by definition limited. Our review concluded that the identification of early "cues of distress" and the easily applied strategies of deep breathing, relaxation, social perception, self-talk, and positive assertion were both effective and within the ability of schizophrenia patients who were at least in partial remission of positive symptoms (e.g., Acosta, Yamamoto, & Wilcox, 1978; Breier & Strauss, 1983; Hawkins, Doel, Lindseth, Jeffery, & Skaggs, 1980; Meichenbaum & Cameron, 1973, 1974; Van Hassel, Bloom, & Gonzalez, 1982). Of particular value at the time was the text of Charlesworth and Nathan (1984), who, among other contributors, described the "scanning for tension" procedure that is reflected in the internal coping approach.

Thus, one of the more important (but difficult) PT components was the internal coping procedure of the intermediate phase. Not only does it require that the patient learn to identify the earliest and least-intensive signals of distress, but also he or she must be able to recognize the process by which these early cues can escalate into prodromes and even minor or major episodes of affective or schizophrenia psychosis (Novacek & Raskin, 1998). Further, in the midst of a stressful encounter, the patient would need to achieve sufficient cognitive distance from the associated feelings so as to enlist a relevant coping strategy. This coping strategy has been difficult for "normal" individuals who are undergoing life crises, but the challenge to a person who is cognitively compromised can at times appear insurmountable. For this reason, the more sophisticated technique of cue recognition and the deployment of adaptive strategies have been reserved to the intermediate phase when patients have achieved some greater stabilization of positive symptoms. In order to facilitate the process, the introduction of internal coping in the intermediate phase should appear as a seamless extension of the broad "scanning" of troublesome events and their prodromal consequences that had characterized basic phase sessions. Neither the procedure, the structure, nor the tone of a session should change noticeably. The process will, however, move progressively from the broad descriptions of being "upset" to the highly specific definitions of the earliest indicators of this distress.

Progression of Cues, Signs, Symptoms, and Syndromes

The first task of internal coping in this phase is to provide the patient with some greater understanding of the likely sequence of events that might lead to an exacerbation of psychosis. Even though it is readily acknowledged that even a characteristic prodrome for an individual patient will likely be as benign as it is a herald of a new episode (see Chapter 4), it appears to be important for the schizophrenia patient to appreciate that awareness of this potential "march of symptoms" is a prerequisite for effective personal management (Bustillo, Buchanan, & Carpenter, 1995; Morley, 1998). And, again, even when precursors have benign consequences, the advantages of self-regulation in difficult contexts can clearly lead to more enjoyable relationships and successful vocational functioning.

Our explanation of this process of progression to psychosis is illustrated in Figure 5.1. While not intended to be a monument to linear thinking, the content of this figure does provide most patients with a cognitive schema that underscores the concept of progression and implies the potential for a successful self-management of schizophrenia by disrupting this process as *early as possible*. Clearly not all, or even a majority of, patients follow a linear progression of decompensation. Every clinician who has worked with schizophrenia patients can recall cases where the patient seemed well stabilized at a treatment session, only to be rehospitalized some 48 hours later. Unfortunately, it is the seduction of probability theory that can lead the clinician to assume that a predictable effect, in a predictable time, will follow a meaningful clinical event, whether therapeutic or toxic. More often, we suspect, the sequence can be a reflection of chaos theory, where a seemingly benign event (environmental stimulus) can

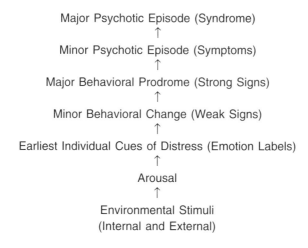

FIGURE 5.1. A schema of progression to psychosis.

quickly lead to a rapid, catastrophic conclusion (psychosis). Chaos theory, in fact, supports rather than detracts from the value of early intervention, even in minimally stressful circumstances. As many as one-half of the major prodromes of psychosis do not result in another episode. In one of our earlier studies, 47% of patients experienced an average of two "mini" psychotic episodes, typically those who lived in highly stressful households, yet relatively few of these minor episodes progressed to a major psychotic relapse (Hogarty et al., 1988). In point of fact, our definition of a miniepisode included positive symptoms of schizophrenia that were not as severe as those seen in a major episode and that subsequently *resolved* in 2–3 weeks with a medication adjustment and/or a psychosocial intervention (often designed to control environmental stimuli), both of which were offered in the context of increased surveillance. But even clear prodromes and minor exacerbations that do not lead to a psychotic episode can destabilize patients, interfere with the performance of resumed roles, and contribute to the demoralization of patients and their loved ones ("Here we go again"). Thus, an early intervention that circumvents even minor exacerbations can be of value in its own right.

Given the requisite distance (in time) from an active psychotic episode that characterizes patients in the intermediate phase, it has been our experience that the majority of them are open to a discussion of this progression, a discussion that is enriched and made highly individual by the patient's own account of past episodes. This discourse becomes particularly meaningful when coupled with the knowledge of environmental stressors and their effects that were gathered by the therapist during a review of clinical records and clinical state. Whether or not patients proceed directly to prodromes, minor episodes, or major episodes, PT assumes that the process has its beginning in the common human response to experience, namely, a *psychophysiological state* that requires *identification* and *labeling* as the precondition for a meaningful affective life and its appropriate management (Schacter & Singer, 1962). A most useful introduction to the topic of early intervention has been the analogy to catching a cold (drawn from our preliminary training manual). Nearly everyone has experienced the physical changes that precede a cold, even before clear symptoms are apparent to an observer. An itching throat, a chill, loss of appetite, or mild fever can be the earliest signals that a cold is imminent and that a prophylactic measure or two might be helpful in containing the full expression of symptoms. Bed rest, plenty of fluids, a reduction of routines, the use of analgesics or zinc lozenges, and perhaps even chicken soup can serve to lessen the ravages of a temporarily disabling viral infection. The thrust of this analogy is to move patients from the *macro-* to the *micro*identification of symptom precursors.

Subjective Cues of Distress

While we shall shortly describe some sources of stress and their contexts that are important to many schizophrenia patients, for now a few truisms need to be acknowledged, primarily the profound individual differences that exist in response to common stressors. These differences appear not only in the magnitude of a disruptive response but also in the patient's own constitutional resiliency and adaptive strengths that have been shaped by prior experience with the stressor and its successful management. Further, individual reactions to a given stressor will range in their expression from distinct physical signs to cognitive signals, altered emotional states, and behavioral styles. Thus, it is neither possible nor desirable to construct a rigid list of subjective cues and their labeling that would apply to all or even most patients. Many texts exist that identify the diverse sources of potential stress for a person and their varied responses (e.g., Charlesworth & Nathan, 1984; Selye, 1976; McKay et al., 1981). It is not surprising, therefore, that the adaptive strategies themselves will need to be similarly individualized, as we shall describe below. Unlike more traditional social skills training approaches that tend to increasingly focus on discrete problem areas for schizophrenia patients or specific deficits that provoke adaptive difficulties (such as initiating a conversation, forming an intimate relationship, or negotiating medication issues), internal coping places less emphasis on the specific nature of a stressor and more on the patient's characteristic response to potential sources of stress, those that arise either externally or internally. Internal sources of stress are quite common among schizophrenia patients, often present as rumination, preoccupation with intrusive ideas, feelings of inadequacy, nonspecific "worries," as well as specific concerns about future functioning. These sources of stress could also be usefully characterized as "phasic" (acute) or "tonic" (chronic), the former representing discrete events (such as receiving a threatening letter from a landlord) and the latter being more persistent and enduring sources of distress, such as living with a critical friend or relative or lacking material resources needed to satisfy basic needs.

Nearly every school of psychotherapy has sought clarification of this personal response to stress with the probe, "How did you feel about that?" In PT, the question is intended to be literal and the response as concrete as possible. The gentle probing and scanning of subjective cues are not intended to eliminate stress or extinguish an affective life since "arousing" challenges are as likely to lead to the rewards of a full and satisfying life as not. Rather, the patient should be encouraged to appreciate these common and often necessary human reactions, but to manage their intensity before distressing feelings escalate beyond control. This primary probe of feelings serves to alert the patient to the fact that there *is* a response to stress, whether consciously acknowledged or not. Patients whose typical response is "I feel OK" can be supported for their coping mastery but calmly queried for any physical, emotional, or cognitive sign that accompanied the stressor. The therapist's goal is not to interpret the unconscious or preconscious symbolic meaning of a cue, but rather to assure the patient that such cue identification is the first step in establishing internal boundaries and thus a sense of self-control. The primary focus again is on the cue and its labeling. Only gradually will the relationship be drawn to the behavioral consequences that follow these cues—and to their management.

When moving from the patient's broad definitions of distress emphasized in the basic phase to the more specific cues of distress, the query is not only intended to direct the patient's attention to their *earliest* expression but also to their *lowest* point of intensity. Patients, for example, might begin with a broad statement of having been "upset" by a friend or close family member who made what was perceived to be an unreasonable request. The deductive probing of *becoming upset* will often lead to the identification of various cues: having been *angry*, perhaps attributed to a *bad temper*, or having *felt like screaming* as a result of being *frustrated* by the demand. The inquiry might conclude with the acknowledgment of very earlier signs such as a *pounding heart* or *finger tapping* when the offending person began their inappropriate request. This example represents a common response to interpersonal conflict (i.e., a series of concurrent affects and attributions). The relatively benign and low-intensity "finger tapping" or some other analogue will often serve as the earliest and lowest-intensity cue.

For patients who experience difficulty with the cognitive processing of emotional states (akin to alixethymia), the therapist should take an active role by introducing examples of possible cues. Tables 5.1–5.4 provide examples of physical, emotional, cognitive, and behavioral cues of distress adapted from various sources (e.g., McKay et al., 1981; Schafer, 1983; Selye, 1974; Charlesworth & Nathan, 1984), as well as from patient reports.

The cues are not graded from earliest to latest in their emergence,

TABLE 5.1. Emotional (Feeling) Signals of Distress

Feeling like hitting someone or something	Fearfulness
Feeling tied up in knots	About the future
Consistent feelings of anger	About others disapproving of you
Feeling "woozy"	About doing something wrong
Feeling like running away or getting away from things	About losing control of oneself
Feeling impatient with oneself or others	That something terrible is going to happen
Feeling out of control	Feeling like you don't enjoy anything anymore
Feeling all "wound up"	Feeling like things are an effort or a struggle
Emotional ups and downs	Feeling like you don't want to face the day
Feeling like crying	Feeling hopeless or discouraged
Feeling like shouting or screaming	Feeling sad, blue, down in the dumps
	Feeling like one is doomed
	Afraid that an accident is going to happen
	Afraid you are dying or going to die

since some patients might identify a cue as appearing relatively early during a progression of signs whereas the same cue could represent a clear prodrome for another patient. Further, some patients might never move beyond broad behavioral cues (such as smoking or drinking more) and others might struggle with accepting a possible relationship between an early "palpitation" and later "flying off the handle." This internal probing of subjective cues will follow an increasingly familiar and natural exchange as the patient moves from one account of recent experience to another, with the therapist commenting on characteristic responses to stressful encounters as these sources of provocation changed in their intensity. Slowly over time, the thread of individual cues will become woven into the fabric of a more readily identifiable and consistent response to stressful life expe-

TABLE 5.2. Cognitive (Thinking) Signals of Distress

Intrusive thoughts	Preoccupation with the same thoughts
Unable to find the right words	Disorganized thoughts
Trouble remembering things	Fuzzy or foggy thinking
Mind goes blank	Thoughts seem unclear
Trouble making decisions	Belittling oneself
Trouble concentrating	Preoccupation with one's health
More easily distracted	Ruminating about real or imagined slights

TABLE 5.3. Behavioral Signals of Distress

Constant arguments
Difficulty falling/staying
   asleep
Easily frustrated
Increased irritability
Jumpiness
Lack of patience
More critical
More sarcastic or
   insulting
Nightmares
Pacing
Picking on other people
Quick mood changes
Rushing around
Staying away from other
   people
Constantly talking

Decreased grooming or
   hygiene
Decreased physical
   activities
Difficulty completing
   tasks
Doing things to
   "escape"(sleep, drugs,
   TV)
Increased medical
   appointments
Increased physical
   activities
Not wanting to talk to
   people
Sleeping more than usual
Smoking many cigarettes

Trouble reading and
   watching TV or
   movies
Trouble sitting still
Using more alcohol or
   drugs than usual
Avoiding social
   gatherings
Eating more
Flying off the handle
Impulsive, spur-of-the-
   moment actions
Irrational actions
Missing appointments
Procrastination
Slow recovery from a
   stressful event
Stuttering/stumbling
   speech

TABLE 5.4. Physical Signals of Distress

Indigestion
Increased sweating
Wet palms
Headache
Frowning or furrowed facial expression
Clenched jaw
Teeth grinding
Lump in the throat
Dry mouth or throat
Muscle tension or pain in neck or
   shoulders
Clenched fists
Finger tapping
Nail biting
Trembling or twitching
Pounding heart
Palpitations
Twitching

Upset stomach
"Butterflies" in stomach
Knot in stomach
Loss of appetite and weight loss
Backache
Chronic fatigue
Frequent need to urinate
Diarrhea
Decreased sexual drive
Foot jiggling
Toe tapping
Difficulty sitting still
Cold hands or feet
Increased breathing rate
Shallow breathing
Shortness of breath
Feelings of pressure or pain in chest

riences. In time, many patients become sensitive to how their pattern of response changes as stressors intensify or wane. Of primary importance is to select a cue or cues that the patient can most effectively couple to a coping strategy that would serve to down-regulate feelings of distress.

Patient "symptom types" also provide a framework for introducing the concept of subjective cue identification. Amotivated, cognitively *impoverished* patients who disavow being stressed can be encouraged to further elaborate the interpersonal, social-vocational, or recreational circumstances in which they withdraw. (Social withdrawal can be a useful adaptation to an overstimulating environment, as mentioned earlier, provided that this form of coping does not evolve into a persistent, characteristic, and dysfunctional way of accommodation.) Conceptually *disorganized* patients can be supported in their efforts to select and focus on a single cue, preferably one that is most easily linked to an adaptive technique, and to ignore the range of associated cognitive, emotional, behavioral, and physical cues that often contribute to the disorganized patient's indecisiveness. Patients with persistent *positive* symptoms, particularly residual paranoia, present more of a challenge. Here the frequent scanning of cues runs the unwanted risk of promoting increased vigilance and hyperarousal. In these cases, awareness of the elementary *signal value* of a cue is encouraged (i.e., a simple indicator that the patient should pause and consider a technique that might either contain or reduce distressing feelings before they further escalate and assume a life of their own).

Finally, as a general principle, physical signs should not be chosen as the most important indicators of distress among patients that either have a known medical disease or suffer side effects of medication that could account for the discomfort, such as extrapyramidal symptoms. (In some patients, physical signs of distress should alert the clinician to the possibility of an undiagnosed medical condition that is in need of further evaluation.) However, there are exceptions to this principle when stress serves to clearly exacerbate the symptoms of a known physical illness—for example, hyperventilation among patients with respiratory or cardiovascular disease, or back or neck pain among those with degenerative disc problems.

DEEP BREATHING AND SIMPLE RELAXATION

Subjective cue identification is not an end in itself, but rather serves as the vehicle for implementing an adaptive response variably described as "resistance" (Selye, 1974) or "the relaxation response" (Benson, 1975). While evidence of efficacy regarding relaxation techniques among schizophrenia patients had been sparse prior to the PT studies, nonetheless a few trials did provide reason for optimism (e.g., Acosta et al., 1978; Hawkins et al., 1980; Van Hassel et al., 1982). Results among psychiatric patients in general have been encouraging (Rickard, Collier, McCoy, & Christ, 1993). During the PT studies, deep breathing and basic relaxation ultimately became the coping strategies that were most frequently endorsed and successfully integrated by patients. These simple strategies (as well as more developed relaxation techniques described in Chapter 6 for the advanced phase) can trace their origins more to the meditation rituals of Eastern cultures and religions than to science, although clear effects on autonomic nervous system functioning have been widely demonstrated in recent years (see Benson, 1996). We introduced these approaches to patients more for their psychophysiological utility than spiritual growth, although the religious belief system of many patients can often be engaged in a way that appears to enhance utilization and efficacy (Benson, 1996). Benson refers to the process as a "remembered wellness" that capitalizes on the patient's and the therapist's personal belief systems and expectations for health.

Rationale

We generally ignore the metaphysical or transcendental reasoning that supports relaxation as well as mechanisms such as "trance induction" or "self-hypnosis" that have been used to explain various meditative exercises. Rather, we prefer a quite popular and empirically based psychophysiological justification. Countless writers have described the process (see, e.g., Selye, 1974, 1976; Benson, 1996), which we briefly summarize for patients. Stress, it is said, activates the sympathetic nervous system (an integral part of the autonomic nervous system) and evokes the evolutionary survival response of "fight or flight." This response triggers multiple body system effects. Principally mediated through the hypothalamic–pituitary–adrenal (HPA) axis, the fight-or-flight response produces increases in hormonal activity (e.g., cortisol, epinephrine [adrenaline], and norepinephrine [noradrenaline]), their biochemical products, respiratory rate, cardiovascular response (e.g., heart rate, blood flow, and blood pressure), digestion, metabolism, and muscle tone, as well as a decrease in slow brain wave activity. (Increased slow brain wave activity is associated with "tranquility.") In fact, stress has recently been shown to affect the neuroplasticity of the hippocampus, including adverse effects on synaptogenesis, reorganization of dendritic structures, and even neurogenesis (McEwen, 2000). Fortunately, there is also a *compensatory* nervous system, the parasympathetic nervous system, that serves to "break" this cascade of organ system reactions. But for those who live with persistent stressors or whose alarm system seems not so easily turned off (a popular explanation offered for the pathophysiology of depression), an array of strategies are available to assist the parasympathetic nervous system in its normalizing functions. Deep breathing and simple relaxation can be the first line of defense, strategies that often serve to underscore the importance of subjective cue identification as well.

Deep Breathing and the Relaxation Response

The *deep breathing technique* is first acquired through didactic instruction that occurs in a neutral (nonstressful) PT session. Once the technique is acquired, early applications are frequently made during PT sessions that "scan" for subjective cues which in turn appear distressing to the patient during the session itself. Ultimately, the intent is to apply deep breathing spontaneously, first when the patient is *alone* and troubled by internally generated distress, and later *with others* in a potentially arousing encounter.

Deep breathing essentially consists of inhaling through the nostrils for approximately 4 seconds, filling the lungs to capacity (and silently counting "in" if preferred), holding one's breath for 2 seconds, and then exhaling slowly for 4 seconds (silently counting "out" if that helps). After pausing for a few seconds, the practice is repeated two additional times. A recent modification that we now apply (Kabat-Zinn, 1990) in our ongoing study includes an instruction that the patient place a hand over his or her belly as a way to reinforce the need to breathe from the diaphragm and to develop a deeper awareness of the *breathing act* itself. It is assumed that both the focus on breathing that serves to distract patients from their distressing cues and the enhanced regulation of parasympathetic functioning work collaboratively to induce a state of relaxation.

Once patients can perform a series of three diaphragmatic breaths during a session, they are asked to practice the routine at home each day for a few minutes in conditions where they are not feeling highly aroused or anxious. Problems that arise in the homework exercises involving deep breathing are identified and addressed in subsequent sessions. Patients continue practicing this breathing technique with therapist coaching for several sessions before the technique is applied in a mild or moderately distressing circumstance. As with all adaptive strategies taught in the intermediate phase, the context in which the technique is applied should initially be minimally distressing to the patient and one that offers the best chance for success. After repeated practice, the clinician should encourage the patient to use diaphragmatic breathing while standing and walking as well as sitting. The process is rehearsed until it becomes as automatic as the identification of distressing cues themselves; it is implemented until the procedure demonstrably leads to a reduction in arousal and a corresponding increase in feelings of calm. Patients are encouraged to monitor their progress by recording their pre- and postbreathing subjective state on a simple linear scale of 1–10, with 1 representing a rarely achievable "perfect" feeling of calm and 10 representing a maximum level of perceived distress. A gradual reduction in numerical ratings serves to reinforce the value of deep breathing. Homework assignments in this phase typically focus on recurrent sources of minor stress, either internally or externally generated.

While the *relaxation response* (Benson, 1974, 1996) is not as easily implemented during actual interpersonal conflicts, some patients also choose to employ it when alone and dealing with internally generated distress. Again, PT provides a choice of procedures designed to gain control, and patients will often select one (or more) procedures that are most acceptable and readily applied. The technique essentially resolves to the selection of a personally meaningful *word* or *phrase* (or repetitive *activity*) that can be as neutral as the word "calm" or as personally relevant as a religious prayer or invocation (e.g., "The Lord Is My Shepherd" or "Our Father Who Art in Heaven"). The selection of a simple word or phrase is once again designed to help patients *refocus* their awareness on something other than their feelings of distress, that is, "giving the brain a time out," as described by Benson (1996). The second step in the process is to *passively disregard* intrusive thoughts, neither entering a self-talk dialogue about the process nor consciously monitoring one's success or failure. The analogy used is akin to simply "staring at a blank wall" while repeating the meaningful word or phrase. For patients who choose the relaxation response, they are encouraged to use the exercise for 5–10 minutes once or twice each day, if possible, and to integrate the relaxation response with deep breathing. The recommended environment in which to practice these exercises is one that is both quiet and allows the patient to assume a comfortable position.

INTERMEDIATE SOCIAL SKILLS

Preparing patients to gain control over the subjective cues of distress through cue identification, deep breathing, and relaxation are essential components of PT. However, their efficacy can be clearly limited in the absence of self-initiated behaviors designed to actively reduce the frequency and/or intensity of the stressors themselves. Some external stressors arise independent of interpersonal relationships per se, such as health or financial concerns that can often be negotiated with therapist or agency assistance. But most others represent *interpersonal* sources of stress found in the work, social, recreational, and family environments, both immediate and extended (Morley, 1998). With intermediate social skills training, the elementary approaches of the basic phase (avoidance and prosocial responses) are expanded to include *social perception* skills and a refined ability to assert oneself as ways to decrease potentially distressing interactions. The social skills of this phase are introduced with the intent of applying them initially in the least conflicted and minimally stressful context. With success, they can ultimately be applied more broadly to avoid or reduce confrontations and disruptions in interpersonal relationships, particularly during advanced phase training. For patients whose primary skill deficits remain visible and disabling, the intermediate phase social skills can be taught while reinforcing and polishing such paralinguistic behaviors as eye contact, the labeling and pacing of speech, and voice tone and quality. Throughout intermediate phase skills training, the clinician will, depending upon the patient's needs and preferences, routinely use repetitive modeling, rehearsal, role-play, and feedback, particularly in situations where the patient appears apprehensive or uncertain as to how to proceed.

Social Perception Training

Social perception is introduced as a skill that is not only needed to initiate but also to maintain relationships at home, with friends, at play, or at work. Much of our social perception training was influenced by the work of Burns (1980). The goals of social perception training are to enable patients to attend to the interpersonal and often nonverbal cues that characterize relationships, to accurately and wisely interpret these cues, and to ultimately craft an appropriate response. Fundamental to effective social perception is the ability to correctly take the "emotional temperature" of the speaker. A failure to do so can significantly increase the potential for a negative and distressing exchange. For example, most patients can recall an experience when they made a simple request of a person who at the time was feeling irritated or frustrated, only to have the conversation result in an argument if not a rude rejection. Had they been able to "read" these emotional cues beforehand, patients might have chosen to "time" their request differently.

We introduce the concept of social perception training by asking the patient to evaluate various individuals in their life with whom they have (or *want* to have) regular contact. The outline for this procedure (which also serves as a handout for patients) is described in Table 5.5. With this schedule, the patient and clinician can carefully evaluate the behavior of a specific individual, seeking overt as well as subtle cues that might serve to indicate the other person's mood and "approachability." Again, the clinician should direct these initial evaluations to the individual(s) with whom the patient is least conflicted and most likely to successfully apply social perception skills. Much like the process of evaluating one's own *subjective* cues, a "scan" is made of the "*objective* cues that might characterize the speaker's emotional state such as anger, frustration, sadness, anxiety, sensitivity, on the one hand, or humor, kindliness, and euthymia, on the other. Other behaviors are also scanned, such as the tone and volume of the speaker's voice, his or her facial expression and gestures, as well as the content of speech—all behavioral cues that might provide an indication of the speaker's underlying emotional state. As with subjective cue identification and relaxation, "emotional temperature taking" also becomes an important homework assignment. Depending upon the intensity and frequency of conflict, the interactions of the patient with the identified individual will often be revisited during subsequent PT sessions, as the contexts that require appraisal and the timing of interactions change.

Closely associated with successful temperature taking is the obvious need to more effectively *listen* to the speaker. Indicating that one is really attentive to the speaker while engaging in conversation is a skill that is not only lost among many patients but also seems deficient at times among a majority of nonpatients. Patients are encouraged to maintain appropriate (but not constant) eye contact while nodding occasionally and to make verbal acknowledgments of the content periodically. The use of clarifying questions and associated comments can also serve this purpose. The value of *empathic listening* is regularly reinforced by the clinician, since it shows the speaker that the patient has indeed heard him or her. Further, it allows the clinician to determine whether the patient has understood the message correctly and conveyed a sense of sincere interest in the speaker's concerns. Empathic listening will best serve the patient by significantly lower-

TABLE 5.5. Taking a Person's Emotional Temperature (Handout)

In order to decrease your likelihood of being stressed and feeling overwhelmed, you might find it helpful to learn how and when to avoid "emotional explosions" by reviewing the following questions:

1. Who has been a "hot" person for you to deal with recently? _____

2. Typically, what gets him or her "burning"? _____

3. What does he or she *do* (that you see and hear) that appears to be "hot"? _____
   _____
   _____
   _____

4. When is the "wrong time" to try and talk to this person about something? _____
   _____
   _____
   _____

5. What happens when this person is "hot" (angry) and you try or want to:
   Just *talk* with him or her? _____
   Disagree with him or her? _____
   Criticize him or her? _____
   Make a *request*? _____

6. When do you know that this person is in a *good* mood? _____
   _____
   _____

7. What happens when the person is "cool" (e.g., approachable), and what is the best way to talk at that time? _____
   _____

8. What can you do to help this person get into a good mood? _____
   _____
   _____

ing the intensity of a potentially negative response from the speaker. At the most elementary level, the patient can simply "parrot" the speaker's statement of mood ("Oh, you feel exhausted today"), or the patient might improve the response somewhat by reflecting the speaker's affect by using different words ("It must be hard to get through the day when you feel so worn out"). However, we would definitely not want the patient to routinely restate the speaker's otherwise coherent ideas, since this interactional style can be annoying, if not patronizing and alienating (see Albrecht, 1979).

Positive Engagement

Correct perception and attentive listening are for naught, however, unless these skills serve to facilitate meaningful and rewarding interactions and to avoid or contain negative ones. Again, from Burns (1980) as well as McKay et al. (1981) and from the clearly successful applications of self-instruction among schizophrenia patients demonstrated by Meichenbaum and Cameron (1973, 1974), patients are taught a sequence of *self-instructions* when approaching individuals whose emotional temperature appears to be somewhat "hot." The sequence is repeated and modeled until it is fairly well incorporated into the repertoire of the patient's verbal skills. The sequence includes the following questions (the replies to which should provide a quick summation of the patient's social perception):

1. "What is this person doing? How is he or she feeling or behaving?"
2. "How am I feeling at the moment about what this person is saying or doing?"
3. "What is it that I need to do here? My choices include (a) *asking* questions to learn more about what the other person is trying to communicate; (b) *show* that I am listening in some way; (c) *say* that I am listening in some way; (d) *say* what I see going on and how I feel about it; (e) *express* my preference about how I would like things to be; (f) be prepared to *repeat* my message a few times; (g) *set limits* on the extent of a negative response ('I can't talk with you now if you continue to ignore me'), and (h) be ready to *leave* for a while, if necessary, until the person cools down."
4. "What can I say to accomplish my goal?"
5. "How do I say it [with what emotions]?"

The sequence not only increases the patient's perception and listening skills but serves to lay the groundwork for the development of conflict resolution and criticism management that will be introduced during the advanced phase of PT for those situations that are highly conflicted (see Chapter 6). Again, this form of training relies heavily on the repetitive use of modeling, rehearsal, feedback, and homework assignments.

Negative Assertion

Negative assertion, or speaking up appropriately for one's own rights, can be a formidable but necessary barrier to overcome if personal relationships are to be maintained over time. While many patients will, in the course of social perception training, come to appreciate that others often feel differently than they do and that such differences are often legitimate and most often deserving of respect, nevertheless patients continue to have the "right" to say no, to change their mind, to hold their own opinions, to protect their own feelings and personal integrity, and to make mistakes (providing there is some acknowledgment of responsibility). But there is a clear difference between appropriate negative assertion in defense of one's rights and the expression of an opinion that appears to be an attacking, aggressive action.

Not infrequently, patients will be aware that an aggressive *response* style can be provocative if it includes name calling, "demanding" in a loud voice, using threats, sarcasm, or criticism, or the inclination toward generalized negative attributions ("always" and "never"). Such a style can be as great or a greater source of stress that is within the patient's control as any independent life event that is beyond the patient's control. Albrecht (1979) has elaborated in detail the components of a stress-generating communication style that the clinician might profitably review, particularly when working with patients who are less overtly aggressive but nonetheless somewhat offensive. Some of these features include constant complaining, failing to negotiate, interrupting the speaker or otherwise monopolizing the conversation, constantly seeking approval, appearing frustrated, diverting conversations before the speaker is finished, using insincere flattery, referring constantly to oneself and one's needs, and even making the speaker feel guilty. We shall comment below on the remarkable similarity between such styles and the social cognitive deficits that might reflect the prepubertal perspective taking and context appraisal deficits of schizophrenia now being targeted in our study of cognitive-enhancement therapy (Hogarty & Flesher, 1999a, 1999b).

A more facilitative style would include the use of "I" statements ("I think" and "I feel"), often made with a calm but firm voice, using moderate affect and appropriate voice tone. Such a style, it should be emphasized, will likely secure the patient's goals far more effectively than a hostile or overly aggressive response. The latter is typically characterized by the use of the pronoun "you" rather than "I" and invariably includes the provocative qualifiers "should," "must," or "ought," rather than a simple

"could." "You *should* do . . . " typically proves to be far less effective in negotiating than the statement "I feel that you could. . . . " In short, close attention to the patient's self-described interpersonal interactions can reveal
whether there is a propensity toward the use of "you," "should," and
"must" (or hostile generalizations), rather than more complimentary
speech. In time, most patients come to appreciate that "I" and "could"
messages will effectively communicate their own preferences, allow for refusal, and better encourage responses from others that alter their behavior.
In the process, the frequency and intensity of stressors will often be decreased.

As mentioned above, ongoing efforts by us to enhance social cognition have obvious relevance to the communication difficulties of many patients. While not used during the formal tests of PT, these observations
and suggestions might prove useful when facilitating relationship formation and maintenance in future applications of PT. Recent work, for example, has underscored the propensity of many schizophrenia patients to
engage in *efficient* speech (as opposed to *polite* speech) that can appear to
the listener as insensitive, blunt, or offensive (Brown, 1996). Not that efficient speech is necessarily "impolite"; rather, it tends to convey only the
basic conceptual elements of a conversation without the requisite contextual details or "softness" that negative assertion, in particular, requires.
For example, when faced with the dilemma of commenting on a proud
chef's new creation that was in obvious need of additional seasoning,
schizophrenia patients most often correctly yet *efficiently* responded, "It
needs salt" (Brown, 1996). *Polite* speech, on the other hand, would be
used to maintain the self-esteem, value and emotional state of the listener:
"Your soup was delicious, very different, and among the best I have ever
tasted. I'll bet it would be truly unique if it had just a bit more salt."
Clearly the latter discourse is "inefficient" in terms of the number of
words used, but remains sufficiently "polite" so as to maintain the relationship and further the opportunity for continued dialogue.

Closely associated with these subtle forms of social deviance (which
have often tended to desocialize patients and distance them from rewarding relationships), is the pervasive difficulty that many patients share regarding a self-perceived inability to *initiate* conversations that might lead
to the formation of desired relationships. Again, Albrecht (1979) provides a useful discussion of communication styles that might facilitate the
initiation (and maintenance) of such relationships. (In our current work,
we focus first on developing a *perspective-taking* competency, as well as the
ability to "read" the informal abstract rules of conduct that govern specific

social contexts, i.e., *context appraisal* prior to the refinement of conversational styles.) But in the PT exercise designed to improve communication styles and to lessen the possibility of interpersonal stressors, Albrecht's suggestions should prove useful. Beyond empathic listening, for example, relationship formation often begins with sharing a bit of information about oneself, including one's values, opinions, and experience. In turn, expressing interest and respect for the other person's values and opinions serves the cause of reciprocity. Being positive and constructive, if one's opinion is sought, is equally facilitative. Verbal and more often nonverbal indicators of acceptance clearly serve to bond a friendship. Indications of equality in the relationship, sincere and appropriate compliments, statements of agreement when possible, the safeguarding of confidences, and openness and honesty are obvious facilitators of relationship maintenance that are too often ignored or deemphasized by patients. Finally, good humor can be the glue that holds a relationship, especially in times of adversity.

We end the discussion of intermediate phase strategies with a reminder that progress is often very slow for many patients, a reality that likely kept a number of patients from graduating to the advanced phase during the time that was available for study. The clinician should not be discouraged with temporary setbacks or with the need to suspend advancement when pressing life problems arise. Time often needs to be spent revisiting basic phase strategies and facilitating their greater integration with acquired intermediate techniques before moving forward. Small steps do lead to greater recovery in the long term, and often this reality provides considerable comfort for the patient and clinician during the slow process needed to increase functioning.

TRANSITION FROM THE INTERMEDIATE TO THE ADVANCED PHASE

We hope we have enabled the reader to gain a greater appreciation of how the components of PT are blended within and between phases and how they logically ebb or flow, depending on the clinical state and strengths of the individual patient. Again, while the therapeutic agenda of the intermediate phase is comprehensive, more than half of our study patients successfully acquired the knowledge and strategies of this phase. Even those who "failed to graduate" to the advanced phase gave evidence of partial mastery, and according to study results realized some greater degree of interpersonal effectiveness and life satisfaction. Those who moved to the advanced phase met the following criteria that once again should be viewed as a set of guiding principles rather than a rigid formula for progression. In the last analysis, it is the clinician's judgment as to whether or not the clinical state of the patient would allow the safe application of advanced phase techniques, once the latter have been reviewed. Overall, patients should be considered ready for the advanced phase of PT if they have satisfied the following criteria:

1. The patient continues to meet criteria that governed entrance into the intermediate phase itself.
2. The patient has a basic understanding of the more common disabilities of schizophrenia (without necessarily subscribing to them), as well as the contribution of stress to a vulnerable person and its association with a possible progression of symptoms.
3. The patient is able to correctly identify or understand at least one distressing feeling and one physical, affective, behavioral, or cognitive (cue) analogue.
4. The patient provides evidence of accurately evaluating (social perception) the volatility of a potentially conflicted situation.
5. The patient demonstrates effective listening skills.
6. The patient gives evidence of the ability to appropriately express preferences, requests, and dislikes as well as to refuse unreasonable requests (assertiveness).
7. The patient demonstrates a degree of stress reduction below baseline, using diaphragmatic breathing or basic relaxation techniques.

As with the basic phase components, the Process Rating Scale (Appendix B) provides micromeasures of these intermediate phase components for monitoring purposes and the determination of advanced phase eligibility.

CHAPTER SIX

The Advanced Phase

Think what life might be for patients who are about to enter the advanced phase of PT. Symptoms are in reasonable remission, and knowledge of their illness has likely increased. Basic strategies for identifying personal prodromes and subjective cues of distress have been woven into a protective cocoon of coping and adaptation, at least one that exists within the more predictable environments of home and clinic. Perhaps a growing sense of self-confidence and optimism has emerged. But now comes the expectation or suggestion of reentry into a fuller community life, and with it an all-too-common feeling of foreboding: "Am I resuming the journey toward a better life, or will this be another invitation to relapse?"

Individuals differ greatly in their approach to this transition, a difference that is often influenced by broad diversity in premorbid competencies, in residual symptoms and deficits, in personality, and in the available support of friends, family, and the health system. On the one hand, some are aware that the coping strategies learned in predictable environments might not be so easily applied in the unpredictable social contexts to which they are drawn. Problems with stamina and motivation and with concentration and memory, as well as fears of rejection and failure, can often be found lurking beneath the surface of stability. Many such patients, often for the first time, will express concerns of a most elementary nature that belie their apparent recovery: anxiety about meeting a new person; how to initiate a conversation, or fears concerning participation in formal or informal gatherings that are unfamiliar. Pressed to elaborate upon these concerns, patients will often indicate an absence of information as to what the appropriate rules or norms of conduct might be in these varied social circumstances. (This latter concern, one of correct *social context appraisal*, is a central focus of our newer cognitive-enhancement therapy approach. However, the seeds of context appraisal were planted in the social perception and assertiveness exercises of the intermediate phase, and patients can be reminded of these previous sessions.) On the other hand, there are patients who revel in a newly found relief from symptoms and in their perceived sense of control and mastery. At times they appear to be "chomping at the bit" to make up for the time lost to illness. Between these extremes are other patients who, no matter how fearful or confident they might be, are painfully aware that the time is running out for continuing residence with family. Rumination about their own long-term survival renders them at least reluctant participants in the transition to advanced phase strategies.

Symptom remission, together with the acquisition of a personal knowledge of vulnerabilities and coping strategies, does not mean that patients have mastered the control of distress and affect dysregulation. To some degree, an emotional upheaval will accompany each new venture into the diverse community contexts of extended family, new or former acquaintances, and academic or vocational pursuits. A more individualized and autonomous application of acquired skills will be necessary, as well as skill in using the sophisticated techniques that will be needed to manage the unpredictable and likely more stressful (and rewarding) challenges of community life. It is for this reason that we established the eligibility criteria needed for entry into this more demanding phase of treatment. These criteria offer assurances that the patient has at least acquired some basic prerequisites upon which advanced phase training can be built. For some who enter the advanced phase still burdened with residual attention and memory deficits, reduced mental stamina, lingering cognitive disorganization, or the amotivation of persistent negative symptoms, their quality of life can nevertheless be improved and the risk of relapse further reduced. Even though competitive employment, independent living, and a rich social life might remain distant goals, the hierarchical steps that involve gradual exposure to community life can keep these objectives in clear view. Along the way, periods of consolidation might be required, but a slow and steady progression along the path to recovery will characterize the process of the advanced phase for all participants, including the more disabled.

The goals of the advanced phase seek to affect a smooth transition from home to community by making the patient's existing adaptive skills more *portable*. Further, the advanced phase attempts to enhance the quality of the patient's social and vocational life through the acquisition and application of coping strategies that are more relevant to the obstacles that are frequently associated with achieving a satisfying community life. Having said that, we need to strongly emphasize once again that the overarching principle of the earlier phases remains constant in the advanced phase as well, namely, to *achieve and maintain clinical stability and avoid decompensation!* It was, after all, the phenomenon of late relapse that fueled the development of PT. If, in the process of achieving the goals of stabilization and relapse avoidance, the patient moves toward vocational success and emancipation, then all well and good. (As described in Chapter 2, such outcomes are indeed possible in that many patients did find employment in the open labor market and a quarter of patients surpassed their own best level of prior functioning.) But these gains clearly remain secondary to the primary objectives of stabilization maintenance and relapse prevention.

This chapter describes how the following components will contribute to the attainment of advanced phase goals:

- *Psychoeducation* will move from more generic information regarding schizophrenia and its associated disabilities to a greater specification of the patients' own vulnerabilities and residual deficits that might impact upon day-to-day ventures outside the home.
- *Internal coping* will encourage autonomous choices in the identification of relevant cues and the selection of available coping strategies. Internal coping will further expand to foster an appreciation of the reciprocity between one's own subjective distress and behavior and the response of others.
- *Progressive relaxation and imagery* will be introduced as the stabilizing strategies that link with internal coping and which can be used to prepare for entry into more stressful and less predictable community settings.
- *Criticism management and conflict resolution* are offered in response to the better-established sources of symptom exacerbation among patients.
- *Social and vocational issues* that might compromise recovery will be described. Successful negotiation of these concerns will clearly serve to facilitate the accomplishments that can be achieved by many PT recipients.

Before describing the details of the advanced phase, we need to acknowledge a reality that might confound application of PT in routine practice. Clearly, patients are not so tidy in their progression of skill acquisition or in the degree to which positive, negative, and affective symptoms remit as our Phase eligibility criteria imply. Many patients, for example, will have resumed social and vocational roles in the community independent of the best judgment of the therapist and without meeting each of the suggested eligibility guidelines. In these instances, the therapist will certainly want to review the strategies and process of the advanced phase, and then select those practice principles that might be relevant for patients who have chosen to follow their own path. If an unfortunate exacerbation arises, more often than not it has been our experience that the patient will become more willing to reenter PT at an earlier-mastered phase. Citing the value of advanced phase entry criteria will often make the next attempt at community transition more successful.

The length of the advanced phase will again depend on the individual patients. Those who were symptomatically stable at admission will likely begin the advanced phase within the first year of PT. For those recovering from a recent episode, few will reach the advanced phase before 12 months. Time in this phase will typically extend from 9 to 18 months.

PSYCHOEDUCATION

In the advanced phase, we have found that psychoeducation is best reserved to the circumstances that impact upon the patient's pursuit of highly personal goals, rather than to be provided in a workshop format. Opportunities to present psychoeducation content typically occur in each advanced phase session. The frequent need to review the concepts of individual vulnerability and of residual cognitive or affective deficits and disabilities will arise when orchestrating the timing of social and vocational initiatives. As mentioned above, this is particularly true for the patient who is motivated to get on with life as quickly as possible. All too often, however, the seduction of symptom remission, as well as the patient's beginning mastery of basic and intermediate coping skills, will also serve to increase family and therapist expectations for performance. This has been true whether or not the patient was eager to proceed with life or was hesitant due to concerns about motivation, stamina, and social engagement.

Central to the advanced phase of psychoeducation is the paradoxical debate about the need for continuing medication that renewed health and confidence often precipitate. In our earlier studies of family psychoeducation and social skills training, and again in the PT studies themselves, the issue of medication compliance sometimes became a contest of wills between the therapist and the patient, particularly among those patients whose clinical state and adjustment were clearly above average during the second year of treatment. In other cases, patients who continued to struggle with amotivation, lethargy, or mental fatigue would often attribute these performance obstacles to medication side effects, with a subsequent conclusion that medication discontinuation was the solution. As mentioned earlier, relapse does not often occur immediately following medication discontinuation; not only is the link missed at times, but the decision to cease medication can be reinforced if relief from residual side effects leads to the patient's "feeling better." For others, medication remains a reminder of the illness and operates against the desire for normalcy. In these cases, a review of schizophrenia pathophysiology, including the important mechanisms of drug action and the notion of a biochemical "imbalance," have proven to be helpful. In more resistant patients, the concept of "harm reduction" can be raised through the sensitive but clear presentation of relapse risk that is associated with medication noncompliance. This risk can be described both in general terms and as a specific "percentage" that is based on the individual patient's own psychiatric history (see Hogarty & Ulrich, 1998, and Chapter 1). Not infrequently, late concerns about medication compliance reveal unresolved issues surrounding denial or adjustment to disability that can be profitably revisited. Once again, the obvious needs to be repeated: the gains achieved will be quickly reversed if the patient suffers a medication-compliance-related relapse. For those patients who do not trust their own ability to maintain an oral medication regimen, the option of fluphenazine or haloperidol decanoate could be introduced as either a primary or supplemental route of administration. (Depot preparations of selected atypical antipsychotic medications are also in preparation at the time of this writing.)

Specific Prodromes

Familiarity with the patient, especially his or her psychiatric history, and the experience gained in scanning for cues of subjective distress should have narrowed the therapist's search for relevant prodromal indicators to a highly individualized set of signs and symptoms. As described earlier, for one patient an increase in suspiciousness or ideas of reference might be paramount, while for another a tendency toward increased isolation might herald a new episode. The stress associated with community integration will often serve to accelerate both the speed of onset and the intensity of subtle cues that had been identified during the earlier protective PT sessions that scanned for subjective distress. The patient can be reassured that prior work on identifying his or her *pattern* of subjective cues will now pay off. A predictability in the emergence and progression of cues that might lead to relapse has been established, and strategies are available to the patient (and reinforced by the therapist) that will disrupt the process of symptom progression. This level of reassurance is crucial for patients who are in the least hesitant or fearful about resuming a fuller life because of the risk of another decompensation.

Drugs and Alcohol

Wider involvement in the community too often means greater opportunities for misusing substances, particularly alcohol and marijuana. Among our own patients, alcohol has typically been the preferred substance of misuse, an observation that has strong support in the literature (Mueser et al., 2000). Patients should again be reminded that the use of alcohol or street drugs among individuals who suffer schizophrenia has a well-documented history of contributing to symptom exacerbation as well as to associated problems with financial security, housing, and the maintenance of valued relationships (Drake & Brunette, 1998). Few patients, according to Drake and Mueser (2000), are able to use these substances even at a moderate level of consumption without encountering serious problems. Nor can they apparently return to a controlled use of alcohol or drugs following a period of serious misuse. Paradoxically, few of the severely mentally ill will develop physical signs of abuse and dependence, precisely because they will rarely achieve this level of use without experiencing a psychotic decompensation. As mentioned earlier, a *hypersensitivity* appears to account for this phenomenon (Drake & Mueser, 2000). Patients should be reminded that their beginning competence in positive and negative assertion acquired earlier will serve as ways to counteract peer pressure to misuse substances. Discussions of these pressures and the rehearsal of assertive strategies should be engaged in as needed. Patients can also be reassured that basic, intermediate, and advanced phase skills should further lessen the problem of personal discomfort surrounding social relationships that might precipitate substance misuse.

While PT did have some beneficial effects on an (unrepresentative) sample of substance-misusing patients, the evidence of efficacy regarding the treatment of comorbidity in schizophrenia, overall, is quite disappointing, at least the evidence derived from randomized clinical trials (Drake, Mercer-McFadden, Mueser, McHugo, & Bond, 1998; Harvassy, Shopshire, & Quigley, 2000). Many authorities feel that motivation toward abstinence must *precede* the successful treatment of substance misuse in schizophrenia and that interventions should be staged to each level of motivation (e.g., Mueser, Drake, & Noordsy, 1998; Ziedonis & Trudeau, 1997; Bellack & DiClemente, 1999). This approach, however, suggests that treatment obstacles might exist for the schizophrenia patient who is unmotivated to discontinue substance misuse. Comprehensive psychosocial treatment for the majority who appeared grounded in the "precontemplation" phase of self-motivated abstinence, for example, might be compromised. Clearly, the staged approach makes sense for nonmentally ill, primary substance abusers (Miller & Rollnick, 2002), but might be less necessary for substance-misusing schizophrenia patients. By definition, comorbid patients have at least engaged with the mental health system for treatment of their schizophrenia. Should the patient's schizophrenia treatment itself be modified to address the shared vulnerabilities that underlie schizophrenia exacerbation and substance misuse, perhaps many of the motivational stages and their related interventions could better become integrated and outcomes improved.

While PT was not originally designed as an intervention for substance misuse, preliminary results among an admittedly unrepresentative subsample of substance-misusing patients did show unexpected good outcomes (see Chapter 2). We feel that this success might have resulted from the simple fact that the pathoetiologies of schizophrenia relapse and substance misuse are very similar. As described by Blanchard, Brown, Horan, and Sherwood (2000), they include vulnerability, stress, affect dysregulation, and poor coping as the precursors to both relapse and substance misuse. What PT has lacked in its development is consideration of the personality or *temperament* dimensions that might dispose schizophrenia patients to substance misuse, namely, *negative affectivity* and/or *disinhibition/impulsivity* (Blanchard et al., 2000). The affect regulation techniques of PT clearly encourage coping strategies other than substance misuse, and the clinician might want to review the temperament characteristics of substance-misusing schizophrenia patients as described by Blanchard et al. (2000) as the basis for selectively emphasizing various PT strategies for these patients (e.g., the cues of dysphoria, pessimism, and demoralization as the precursors to symptom exacerbation *or* substance misuse). Our studies of PT that attempted to regulate affect and enhance coping strategies and self-esteem have indicated that positive effects on substance misuse among many patients do follow the application of existing PT strategies, even in the absence of a preintervention motivation toward abstinence.

Coping Strategies

Finally, in keeping with the format of the intermediate phase, psychoeducation should include a comment on the yet-to-be-acquired skills of the advanced phase such as the use of progressive relaxation, imagery, criticism management, and conflict resolution, including rationales for their use. Issues that facilitate or obstruct a successful resumption of social and vocational roles (discussed below) can be summarized. This personal education can be enriched by a review of the obstacles and the successes that were associated with previous occupational and social roles that the patient held in the community. Subjective responses to these prior experiences will be a focus of other advanced phase techniques.

INTERNAL COPING

It is one thing for patients to appreciate the cues of distress and their signal value for applying coping strategies that might significantly lower personal discomfort. It is quite another for them to determine the relative efficacy of these techniques in novel contexts that often arise spontaneously, and to acquire a facile way for their implementation in day to day life. More importantly, achieving a level of stress relief without some appreciation of how one's feelings and subsequent behavior affect others could lead to the unhappy situation of having done little more than to have crafted a "relaxed incompetent", in the words of Bandura (1969). In the advanced phase, internal coping attempts to raise awareness of subjective state and skill implementation to a level of maximum efficiency and social competence that is appropriate to a patient's existing strengths and liabilities. In some ways, this process reflects elements of S. Semrad's analytically oriented component (cited in Fenton, 2000) wherein the therapist assists the patient in forming a greater awareness of helpful and unhelpful coping strategies through the review of past experiences and painful affects. This phase of internal coping is also as close as PT is likely to come to the "insight-oriented task" of Fenton's (2000) flexible psychotherapy for schizophrenia, that is, to "improve the capacity for intimacy and productivity" (p. 65). In our experience, formal attempts at insight develop-ment are reserved to a subsample of patients who qualify for advanced phase treatment.

Selecting Cues and Strategies

A useful introduction to the topic of selecting subjective cues and strate-gies is the analogy of the "community as a laboratory," a place where one can monitor subjective state and test coping strategies. The patient and therapist will be like sleuths that explore past and present circumstances that served to dysregulate the patient or cause emotional suffering. What were previous jobs like? How did the patient relate to a supervisor or coworkers? Did difficulties arise around accepting "orders," following in-structions, or maintaining job stamina and a routine? Did problems in at-tention and concentration, or working memory, interfere with the perfor-mance of expected tasks? Were coworkers supportive or critical? What were the most uncomfortable circumstances encountered when relating to coworkers: cooperating on a task, negotiating a difference of opinion, or initiating and maintaining "small talk"? In social relationships, did con-flicts arise around inequality in the relationship, submission to the prefer-ence of others, failures to compromise or negotiate, perceived pressure from family or peers to conform to expectations, and difficulties in accept-ing and responding to criticism, or even in accommodating positive sug-gestions? The review of past encounters in the community can provide a more clear focus on the patient's affective state and the associated cogni-tive, physical, and behavioral cues of distress encountered during these experiences. (The process of review, rehearsal, and in vivo social and voca-tional simulations is discussed below in greater depth.) Next, a relation-ship can be delineated between these prior responses and the subjective cues that had been identified in earlier PT sessions. Is there a pattern of re-sponse, or do some subjective cues tend to arise only on the job, or only with an authority figure, or with a certain friend or family member? The intent here is not to overly sensitize the patient to every nuance of feeling and behavior experienced during an interpersonal encounter, but rather to erect a broad experiential stage for the evaluation of the social and voca-tional contexts in which the patient had typically felt uncomfortable or perplexed.

This patchwork of responses to past vocational and social experiences can be organized around a few selected probes. The question "What worked for you?" can provide the opportunity to reexamine and reinforce the patient's own useful *autoprotective* strategies. One patient, for example, who feared conversations with strangers during the bus ride to an earlier job had taken to using a headset and music, together with a comic book, as ways to lessen the feelings of disorganization as well as the fear of uninvited conversation. Similarly the query "What didn't work?" can lead to a better appraisal of the need for a new strategy. More importantly, the review of past encounters allows the patient to independently begin to choose among the acquired coping strategies of the earlier phases. The question "Given what you know now, is there anything that you would do differently if faced with the same situation?" will often open the door to a reexamination of those adaptive strategies that had been successfully applied in the less stressful situations (and at the earliest point of feeling distressed) of the earlier PT phases. In short, given the strategies already acquired (and those about to be learned), the patient can become increasingly self-directed in the choice of options that might be more effective than prior forms of coping in potentially stressful situations. For patients who found them useful in earlier phases, modeling, role-play, and the rehearsal of new or potentially troublesome encounters could continue.

The metacommunication of internal coping in this phase is to encourage an *anticipatory* stance toward those situations that might likely be distressing, as well as a bit of foresightful planning as to which strategy might be usefully employed. As the treatment plan (the patient's goals) is slowly implemented in the areas of vocational training and placement as well as excursions into family and nonkinship social networks, the "scanning" done at the start of a PT session should follow a predictable routine: (1) the success or failure of recent transitional experiences, (2) the associated feelings of personal comfort or distress, and (3) the nature and outcome of the adaptive strategies that were chosen. Throughout these reviews, the therapist will want to reinforce the successes made and to encourage an increasingly autonomous selection of coping options in situations that had not been successfully negotiated. The goal for the patient is better management of the relationship between his or her internal affective state and the potential provocation from a specific environmental context.

Behavioral Reciprocity

The process of internal coping to this point has been primarily patient centered since it relied on the identification of subjective cues, the events that trigger them, and attempts to abort an escalation of symptoms. Internal coping now moves to consider the effects of the patient's subjective state and coping behaviors on the feeling and behavior of others. The guiding principle for the management of this behavioral reciprocity has been grounded in a rich social work tradition, perhaps beginning with Mary Richmond's *Social Diagnosis* in 1917, but greatly enhanced in the supportive psychotherapy approach described by Florence Hollis in her 1964 classic, *Casework: A Psychosocial Therapy*. Hollis refers to the process of behavioral reciprocity as a "reflective consideration" that occurs in the context of other casework components such as the sustaining supportive relationship, directive action by the clinician (e.g., advice giving and advocacy), and the opportunities for ventilation. The awareness of *one's own* subjective state that had been fostered in previous phases can now facilitate the transition to awareness of *other* people's internal states. Most patients can come to appreciate that others share the same fears, pleasures, needs, and opinions as they do, and are very often just as uncertain as to how to cope and respond.

In PT, reflective consideration involves (1) helping the patient to appreciate that his or her affective, cognitive, and physical state as well as subsequent coping behaviors impact upon the feelings and behaviors of others in a positive or negative way; (2) enhancing the patient's ability to correctly interpret the verbal and nonverbal cues from others; (3) understanding that there will be either undesirable or positive consequences for the patient, including the advancement of the his or her own self-interest; and (4) learning to alter one's coping behavior, if necessary, in a way that sustains acceptance and approval and thus the opportunity for continued positive interaction.

Reflective consideration, as Hollis describes, can exist independent of the insight development and clarification techniques that otherwise characterize more psychoanalytic approaches. It focuses on the realities of the patient's behavior and the available information that supports a reciprocal response from others in the patient's environment. In sociological terms, this reflection can be viewed as an exercise in "perspective taking," namely, the correct identification of the likely feelings, thinking, and response of another person to one's own behavior. A useful probe that illustrates the patient's level of self-awareness is the traditional "if . . . then" self-coaching proposal: "If I say [such and such], then my [friend, relative, coworker] will likely [feel, think, behave] in the following way." For the relatively few patients who are clueless as to the effect of their behavior on others, the clinician can directly describe the effects that have been previously discussed or observed, or ask the patient how he or she might respond if faced with similar behavior from someone else. Hollis suggests the use of rhetorical-like questions that will guide patients to a more correct understanding of the effects of their own behavior on significant others. These queries, which are designed to foster self-awareness and perspective taking, can frequently serve as opportunities to enhance more realistic social and vocational expectations held by the patient. Reflective consideration of the response from others can also counter incorrect appraisals of self worth, "all-or-nothing" polarized thinking, as well as the tendency to catastrophize the consequences of an interpersonal encounter or vocational initiative. For some patients, an absence of insight might be corrected by feedback from the clinician regarding the effects of the patient's behavior, but for others this seeming insight deficiency might often serve as a defense against strong and potentially disabling affects or a perceived assault on self-esteem. In the latter instances, the application of supportive therapy principles described in Chapter 3 can be most helpful.

Failures to correctly interpret feedback from others could, of course, be secondary to the distortions and misinterpretations that accompany residual paranoid thinking, cognitive disorganization, concreteness and rigidity, or deficiencies in the mental stamina needed to actively process information. An autistic-like preoccupation with internal states can also detract from the patient's awareness of others. In these instances, a sensitive restatement of the patient's own account of interpersonal interactions can be helpful, with descriptions of the other person's likely feeling and thinking being clearly but sensitivity articulated by the therapist. Conversely, many patients have difficulty repressing their own inappropriate verbal and nonverbal messages, as is common among disorganized patients who often fail to appropriately self-edit, or whose limbic arousal leads to familiar, trusted, but socially offensive displays of emotion. Training exercises designed to better regulate the limbic–frontal equilibrium that underlies age-appropriate social cognition are currently under development. But basic psychoeducation regarding limbic dominance and affective displays that can become a source of discomfort to others, as well as the consequences of poor impulse control, can be confidently described (see Taylor & Cadet, 1989). When failures to appropriately repress affect lead to irritability or anger in the other person, the techniques of conflict resolution described below can often be helpful.

In extreme cases, the reality of behavior consequences to self and others is clear, as when a patient might move to terminate an intimate relationship or impulsively quit a job. In others, however, the effects of one's affective state (a frown, a clenched jaw, a look of detachment, or irritable tone) might not be so obvious. Annoyance, frustration, and ultimate dis-

tancing by others that precludes opportunities for continui
ary") socialization is often an unwanted consequence. Ag
questioning can lead the patient to a better understanding o
ae, all the better. Otherwise, for those who are less insight
logically minded, a sensitive but simple description will often suffice as indicated above. Finally, it should be emphasized that the use of more
effective and appropriate coping strategies that accompany the process of
internal coping (see below) can serve to circumvent negative affects and
unwanted responses in others, as well as foster the attainment of the patient's own social and vocational goals.

PROGRESSIVE RELAXATION AND IMAGERY

The intent of the advanced phase is to successfully negotiate an increasing
exposure to the "real world" and the gradual assumption or resumption of
roles related to interpersonal, social, and vocational activities. However, as
mentioned above, many patients will continue to be apprehensive or unsure about their ultimate success in applying basic and intermediate phase
coping strategies. After all, the therapist's office, or even carefully selected
encounters in the home, are not the equivalent of life in the community.
Thus, treatment in this phase will attempt to reinforce and strengthen the
less complex techniques of deep breathing and simple relaxation that most
patients should have successfully mastered in the intermediate phase. If
nothing else, the advanced phase exercises will often serve to increase confidence and/or provide a safety net for patients who might falter in their
attempts to achieve more active engagement using coping strategies that
had already been acquired.

The relaxation field has grown dramatically since the inception of PT,
and most bookstores and libraries now stock many detailed and expert
texts that the PT clinician might want to consult. In fact, it is no longer
unusual to find the principles of advanced relaxation and imagery being
taught as components of the clinical core curriculum in many graduate
programs, often techniques that are targeted to mood disorders and the
"worried well." Some useful relaxation tapes include those of Budzynski
(1974) and Sippel, Tubesing, and Halpern (1982), as well as the guided
imagery tapes of Naparstek (1993). When PT was first designed, we relied heavily on the texts of Goldfried and Davison (1976) and Bernstein
and Borkovec (1973). Here, we can provide but a circumscribed overview
of these relaxation techniques together with a statement on the induction
principles that many authorities feel ensure an effective application. We

begin with a caution or two from Schafer (1983) and Selye (1974) to the effect that few of us can master each and every stressful situation successfully. Thus, potentially provocative contexts and issues need to be prioritized and choices made by the patient as to which ones deserve a response. We have, as Selye (1974) reminds us, a finite "deep adaptive capacity" that should not be depleted on nonessential issues or even exhausted on enduring sources of stress. Better to change the venue to aspects of relationships and roles that offer personal rewards, without becoming overwhelmed in the process.

Regarding the exercises themselves, the clinician should become intimately familiar with and skilled in their application. The therapist should listen to a relaxation tape, segment by segment, over several sessions, for example, noting whether the content might be intolerable or difficult for a specific patient to master. Advanced relaxation, it should be noted, is simply an extension of the patient's own self-calming activities that include deep breathing, appropriate withdrawal, or other autoprotective strategies (taking a walk, listening to music). Patients should not be encouraged to perform exercises that are beyond their ability. A 5-minute deep-breathing exercise is far better than a half hour of systematic muscle relaxation when the patient cannot maintain focus. Reviewing tapes or scripted routines with the patient allows the clinician to tailor relaxation exercises to the patient's interests and needs. Frequently the clinician will want to make a tape that is uniquely tailored to the individual patient's needs and interests. If relaxation and imaging audiotapes prove useful for patients, they can either be purchased commercially or actually made by the clinician. (However, we generally have not used the voice of the PT therapist, but rather that of another clinical colleague who might have volunteered to record a relaxation script.) Patients need to be given a rationale for using advanced relaxation and imagery. As in the intermediate phase, we review the rationale offered, including the role of autonomic arousal in stressful situations (e.g., sweaty palms, increased blood pressure, or muscle tension) and the indirect way that advanced relaxation can reduce arousal through the release of muscle tension. Reduced muscle tension further allows for increased attention to other matters, including pleasurable ideation and even a foresightful plan for dealing with the potentially stressful situation itself. Some patients might have been captured by popular self-help books that claim to unequivocally achieve "recovery," "cure," or "total healing." We dispel these myths and indicate that we use advanced relaxation simply as a way to reduce autonomic arousal in order for the patient to feel more in control and empowered regarding internal states.

Paradoxically, some patients might feel that "letting go" of muscle tension might invite a loss of control or might become a source of seduction for patients whose gender is different than the therapist (Goldfried & Davison, 1976). In such circumstances, patients should be encouraged to keep their eyes open during the exercises, assume a comfortable position in a chair (as opposed to lying down), and be clearly informed that they can stop the exercise whenever they feel uncomfortable. Goldfried and Davison (1976) indicate that greater control most often follows the "letting go" of muscle tension. They use the analogy of "floating in water" where relaxation (letting go) actually sustains body buoyancy against the competing force of gravity.

Progressive Relaxation

Most patients have found progressive muscle relaxation intrinsically appealing. Often exposure to the training procedure is enough to quiet doubts about its efficacy. The therapist should begin by demonstrating how a muscle group can be tensed and relaxed, being mindful of those with physical ailments that could be adversely affected (e.g., those with arthritis, tendinitis, or back pain). Voice tone should be soft, soothing, and somewhat slow in order to encourage relaxation. Patients should be reassured that they will not be "tested" for perfect performance and that the exercises themselves should not become a burdensome chore. Rather, they should approach progressive relaxation training much like someone interested in acquiring a new skill such as riding a bicycle, driving a car, or hitting a ball. The idea is to perform the exercise with repeated practice until it becomes part of one's "motor memory" and can be acquired automatically and applied spontaneously during daily activities, especially those that might be potentially stressful.

Essentially, the exercises encourage the patient to systematically tense various muscle groups with moderate strength for a few seconds, then let go or relax, with 5- or 10-second pauses and deep breathing interspersed. A detailed script of an induction process can be found in Goldfried and Davison (1976, pp. 88–94). The clinician typically begins by having the patient first clinch the left fist and then let go, followed by the right fist. The exercises progress to the tensing and relaxation of each of the biceps, the shoulders, the muscles of the face, neck, chest, stomach, lower back, hips and buttocks, legs (including thighs, knees and calves), and concluding with ankles and toes. The goal here is to have the patient experience the dramatic differences between muscle tension and the calming sensations that follow muscle relaxation.

Patients are encouraged to practice these tension-release routines at home at least once each day for at least 10 minutes. The clinician can assist the patient in deciding when and where the practice might be most beneficial. Eventually, the exercises are reduced to a smaller number of muscle groups that the patient has mastered and prefers, and from which a clear sense of relief has been experienced. The scale used previously for monitoring the effects of deep breathing can again be employed for the muscle tension release exercises as well: a pre/postexercise rating, where 0 is equal to no tension and 10 represents extreme tension. Once the patient has clearly achieved a level of relaxation using the shortened tension-release procedure, the systematic tensing of the muscles themselves is gradually eliminated and the patient is asked to simply *recall* the physical and emotional sensation that had been associated with tension release, often with the tensing and relaxing of a single preferred muscle. It is this "recall-relaxation" phenomenon that patients should be encouraged to use in community encounters that might provoke anxiety or other subjective cues of distress. The clinician will need to revisit the tension-release routine for specific muscle groups if the patient has experienced difficulty in achieving relaxation using the recall method. When the patient has tried unsuccessfully to use the procedure during an actual anxiety-provoking encounter, the clinician should return to the technique of having the patient imagine a provocative exchange (e.g., someone criticizing him or her) and then attempt relaxation during the PT session. Patients often need to be reminded that the benefits of progressive relaxation are not always noticed initially but do become quite apparent with extended practice.

Guided Imagery

Unlike progressive relaxation that is designed to be employed during actual or anticipated stressful encounters, imagery is a technique that some patients will find useful as an aid to achieving a deeper level of relaxation overall. As such, imagery is a private, self-directed exercise. Only the procedure itself will be guided by the therapist according to the patient's interests, needs, and ability. It can be offered as a tool that compliments the patient's self-calming strategies such as taking a walk, listening to music, deep breathing or carrying cards with self-assuring statements ("I am safe," "I am in control of my feelings," "I can handle a difficult situation"). As in the intermediate phase, it is important that the patient learn that the therapist is not promoting a specific religious, spiritual, or metaphysical belief system.

While patients will initially vary widely in their ability to envision images across diverse sensory modalities, we have observed that this capacity can be developed among many schizophrenia patients. Imagery is explained as a mental picture of something that is not physically present. The procedure can be introduced by asking patients what everyday objects give them pleasure and, if they close their eyes for a moment, whether they can create a mental image of the object. For those who experience some difficulty, they can be asked to imagine the number of windows in their home or apartment that allow in strong sunlight. The clinician might begin by walking the patient through a familiar scene:

> "Close your eyes for a moment, relax and think about your kitchen. Open your refrigerator door. Can you visualize the contents of your refrigerator? Can you feel the puff of cool air when you open the door? Now find a ripe and juicy apple. Take it into your hand and feel the waxy skin. Look at the warm red color. Now close the refrigerator door and listen to the click. Scrape the skin of the apple with your fingernail. Bring the apple to your nose and smell the aroma. Take a bite. Taste the sweetness and the texture. . . . "

Imagery exercises, like the deep-breathing and progressive relaxation routines, can be rated on a scale of vividness (0 representing no sensory recall and 10 being vivid, and involving the senses of sight, smell, hearing, touch, and taste). The ultimate goal of imagery is to have the patient develop his or her *own* pleasant images, whether they be scenes (lying on a beach), sounds (waves breaking or birds singing), colors (an enjoyable painting or photograph), touch (warm ocean breezes), or other past experiences that the patient has recalled as having been peaceful, calming, and relaxing. If a patient is unable to do this, standard scenes can be suggested (e.g., waves rhythmically breaking and receding on a beautiful beach). These principles of relaxation have been outlined in the report of Zahourek (1988), and we emphasize the point that the images recalled are completely within the patient's power to evoke or terminate. These guidelines also influence clinician instructions to the effect that when exercises are terminated at home, the patient should open his or her eyes slowly, take a deep breath, and become fully oriented to time and place. We suggest that patients create their own "safe place" for practicing these exercises and to maintain a journal of their experiences, including the context and the time or day that the exercises were practiced and the level of success achieved.

Any discomfort with an exercise should be discussed in the subsequent PT session. While it is desirable to have as many senses as possible incorporated into the mental image, the therapist should assure the patient that evoking even one sense is better than none and that no one sense is better than any other. Eventually most patients create their own relaxation routine using deep breathing, the "relaxation response," progressive muscle relaxation and imagery, selectively or in an integrated fashion that reflects their preference, individual circumstances, and efficacy. Recent professional reviews of the imagery process can be found in Miyashita (1995) and Hoffart and Keene (1998). Hyman, Feldman, Harris, Levin, and Malloy (1989) also provide an overview of relaxation training efficacy in various clinical populations. The relaxation audiotapes of Budzynski (1974) and Sippel et al. (1982) and the guided imagery exercises of Naparstek (1993) have been found to be useful by our own PT clinicians.

CONFLICT RESOLUTION AND CRITICISM MANAGEMENT

Few human experiences have been shown to have as serious an effect on the clinical stability and social adjustment of schizophrenia patients as critical and hostile comments (Leff & Vaughn, 1985; Kavanagh, 1992). Such effects also adversely impact the outcome of other psychiatric and medical disorders. Unlike discrete life events (e.g., loss of a job or having an accident), poorly managed criticism can become an enduring, negative-reinforcing characteristic of a close relationship. Criticism can underlie persistent elevations of arousal, provoke cognitive and affective symptoms, and otherwise contribute to an unhelpful adaptation such as chronic withdrawal, social isolation, and passivity. For this reason we have added some "tried-and-true" behavioral techniques to the advanced phase of PT that were designed to either forestall negative interactions or to manage such encounters when they arise unexpectedly and cannot otherwise be avoided. The latter circumstances are particularly common among advanced phase participants who seek a more active engagement with others in and out of the home. Behavioral approaches to conflict resolution and criticism were well described in the literature prior to the initiation of PT. We have relied heavily on the Novaco (1976) and Meichenbaum and Novaco (1985) anger management and stress inoculation approaches, the Meichenbaum and Cameron (1973, 1974) self-instruction technique, and the Burns (1980) criticism management technique during the implementation of PT, as well as in the following descriptions of their application. However, we caution the reader that these techniques do not constitute a fast track to behavior therapy proficiency, but rather serve the specific goals of circumventing or more effectively negotiating a negative interaction.

Conflict and criticism management should be seen as a progressive strategy that characterizes all phases of PT, the complexity of which bears a very close relationship to the patient's clinical state, especially those encounters that the patient can successfully negotiate as symptom remission and stabilization fluctuate. In the basic phase, simple avoidance and prosocial positive comments were primary strategies. In the intermediate phase, the appropriate use of positive and negative assertion was emphasized, especially in relationships with household members. Now, close and unpredictable encounters of an extrafamilial nature, as well as more spontaneous interactions with family members, will often require a greater negotiating skill. However, patients should not lose sight of the efficacy and appropriateness of earlier phase techniques that can continue to serve a valuable function in the advanced phase.

Preparing for Conflict

Unfortunately, persistent negative symptoms can often lead others to confuse amotivation, blunted affect, and alogia with willful defiance. Concrete thinking and social cognitive deficits will also frequently invite a critical or hostile response from others. "Reflective consideration" of one's behavior and its effect on others should help, but the most interpersonally sensitive patient will often fall victim to an unwarranted and often destabilizing verbal attack from time to time. Throughout the preceding phases, the use of self-coaching statements characterized many of the internal coping, relaxation, and basic social skills strategies. The therapist will now want to facilitate a greater online mindfulness in the patient when approaching a potentially negative interpersonal encounter by continuing to encourage the use of self-instructions. Making a distinction between *helpful* and *distressing* self-instruction should become the first order of business. Examples of the former include the following: "I should pause now and think about what I need to do"; "I can handle this"; "I can take a deep breath"; "There is no need to get worked up and anxious"; "I've been through this before and I can get through it again." Conversely, "distressing" self-instructions are also common and a brief appraisal by the therapist can usually identify the patient's own repertoire of unhelpful self statements: "I'll never be able to handle this"; "There go all my plans"; "Things never work out for me."

For patients preparing for, confronting, and coping with a real or an impending provocation, Novaco (1976) suggests a number of useful approaches that include a plan of response. The first is to employ those self-calming techniques that worked well in the past and/or that were learned in the earlier PT sessions (e.g., "I can focus on my own relaxation response"; "I can take a deep breath"; "I can tense and relax a muscle"). The second represents a set of self-instructions as reminders to stay calm and in control and not to take the offense personally. Patients are cautioned not to assume what the critic is implying and therefore not to jump to conclusions. They are encouraged to reflect on the fact that if they lose control they are likely to lose out. Reminders of past success and acquired skills can serve to boost confidence. Foremost, the subjective feeling of distress (one's "cues") unequivocally indicates that the patient needs to do *something,* an action that can range from employing an acquired relaxation technique to cooperating or even using appropriate negative assertions. The latter represent the now familiar "I" statements from the intermediate phase that indicate how the patient feels about the criticism ("I feel that . . . "), what the patient thinks the critic is doing ("What I hear you saying is . . . "), and what the patient would rather have the offending party do or say ("I prefer that you not yell at me when you want me to do something"). Social perception skills (emotional temperature taking) learned in the intermediate phase can often influence the selection and timing of the most appropriate "I" statement. For patients whose confidence waivers or who uncertain as to the natural flow of conflict resolution, the modeling, role-play, and rehearsal of recent provocative encounters should be initiated and practiced until the patient is comfortable with the routine and confident about its successful execution. Rewarding oneself with congratulatory statements is a final but essential reinforcement of the successfully negotiated provocation (Novaco, 1976).

Managing the Criticism

The clinician should indicate that there are four steps that will be used in approaching and responding to a criticism: (1) estimating the tone of the criticism, (2) briefly assessing the critic's perspective, (3) determining whether the criticism is valid or invalid, and (4) generating a response.

Regarding tone, the patient should appreciate that a "high" critical tone will likely exact a greater price in terms of personal distress than a "low" tone. Skill in distinguishing tone is therefore crucial. Otherwise, the patient could overinterpret or overrespond to a benign though valid and largely inconsequential remark by incorrectly implying that the comment is hostile. Conversely, misreading the intensity can lead to increased anger, sarcasm, or censure by critics if they feel that they have not been "heard." In a highly stressful criticism, the *tone* is characteristically intense, the *volume* loud or high pitched, the *content* hostile (global or pejorative), and the *context* typically one that occurs in the presence of others, with little or no chance for escape. In minimally stressful encounters, the tone of the critic is more often subdued or monotonic, the volume soft or low, the content specific, time limited, often constructive and reasonable, and the context typically private (one on one) with escape possible and public embarrassment minimal. It is often wise for the clinician to model criticisms of varying intensity until there is assurance that the patient can accurately differentiate between a high and a low distressing criticism. Examples of perceived criticisms should be drawn from the patient's recent life experiences, and the patient should be encouraged to rate them for their high- or low-stress potential.

When calculating the nature and intensity of a critical comment, the patient should be counseled to consider where the critic is "coming from" (i.e., an exercise in perspective taking). A message is given that critics will most often lower their intensity level if they feel that their message is understood, whether valid or not. This can be a most difficult task when the critic is emotionally distraught. The patient need not agree with the criticism; rather, the important issue here is to develop some greater appreciation of *what* the critic's concern might be, *why* the critic is at a particular level of intensity, and *when* this intensity is likely to be greatest. If a critic were to offer the generalized criticism, "You screwed up again," it is appropriate and necessary to ask for more information: "What is wrong?"; "Why are you so upset?" Benign and empathic inquiries that guide the critic's identification of the source and nature of concern will usually leave the patient with a better understanding of what the critic believes has gone wrong: "I know you think that I screwed up"; "I realize that you are upset"; "You are angry because the freezer door was left open and the ice cream melted." In the process, the critic will likely become assured that his or her concern is being recognized and understood. However, an important caveat to perspective taking is necessary when a quick assessment indicates that personal safety is in jeopardy, either by threats of physical harm or verbal abuse. Again, appropriate negative assertion ("I" statements) and withdrawal will take precedence over perspective taking: "I'm not going to talk with you if you call me names. I'll listen if you have a complaint, but I need to leave if you continue to [yell, threaten, name call] and talk with you later when things cool down."

Determining whether the criticism is valid and reasonable or invalid and unreasonable, together with a set of appropriate negotiating strategies, are the final but most crucial components of criticism management. A criticism is judged to be *valid* and *reasonable* if it correctly identifies a *specific* act of omission or commission and does so in the "low stressful" manner described above. It is *invalid* and *unreasonable* if it is either wrong or the criticism is offered in the high-intensity mode that includes generalizations of behavior ("You never"; "You always") or of character ("You're an idiot . . . , lazy . . . , a jerk . . . , a bum").

Dealing with valid and reasonable criticism simply involves having the patient seek information about the necessary details, apologize if the criticism is correct, form a plan, and begin to implement it (Burns, 1980). Burns also cautions that patients are not expected to be perfect and, if one's immediate solution is not acceptable to the critic, then an inquiry as to what would be preferred is appropriate.

Invalid criticisms, particularly those that are pejorative and reflect a generalized hostility, are more difficult to negotiate. The process involves having patients ask themselves whether they are able to *stay* and *respond* or whether they should *leave* the situation for the time being. (Again, the latter should be executed as tactfully and politely as possible.) Patients who feel up to negotiating the invalid criticism will need a substantial amount of coaching and support. The goal for patients is to *set limits* on the invalid and unreasonable criticism if they choose not to terminate the encounter. Patients are reassured that their acquired techniques will serve to help them exert some level of control over a potentially distressing interaction.

The *practice* induction for managing invalid criticism is somewhat hierarchical in nature and should begin with a simple (and usually ludicrous) criticism that will tend to put the patient in a game-playing mood (e.g., "You are the cause of every problem ever faced by mankind"). Patients should be encouraged to generate their own silly criticisms and practice responses before moving on to erroneous specific criticisms, global criticisms, or permanent characterizations of personality. Patients can also be counseled about other behaviors that can quickly escalate to generalized hostility, such as ignoring someone or being ignored, speaking or being spoken to sarcastically, or giving or receiving "digs."

The approach to limit setting first employs the use of empathic remarks designed to defuse the critic's intensity ("I'm sorry to see you so upset"). Second, patients should be cautioned not to argue about the validity of a false accusation or otherwise enter into a protracted defense. Third, the patient should ask specific questions about the critic's complaint (without agreeing with the criticism itself). Fourth, the patient can show (e.g., by nodding or maintaining eye contact) that he or she is indeed listening and trying to understand the concern as the critic sees it ("I know you think I'm a . . . "; "I hear you when you say . . . "; "It is clear that you think . . . "). Fifth, the patient should use one or more responses that indicate that he or she has heard and understood the critic but *does not agree* with the criticism ("I'm sorry that you feel that way, but I don't agree"; "I know that is how you see it, but I have my own understanding"). Finally, the patient can volunteer his or her plan for overall change (e.g., the treatment plan) where indicated, and ask what changes the critic would like to see. If possible and appropriate, the patient can attempt to negotiate a compromise by offering a realistic accommodation that can be implemented in a reasonable period of time.

SOCIAL AND VOCATIONAL ISSUES

General Concerns

Throughout this text we have commented on the not-so-obvious cognitive deficits that characterize schizophrenia during the recovery phase. Unfortunately, workers in the rehabilitation field (including vocational counselors, placement officers, and field supervisors), too often equate schizophrenia disability with positive symptoms of the illness or with associated impairments of affect. Less frequently acknowledged are the constraints against social and vocational recovery that are represented by cognitive dysfunctioning. Even today, the policy of many public rehabilitation agencies will often require *full-time* training, placement, employment, or schooling in order for the patient to qualify for rehabilitation benefits. Not only does a reduction in mental stamina and energy continue to characterize most patients who have achieved a symptomatic remission, but problems with the speed of information processing, distractibility, concentration, working memory, and problem solving (especially indecisiveness and ambivalence) often persist. In fact, a recent study has indicated that problems with working memory load, as opposed to abiding difficulties with attentional vigilance, lead to symptom exacerbation in stressful situations, for example, in the context of interpersonal criticism (Rosenfarb, Nuechterlein, Goldstein, & Subotnik, 2000).

Against this background of covert cognitive deficits are the rudimentary requirements that characterize most jobs. Beyond appropriate appearance and personal hygiene, the "mental status" of a worker today requires a modicum of cognitive organization and flexibility, some skill in abstraction regarding the rules of personal conduct and task performance, the ability to concentrate and to keep the essential details of a task in mind for extended periods of time, and a minimum capacity to exercise appropriate social judgment in the workplace setting. Compatibility with coworkers, basic conversational skills, the ability to reciprocate and communicate clearly and the willingness to accept guidance, instruction, and criticism and to avoid unnecessary confrontation are all minimal expectations needed to secure and maintain competitive employment or even a volunteer position. Added to this is the quality of task performance itself: maintenance of a schedule; persistence; focus; regularity of attendance; endurance; timeliness of task completion; quantity of work produced; the ability to withstand pressure and to work safely. Jobs that involve interaction with the public demand even greater social cognitive abilities such as empathy, sensitivity, listening, and negotiation skills. (It is well to keep these abilities in mind when considering whether the patient is *disabled* and eligible for Social Security benefits [see Chapter 3].) Thus, therapist, family, and patient initiatives to resume work or formal education need to balance these realities of the vocational world with the capacities and disabilities of the patient, and to do so in the context of a rehabilitation plan that includes provider and employer sensitivity to these competing requirements. As we have emphasized in the past (Anderson et al., 1986), the formula for a successful social and vocational recovery often includes a number of commonsense approaches that acknowledge the reality of subtle cognitive deficits: breaking a long-term goal into its component parts that can be achieved in an incremental, stepwise fashion; temporarily revising expectations for full-time schooling, employment, or social engagement; maintaining flexibility as to progress (a setback is not a failure but an invitation to temporally revise the rehabilitation plan); and monitoring work or school performance for intermittent shifts in cognitive functioning that might be associated with occupational demands. Initially, at least, these approaches will often lead to part-time work or school, a setting that requires only a modest degree of social interaction, and a work or training environment that is supportive.

Advanced phase placement does not necessarily imply a superior premorbid adjustment among participants or the presence of highly sophisticated social and vocational issues that need resolution. Rather, patient background characteristics often reveal only modest work accomplishments. Indeed, the concerns of most patients who are about to institute social and vocational initiatives are quite basic. Many have no work history, or a spotty one at best. Former friends (or employers) have often moved on, and the need to reinstitute social contacts carries with it a host of issues: how to begin; what and how much to share about one's interim history; and the ubiquitous but unhelpful comparisons to the accomplishments of peers, siblings, or even to one's own highest premorbid functioning. (For these disheartening comparisons, we again encourage the use of the "internal yardstick" that compares the patient's own progress over time, rather than contrasts the performance of self to others.) Among patients who are anxious to pursue competitive employment, the range of common concerns expressed can also be disarming: how does one interview for a job, respond to criticism or praise by a supervisor, refuse unreasonable requests, negotiate a wage or pay raise, or deal with authority? Whether the patient should rely on rehabilitation agencies (which acknowledge a mental illness) or seek employment independently is also a frequent concern. If resumption of formal education is the goal, issues regarding the type and number of classes to be pursued, the cognitive demands of study, the preferred types of study habits, and test anxiety are not uncommon. A major issue often involves determining a course of study that leads to an attractive career opportunity that the patient feels able to successfully master. Beneath all social and vocational pursuits are even more basic concerns; how to initiate a conversation, make a friend, cope with possible rejection or failure, and even maintain "small talk."

The patient can be reassured by the general approach that the advanced phase will take to these concerns: (1) there will be a review of past experiences including an assessment of what did and did not work; (2) there will be an appraisal of "subjective cues" (affective, cognitive, physiological, and behavioral) in these social and vocational contexts; and (3) through practice simulations, a selection of one or more of the PT coping strategies will be made for situations where previous attempts at coping were unsuccessful. Social and vocational ventures will be viewed as "trials" or "beginning steps" that will yield important information regarding residual strengths and limitations, including what can be successfully pursued and what needs to be either avoided or approached differently; that is, the community will primarily serve as a laboratory where newly acquired skills and mastery can be tested.

Specific Concerns

Once again, social and vocational attainment in the advanced phase seeks a process for making the acquired coping strategies of earlier phases more *portable* (i.e., a transfer of skills from the predictable and more protected environments of home and office to the unpredictable and often stressful challenges of community life). In many cases, it will become apparent that familiar and predictable stressors do not always adequately prepare the patient for the unpredictability of community encounters. We therefore approach social and vocational initiatives in a progressive fashion: (1) a review of the patient's past social and vocational history as the basis for a plan of action; (2) a discussion or actual role-play and rehearsal of previous social and vocational encounters that were distressing; and (3) actual in vivo encounters that the patient has made between sessions as the foundation for review and further practice, if needed. During the basic phase, the treatment plan sought to incorporate the patient's own broad social and vocational goals. In the interim, however, these goals might have changed as awareness of vulnerability and adjustment to disability have increased. For those now ready to resume the quest for a more fulfilling social and vocational life, these personal goals need to be revisited in greater depth, preferably over a series of sessions.

Social and Vocational History

For many patients, perhaps a majority, performance difficulties with work or school have been associated with the initial appearance of psychotic symptoms: beginning college or flunking a course; starting a job, joining the military; getting fired or demoted. Difficulties in forming and maintaining new relationships beyond the family might also have been common. As described by us elsewhere, problems in social cognitive development might have underlain the difficulty experienced in successfully negotiating these milestones (Hogarty & Flesher, 1999a). It is therefore not enough to simply inquire about friendships, the tasks and duties of a past job, or the types of courses and the grades achieved in school. More pertinent to the task of community transition is the therapeutic challenge to identify the subjective distress that accompanied work, school, or social demands and the contextual triggers that led to the patient's dysregulation and symptom formation. The history of jobs, duties, salary, courses, grades, and friendships largely serve as a format for the probing of subjective cues of distress and related coping styles. We have found that the following probes often elicit the type of information that ultimately permits a greater portability of acquired skills:

1. The first probe explores the quality of relationships that the patient had with various supervisors or teachers: ("How did you like _____, and how did he or she like you?" Many patients will try to put the best face possible on these relationships, and it is important not to strip defenses or lower the patient's self-esteem during the exploration. The therapist will need to determine whether the patient became dysregulated by a particular supervisory style (e.g., one that was critical or overly demanding) or with "authority figures" in general. Were positive and negative experiences with specific supervisors or teachers common among other coworkers or students, or were they unique to the patient? Most importantly, the cues of dysregulation that arose when dealing with authority should be identified by the therapist as stressors that likely affected the patient's ability to work or learn. The identification of a potentially relevant strategy or two from the prior and current phases related to social perception, perspective taking, assertion, or criticism management can be made.

2. The second probe is similar in that it focuses on the relationships with coworkers and fellow students and can be broadened to include significant others outside the home with whom the patient had been involved socially (e.g., a boyfriend, girlfriend, or former school friends). Again, the clinician will want to look for common thematic provocations initiated by the patient or other persons and for the subjective feelings that accompanied these encounters. Did the patient feel appreciated and admired, or taken for granted, ignored, and even rejected? Did the patient have difficulty attempting to interpret the rules of appropriate conduct in different social contexts or what others expected? How did the patient feel when engaged in close relationships? What were the circumstances within which affective dysregulation arose? Patients can be asked to recall their already identified "cues of distress" and queried as to whether there were times in previous relationships at work, school, or socially when these *same* cues were present? As above, the discussion can lead to a review of potentially useful coping strategies already acquired.

3. Another critically important probe seeks to determine whether constraints on a patient's mental stamina and/or physical energy existed in prior social and vocational endeavors. Inevitably, distress and dysregulation will more likely arise when the patient's activity level exceeds a personal reserve of stamina and energy. Understanding the nature of voca-

tional and educational demands in relationship to the patient's threshold for mental and physical endurance will not only heighten sensitivity to occupational stress but also serve to guide the patient's selection of a job or type of course, as well as the number of hours each day and of days each week that will be committed to these activities. The same applies to social and leisure pursuits. Late hours, disrupted sleep, or an inordinate number of social activities can lead to the same feelings of fatigue that are exacted by a vocational or academic schedule that exceeds mental and physical capacity. Equating fatigue with the increased probability of dysregulation can both serve a signal function of distress and indicate the need for a coping strategy that will control excessive social and vocational demands (e.g., negative assertion, negotiation, or compromise).

4. As indicated earlier, a probe for specific symptom experiences that occurred in the context of work, school, or social role performance is also important. This review may well serve to *desensitize* the patient to the often fearful and unpredictable breakthroughs of prodromal or formal psychotic symptoms. Even for patients who continue to harbor delusional thinking about supervisors, coworkers, teachers, fellow students, or intimate acquaintances, the connection between social and vocational stressors, internal dysregulation, and symptom manifestation can be reassuring. This is particularly true for patients who now realize that they possess the skills that can control an otherwise chaotic progression of symptoms. In the cognitive-behavioral therapy sense, a seed of doubt can be planted in the form of an alternative explanation for the distressing thoughts and feelings that arise in social and vocational contexts.

5. Expectations for social and vocational performance, both those held by the patient and by the family, should be revisited. Earlier in treatment, expectations had deliberately been revised and often lowered, but with symptom remission and a greater sense of control, expectations for role performance might have escalated, perhaps unrealistically. In many cases, these revised expectations will pass unnoticed by the therapist unless they are specifically probed. It should be shared with the patient (and with family members when appropriate) that not all social and vocational stressors arise from community encounters; rather, a significant amount of stress can be traced to self- and/or family-generated expectations for social and vocational attainment. We recall the wise counsel of Selye (1974) to the effect that people should choose their stressors, so to speak, in the cause of conserving resources and maximizing personal rewards. Pushing oneself, or being urged toward social and vocational activities that exceed cognitive ability and stamina, will quickly exhaust the effectiveness of ex-

isting coping abilities, in our experience. A review of personal vulnerability, including the components of disability taught earlier, is appropriate. Family expectations that are alleged to be excessive according to the patient's account need to be confirmed independently through family contact. If a discrepancy exists between the patient's report and the family's actual expectations, it should be determined whether this is simply a misunderstanding on the patient's part or a projection of unrealistic goals, either of which requires a therapeutic response.

6. Finally, the review of expectations should lead to a more realistic appraisal of the patient's social, vocational, or educational goals. The preceding probes, together with earlier phase experiences, will likely have redefined initial goals once the realities of personal ability and disability have become better appreciated. For most patients, the goals that led initially to "joining" and formation of the treatment contract will have become tempered. The focus now is to guide the patient away from highly specific and often rigid or fixed goals through the encouragement of "divergent thinking" (i.e., entertaining multiple paths to a goal). For example, if the stated vocational goal of a patient who had some formal preillness training in computer science is to work as a programmer for a specific company in a specific part of town, then a sensitive illustration of the difficulties that might be encountered in pursuing this goal should lead to the conclusion that such a narrow and fixed objective could prove to be unattainable. Reframing the goal to include a job that pays decently, is relatively easy to access using public transportation, offers personal rewards, compliments the patient's training and interest, and ideally (though not necessarily) involves computers makes the goal far more attainable. (For example, a volunteer position tutoring high school students in computer usage might be the first step to part-time employment as a computer troubleshooter for a local company.) Throughout the subsequent implementation of the treatment plan, the therapist should refer to these revised and more realistic social and vocational goals.

The history review would not be complete without a comment on the significant minority of patients who remain *unmotivated*. Paradoxically, many of these patients are prepared and "interested" in a fuller social and vocational life, yet lack the drive or energy needed to actually formulate and implement a plan. In these cases, there is a useful "metamotivational" probe that can be used which involves asking patients whether they are "motivated to become motivated." Becoming motivated involves the routine performance of simple tasks (often extensions of task assignments from the basic and intermediate phases) that contain the potential for being self-rewarding and reinforcing. Further, patients can be encouraged to reward themselves (e.g., watch a favorite TV program, or read a popular magazine) if they complete a task that has no apparent and immediate reward. Our experience has been that minor rewarding behaviors (and the identification of the associated state of self-satisfaction) are often cumulative and progressive. The self-expressed desire to become motivated then becomes the reference goal throughout subsequent discussions of the social and vocational rehabilitational plan.

Addressing Common Social and Vocational Dilemmas

The behavioral principles of role-play, rehearsal, and feedback might leave many "dynamically" trained clinicians feeling that these techniques represent an unnatural, programmed approach to the otherwise spontaneous experiences of an unpredictable life. So too, many advanced phase patients are not inclined to pursue a rehearsed approach to the unique and spontaneous day-to-day experiences that add meaning (or stress) to their lives. In our opinion, formal behavioral skills approaches have had their greatest value (and demonstrated efficacy) among the more impaired and disabled subsamples of the severely mentally ill. However, those who have achieved a good remission of symptoms, when coupled with a premorbid history of accomplishment, are often more inclined to want a sensitive but candid discussion of various problem-solving alternatives to social and vocational dilemmas. These exchanges can, however, include advice as to how an interaction might best unfold in the absence of formal instruction that includes role-play, modeling, and rehearsal. Thus, the process used to address the common "pressure points" of social and vocational interaction will vary from patient to patient, according to preferences and need. For some patients, the anticipatory anxiety surrounding these pressure points will clearly necessitate the formal use of modeling, role-play, and rehearsal, especially in conditions where the patient has only one chance at creating a good first impression. For others, a sensitive discussion of the issues, including problem-solving alternatives, will suffice.

The most common social and vocational dilemma is subsumed within the issue of *what to say* or *not to say* about one's illness and interim history, especially among patients with a recent hospitalization or who have been housebound for a period of time. The issue arises when patients are meeting new or former acquaintances and extended family, going on a job interview, or applying to school. The necessity of having to self-account is often sufficient to precipitate dysregulation itself. Indeed, some patients resolve the dilemma by avoiding potentially revealing encounters altogether. Others might embark on a fanciful rumination about role performance that is more befitting an earlier age or developmental period. The therapeutic task becomes one of convincing the patient that the best approach is to try to *finesse* self-disclosure according to the circumstances of a given social context. The concept of finesse, however, can itself be intimidating, especially for the many patients who tend to give a morally literal account regarding the "truth" of their recent history. (Often lost in this response is an appreciation of the fact that a majority of patients can actually project confidence when commenting on their accomplishments and abilities, and most in fact do remain calm during these exchanges.)

The general approach to dealing with self-disclosure is to encourage patients to "put their best foot forward," a formidable task for those who tend not to take the initiative or otherwise act as passive processors of social information. The clinician can begin by helping the patient to format the message they want to communicate and what they hope the result of the encounter will be. Patients are reminded that they have control over what they choose to share and that prudence should be used in volunteering the details of a psychiatric history. Rather, emphasis should be placed on sending positive messages. In the job interview, for example, the use of finesse will have the patient steer the conversation in the direction of why they want to work for this particular employer in this particular job.

If there is a direct question asked about psychiatric history, patients need not discuss diagnosis or symptoms, but can acknowledge the reality of their history and calmly state that their doctor believes that they are now ready to work, the legitimacy of which can typically be confirmed by the employer, if desired. (Today, it can be illegal for potential employers to directly inquire about a patient's medical history.) In reality, most patients who pursue employment do so through the office of a rehabilitation program and the job developer has typically prepared the potential employer for the abilities and disabilities that a particular applicant will bring to the position.

The patient is not only encouraged to project interest and ability but to *shift* the focus of responding back to the interviewer. The more questions a patient asks about the job (e.g., its attractions and challenges), the less time the patient will need to spend in the hot seat. The goal is to ask open-ended questions that lead the interviewer to share more information about the position. These questions and follow-up inquiries not only indicate interest on the patient's part but can help improve the patient's listening skills as well. Gaps in employment history can be acknowledged, but the interview can be quickly turned to the patient's eagerness and readiness to return to the workforce. The expression of willingness to "go the extra mile" in order to do the job properly is often very helpful. If there have been interim volunteer experiences, these should be noted and described in a positive fashion. Simply having questions available and a plan of response are themselves reassuring, but they become most useful when coupled with learned calming strategies acquired prior to the interview. The process of being active and positively assertive should be discussed (or practiced) until the patient feels comfortable and confident in facing a job interview. Issues of salary and increases are best avoided in the initial interview; the patient can always turn the job down if an unacceptable offer is made. The experience of having applied for a position, successfully or not, can be viewed both as being useful and as laying the foundation for subsequent interviews.

The approach to other potentially distressing first encounters is similar, including the initiation of conversation (including "small talk") with new or former acquaintances and extended family members. The process includes first asking *general questions,* then *listening* attentively to the answers, followed with another *relevant question,* all the while being *supportive* of the respondent (e.g., "That's very interesting"; "It must have been hard for you"). In reality, patients will rarely use the entire repertoire of coping strategies, open-ended questions, or supportive comments that were reviewed in anticipation of these first encounters during discussions or actual practice simulations. However, knowledge that such resources are available and easily accessed is often sufficient to reduce the anticipatory dread associated with these initiatives.

"Real-World" Experiences

Most patients will enter the employment arena through an Office of Vocational Rehabilitation and its contracted agencies, many of whom offer additional resocialization experiences. Too often, however, therapists tend to view government-supported rehabilitation programs as unnecessarily regimented, overly demanding, or focused on narrow goals mandated by the funding sources. Rehabilitation specialists, in turn, might sometimes feel that therapists are naïve as to the demands of the workplace. When patients stumble during rehabilitation, including setbacks attributed to poor social judgment or fluctuating cognitive deficits, they are often referred back to the clinician for "more therapy." In order to minimize this potential "tug of war" for patients, we pursued local resources that could provide volunteer "in vivo" social and vocational opportunities prior to referral to formal rehabilitation programs. (PT therapists were not job-finding, training, or placement counselors.) Through the good offices of our hospital volunteer program, the generosity of its human resources department, and the willingness of various clinical and research program directors, numerous volunteer positions became available where patients could test their instrumental skills, stamina, and learned coping strategies. Supervisors were most often eager to receive guidance from the therapist and to provide feedback regarding patient performance. Volunteer experiences then became the substance of subsequent PT sessions where a review of progress, use of coping strategies, and achieved outcomes could be discussed and, if necessary, solutions to interpersonal problems modeled and rehearsed. It was not that we were uniquely "blessed" with such relevant resources; rather, with a modicum of energy we feel that most therapists can readily identify a number of volunteer or transitional work opportunities in their own communities. The initial effort required might be relatively substantial, but the investment will pay dividends for current and future patients over a period of many years. Therapists have often been pleasantly surprised at the number of community programs that welcomed patient volunteers. (We are aware of the priority placed on the "supported work" approach today, in which a number of our patients have also successfully participated. However, the dropout rate remains high in many of these programs, which we feel can often be traced to the deficient social cognitive skills, coping strategies, and residual disabilities that PT addresses.)

The ever-changing, novel, often unexpected, and spontaneous encounters in these vocational and social contexts sometimes will often bear only a modest relationship to the themes of distress and coping that had been identified in the review of past experiences. Social skills and internal coping strategies that had been practiced in the somewhat contrived interpersonal encounters that were modeled and rehearsed in the office often seem difficult to integrate when the contexts and the players, as well as the type and degree of dysregulation, vary in real-world settings. The PT window to the actual vocational functioning of a patient most often came through the patient's work supervisor. In most instances (other than the fewer cases where patients independently acquired positions on their own), patients were open to therapist contact with a supervisor. Supervisors, in turn, came to highly value and welcome the therapist as a resource. Many supervisors would initially begin with a volunteer patient in a somewhat cautious manner, not knowing what to expect, and at times they were fearful that any criticism or demand would do irreparable harm to the patient. Others were hesitant to include patients in the social activities of the workplace (e.g., a birthday celebration) for fear of making the other staff "uncomfortable." In these instances, the therapist needed to reassure the supervisor by demystifying the realities of recovery from psychosis. While the harshness of a military boot camp was clearly to be avoided, an unrealistic, undemanding, and overly accommodating environment would also not be instructive or facilitative of eventual independent employment.

Through regular contact between the therapist and the supervisor, the realities of patient performance and coping in novel contexts can be exquisitely appreciated. At times, the supervisor can be redirected in his or her relationship to the patient, but more often the integration of relevant internal coping strategies can be better targeted to the realities of the patient's behavior in actual work and social settings. For example, one patient who appeared well prepared for work and coping nevertheless tended to make her coworkers uncomfortable by her silence in an otherwise engaging and highly interactive environment. The PT sessions subsequently focused on this patient's assertiveness skills, which had seemed less relevant in earlier phases. Conversely, another patient was viewed as being overly talkative and distracting to coworkers in a work environment that required close attention to detail. Subsequent reviews during PT sessions revealed that performance anxiety led this otherwise gracious patient to an escalation of affect in the face of newly assigned tasks. Internal coping shifted to the reexamination of relevant relaxation techniques that had not been sufficiently emphasized. In yet another instance, internal coping strategies had focused on the patient's previous failures to negotiate what had been perceived by him as unreasonable supervisory requests. In the past, the patient's anger had quickly led to conflict and ultimate dismissal. In the volunteer position, however, the patient had simply chosen not to perform a task that he considered to be unreasonable, doing so without consulting the supervisor. Coping strategies thus shifted from the control of affect escalation to appropriate assertion and negotiation. Reinforcement of these desired behaviors by supervisors have tended to increase the motivation of patients to acquire the requisite coping strategies needed to survive in their particular work setting. Many of the unforeseen inconsistencies between prior social and vocational difficulties and the reality of a current placement will be lessened as the therapist becomes more experienced in calculating the relative advantages and disadvantages of a specific work environment as they relate to the strengths and vulnerabilities of a given patient, that is, the process of determining the best "environment–patient fit."

Invariably, the first volunteer experience is the most difficult to manage. Anticipatory anxiety is highest in the patient, the need for reassurance most constant, and the challenge to integrate learned coping skills with actual work and social experiences the greatest. Sharing information about the physical characteristics of the proposed work environment, what the coworkers will be like, as well as the expectations of supervisors (together with a preplacement visit) can contribute greatly to patient comfort. These social and vocational simulations should continue in the volunteer role until the real-life integration of PT strategies and the demands of the work, school, or social environments have been comfortably engaged. Most graduates of the advanced phase, when faced with potentially distressing interpersonal encounters, will have acquired the process of integration to the point of it being "second nature." In its simplest form, this process involves (1) assessing the situation, (2) checking one's feelings or other subjective cues, (3) applying an internal coping strategy, (4) deciding what to do, and (5) responding appropriately.

In closing, it should be mentioned that not all advanced phase patients will become candidates for these in vivo social and vocational experiences. Some will continue to become dysregulated quickly by novel encounters, and the challenge for them will be to remain symptomatically stable and out of hospital. In these cases, social encounters will be reserved to relatives and acquaintances with whom the patient is comfortable or to structured resocialization experiences. Other patients will prefer to negotiate social and vocational initiatives on their own, and these patients can simply be supported in their achievements. If difficulties arise, the latter patients can be invited to discuss or rehearse alternative ways to manage social and vocational challenges. Most patients who participated in the in vivo experiences were eventually successful in improving instrumental and express role performance as described in Chapter 2. Many actually become highly valued members of the volunteer work settings, and many of these proceeded to either paid employment or the pursuit of a formal education. The astute observer will note that later advanced phase approaches began to address what ultimately proved to be the more important "rate-limiting" factors to a meaningful social and vocational life. These included the elements of perspective taking, social content appraisal, and social judgment. It was these rate-limiting factors and related deficits in social cognition that gave birth to our current initiative represented by the de-

velopment and testing of cognitive-enhancement therapy, a most promising poststabilization "recovery phase" intervention for the increasingly
large number of patients who are now able to acquire a qualitatively better
remission of symptoms through modern pharmacological advances. Overall, most graduates of PT, including the less successful cases, felt empowered by the strategies that provided a greater mastery of illness. A significant majority felt that the quality of their lives had much improved. For all
but the small minority (12%) that most often suffered persistent and un-
relenting symptoms of schizophrenia, life following PT was distinctly
better.

POST-PT MAINTENANCE

Once patients are able to achieve an optimal exposure to and mastery of
one or more PT phases, the clinician will be faced with questions related
to maintenance, primarily the frequency of contacts and the content of
subsequent sessions. Such concerns must be addressed with the realization
that for all but a small minority of poorly characterized patients, schizophrenia will be a lifelong concern. Next, in the final chapter, we propose a
role for PT that accommodates both the stage of illness and the level of residual disability. The "algorithm" describes the nature and frequency of
maintenance PT sessions in the face of either interim relapse or continuing
stability, according to the level of disability. For those with severe and
persistent disability, the addition of other necessary interventions such as
cognitive-behavioral or skills-training approaches are recommended. For
PT graduates with mild or moderate disability, cognitive rehabilitation
strategies appropriate to the poststabilization recovery stage are suggested. Among successful PT cases, weekly sessions for at least 1 year are
recommended, especially for patients who continue to seek a more fulfilling community life where newly acquired strategies will routinely be
tested and in need of periodic review. Should interim symptom exacerbations occur, clinicians need not restart PT from the beginning; rather,
they can simply return to a review of the phase-relevant interventions that
were appropriate to the source(s) of destabilization. Even for the unequivocally successful patient, monthly-to-quarterly status reviews will provide
the safety net needed to pursue life goals confidently and with the assurance of continued health. Appendix B provides a set of guidelines for
monitoring advanced phase progress.

CHAPTER SEVEN

Toward a Psychosocial Treatment Algorithm

Following a publication that described our latest treatment initiative on cognitive-enhancement therapy (CET), a colleague asked (a bit sarcastically) whether PT and family psychoeducation were now "passé." While the question initially provoked a cavalier response, a moment of reflection led to the realization that this seemingly facetious query did contain what would likely become *the* challenge of the new millennium to mental health providers faced with delivering care to the seriously mentally ill: how to select, integrate, and implement demonstrably efficacious psychosocial treatments, according to the diverse needs of patients. (The short answer to our critic was that PT is a strategy best suited to the stabilization phase of illness, where prophylactic techniques hold the greatest value; CET is more appropriate to the later recovery phase of illness.)

Treatment algorithms that provide a blueprint for the prescription of various *psychopharmacological* agents for schizophrenia and affective disorder patients have proliferated in recent years. Many are well known to the readers of this volume, and all have followed a fairly predictable "decision tree." Models differ essentially in the choice of a first-line medication based on symptom severity, second line alternatives, and third-line augmentation strategies for partial or nonresponders. In schizophrenia, for example, a popular model (Pearsall et al., 1998) begins with the selection of one of the new atypical antipsychotic medications for moderately ill patients. If the patient has an incomplete response, then the dose is increased every 3–5 days until the maximum is reached, following which the dose is maintained for 3 weeks. If the patient still does not respond adequately, another antipsychotic drug is chosen that follows this same sequence. (At this point, other models might include haloperidol or fluphenazine decanoate.) If symptoms persist, the patient is then placed on clozapine. In most models, a suboptimal response to clozapine serves to introduce augmentation strategies, such as the addition of a typical or an atypical antipsychotic medication, or lithium or an anticonvulsant. If all else fails, electroconvulsive therapy is the treatment of last resort. The medication algorithm thus varies little among different models and depends on relatively few patient characteristics: an accurate diagnosis; sometimes the severity of presenting symptoms; and a criterion of response, including symptomatic remission and/or the tolerability of side effects.

Now consider the challenge in developing a psychosocial algorithm using treatment components that have been shown to increase the efficacy of "warm medication" by 50% or more. The "decision tree" would similarly include diagnosis, symptom severity, responsiveness, and tolerability (i.e., the intervention would not provoke symptoms or otherwise destabilize the patient), similar to the algorithm for medication. However, the model would also need to accommodate the following dimensions: (1) the type of setting (e.g., inpatient, partial hospital, community residential, or outpatient); (2) the phase of illness (e.g., acute, stabilization, recovery, or postrecovery); (3) the level of functional disability (e.g., low, intermediate, or high); (4) the type of requisite service delivery system (e.g., case management, a psychosocial rehabilitation center, or the Program for Assertive Community Treatment [PACT]—with or without supported work, education, or housing); (5) caseload size and frequency of contact; and finally (6) the type of psychosocial treatment itself. (It is no surprise, therefore, that such complexity has constrained "public health model" effectiveness studies in the mental health field.)

That only one well-conceptualized psychosocial treatment algorithm is available, to our knowledge, should come as no surprise: the "Expert Consensus Guideline Series: Treatment of Schizophrenia," developed by McEvoy et al. (1999). The litany of services and psychosocial treatments recommended for schizophrenia patients in the American Psychiatric Association's publication "Practice Guidelines for the Treatment of Patients with Schizophrenia" (1997) is not so much an algorithm as it is an anthology of diverse services and treatments that are felt to help a person with schizophrenia, offered without priorities and often independent of efficacy evidence. Such exhortations tend to complicate the formation of a relevant and well-justified algorithm, and they also run the risk of ultimately providing little or nothing to patients, since the implementation of all-encompassing recommendations may not only be overwhelming for administrators but economically unfeasible as well. However, even the Expert Consensus Guidelines contain some limitations. While they do reflect the priorities of "psychosocial treatment experts," this leadership group was clearly handicapped by the categories that were available for rating and the forced-choice nature of responses. It nevertheless serves as an historical undertaking, given the hundreds of therapies and contradictory theories that characterize the field of psychological and psychosocial treatment. Since the present author served on the editorial board that drafted the questions used to form the psychosocial treatment guidelines, he bears a certain responsibility for the incomplete results—and hence an associated obligation to reconsider a "best practice" approach to the implementation of empirically supported psychosocial treatments.

SOME LIMITATIONS OF THE EXPERT CONSENSUS GUIDELINES FOR SERVICES AND PSYCHOSOCIAL TREATMENT

We shall begin by taking a moment to review both the task placed before the psychosocial treatment experts and the results of their effort, as an introduction to the more narrowly drawn evidence-based guidelines that we suggest for psychosocial treatment. The questions rated by the experts relied on a scale of 1–9, where 9 represented the "extremely appropriate" treatment of choice; 7 or 8 indicated a "usually appropriate" but nevertheless first-line treatment; 4–6 represented a second-line treatment of equivocal importance; and scores of 3 or less represented clearly inappropriate treatments. The experts were instructed to base their ratings on their experience in treating schizophrenia, even though the important clinical questions had not been "adequately addressed or definitely answered" by necessary research. While different groups of experts rated medication guidelines, policy issues, and psychosocial treatments, we shall focus on the psychosocial guidelines. In addressing the psychosocial treatment needs of schizophrenia patients, various interventions, service delivery systems, staffing intensity/frequency of recommended contacts, and residential settings were rated. In this overview we shall focus primarily on the service delivery systems and the types of interventions that were recom-

mended. Further, these same questions were asked for each of four relatively distinct patient groups: (1) the first-episode patient, (2) the severely
impaired and unstable patient, (3) the moderately impaired and intermit-
tently stable patient, and (4) the mildly impaired and often stable patient.
As if this process were not sufficiently complex, the types of services,
interventions, settings, and residences of the four patient groups were
evaluated for each of three phases of illness: during an acute episode or exacerbation, during the early postepisode resolution phase, and during
maintenance.

Our overall impression of the more important recommendations is
next offered, followed by a brief commentary on the recommendations
themselves. First-line *service* recommendations were relatively few in number, perhaps a reflection of the current managed care environments that
limit reimbursement streams to only a few needed services. The *interventions* were largely generic recommendations that seemed not to bear a
close relationship to the cognitive, affective, social, and vocational impairments and disabilities of schizophrenia patients. Often these interventions
themselves represented services rather than treatments. Perhaps the circumscribed number of interventions rated and the fewer high recommendations made were themselves a concession to the legions of advocates
that would likely have championed their own preferred therapeutic approach had the door to psychological interventions been opened more
widely. Lastly, but of great importance, the guidelines provide little for
the "mildly impaired" and often stable patient, recommendations that ignore the treatment responsiveness of these patients and the inherent risk
that many will become more dysfunctional without appropriate psychosocial treatments.

Regarding services, although the recommendations were few, the options available for consideration were also relatively few. Examining the
distribution of expert evaluations for each question (pp. 57–68 of the report), the service system *MD appointments in conjunction with a non-MD
outpatient clinician* was the overwhelming first-line choice for a service delivery system for all four patient groups during all three phases of illness.
(*Assertive community treatment* also qualified, not surprisingly, for the severely impaired group.) *Case management* found prominence as a first-line
treatment in the early postepisode and maintenance phases for all patients
(surprisingly for first-episode patients as well), except for the mildly impaired. *Rehabilitation services*, to the chagrin of most mental health researchers, found a first-line endorsement only for the moderately impaired
patient during the maintenance phase of treatment. The services of the

psychosocial rehabilitation center and their psychiatric and vocational rehabilitation programs, the partial hospital program, and the day treatment center achieved little prominence and were variably rated as second- or third-line choices. One could only speculate about this apparent neglect, but relative unfamiliarity with the components of various rehabilitation, partial hospital, and the day treatment programs, when coupled with the training requirements of providers and the associated cost, might have contributed to the lower ratings. Service systems that received a "star" (defined as a first-line "9" treatment by more than 50% of the experts) were reserved *to assertive community treatment* during the acute and postepisode phases for the severely mentally ill, as well as to case management services for this group in the recovery phase. Otherwise, *MD appointments in conjunction with a non-MD clinician* achieved this highest status for severely impaired and moderately impaired patients, but only during the acute phase.

Regarding the interventions themselves, these fared somewhat better than service systems. Beyond some commonsense, generic prescriptions, however, the few well-studied and demonstrably effective interventions that were available for rating often failed to qualify as first-line treatments of choice. Topping the list of recommended interventions was *collaborative decision making with the patient*, not so much an intervention as a philosophical posture that might speak volumes to patient advocacy efforts that resist unilateral decision making by professionals. While not strictly defined in the glossary of terms (p. 21 of the report), this recommendation leaves one to ask about the potential for questionable decision making, if "collaboration" reflected the narrowly conceived "strengths model" discussed in Chapter 5. Unrealistic patient (or family) expectations for social and vocational goals described earlier in Chapter 6 might also qualify a number of collaborative decisions. Otherwise, *medication and symptom monitoring* (including *assistance obtaining medication*), were among the highest and consistently rated recommendations for all patient groups across phases of illness, recommendations that only loosely qualify as psychosocial treatments per se. So too for *patient and family education* (except for the severely ill patients in the acute phase), a first-line recommendation that at least has supporting evidence in the literature. *Assistance with obtaining services and resources* (seemingly a case management function) was the last uniform first-line intervention recommended, although mildly impaired patients were excluded. The remaining first-line treatment recommendations were reserved to a specific group or phase(s) of illness. For example, first-episode patients were the exclusive candidates for *supportive, reality-oriented individual therapy* in the postepisode and maintenance phase, leaving one to wonder whether other patient groups were felt not to profit from supportive therapy or whether the treatment was not worth the cost (i.e., therapeutic nihilism). *Training and assistance with activities of daily living* as well as *cognitive and social skills training* (in the maintenance phase) were also exclusively reserved for the severely impaired patients. Moderately impaired patients received their complement of these first-line recommendations, but mildly impaired patients received fewer. Recommended for both of these latter groups was *peer support/self-help groups* during the maintenance phase, a recommendation that appeared to be something of a "Bye now, . . . see you later" concession to these uncostly yet distinctly untested interventions. *Group therapy* received little endorsement, as did *supervision of financial resources, involuntary outpatient commitment,* and—not surprisingly—*psychodynamic psychotherapy*. Thus, the mental health interventions were most often variations of services, and these interventions were, in turn, sometimes grouped into one category (e.g., cognitive training and social skills training). Ignored in the process is the fact that these are two very different treatment approaches that can differ in terms of theory and method (e.g., developmental vs. behavioral) as well as treatment objectives. With the few exceptions noted, the recommended interventions rarely differed among the four patient typologies or the stages of illness. However, the greatest concern to us was the inclination of the experts to *decrease* the number of first-line interventions as impairment and disability lessened. First-episode patients did not always suffer from this "less is more" philosophy, but clearly the mildly impaired and often stable patients did.

The "squeaky wheel" approach to treatment allocation is, of course, prone to many problems. Most evidence regarding psychosocial treatment responsiveness and optimal recovery of function favors the less impaired and better premorbid patients in our opinion. This was clearly the case with PT, as described in Chapter 2, where the more symptomatic but somewhat less impaired did best. Most moderately or severely impaired patients began their psychiatric history as "mildly impaired." It would take many, many years of observation and follow-up before a clinician could correctly conclude that the seemingly "mildly impaired and often stable patient" would maintain this mental status over time. Too often, a seemingly stable course can take a disastrous turn, particularly when substance abuse enters the equation, in the absence of an appropriate intervention. Social and vocational *potential* is rarely achieved without psychosocial treatment. Were services and interventions to be withheld early in the course of illness, the opportunity for a significant *prevention* of long-term and persistent impairment could be lost. We gratefully note that the recommended frequency of contact for most patient groups in the different phases of illness was appropriate (one to four times a month as needed for the moderately impaired patients, and as high as one to five times a week for severely impaired patients). But no first-line recommendation for frequent contacts accrued to the mildly impaired patients. The recommendation for high caseloads (greater than 50 patients) and contacts every 2–3 months or less frequently appeared to be the recommended norm for this group.

When the mildly impaired (including the first-episode) patient is initially seen, it is well to remember that for most patients schizophrenia will be a lifelong illness. Functioning might return to premorbid levels for some patients, but it is rare that mild cognitive impairments (e.g., trait characteristics) ever disappear. These residual deficits can quickly escalate to state characteristics when patients become overly stressed. As we have described earlier, there is no "cure" for schizophrenia, only an arrest, much like what happens in the course of tuberculosis treatment by drugs such as isoniazid. At the present time, and certainly in the coming years, the wave of new atypical antipsychotic medications will do much to increase the number of mildly impaired and often stable patients. Do we then deprive these patients of needed interventions that enhance and sustain social and vocational functioning because they appear to be doing "pretty well" with a new medication, do not make costly demands on the service system, and otherwise serve the administrative need to fill low-surveillance caseloads? In a career that now spans many decades, the present writer is convinced that the overwhelming number of "mildly impaired" patients are simply doing better but are not necessarily well at any given time. It is the mildly impaired patients that are most likely to take on the greater challenges in the social and vocational areas, and so experience more potentially destabilizing crises. These patients need to be optimally prepared and intensively supported during these transitions. Ultimately, we need to capitalize on the potential of these patients for work beyond a minimum-wage job, housing beyond a substandard residence, education according to ability, and meaningful relationships beyond informal "acquaintances." Realizing the fullness of a patient's potential requires the application of highly specific and demonstrably effective interventions. The history of psychiatry, if large catamnestic and long-term treatment studies are any clue, leads firmly to the conclusion that society will either "pay now—or pay later" in terms of treatment costs, and probably at a greater and inflated price over time.

A PROPOSED PSYCHOSOCIAL
TREATMENT ALGORITHM

In the Cartesian spirit that a false premise will at least serve to stimulate more correct thinking, we offer the following psychosocial treatment guidelines as a way to better serve the needs of *all* schizophrenia patients. Ideally, these treatments would become core components of various service delivery systems, except that some, by definition, will be directed to the more disabled patients (e.g., assertive community treatment and case management). What we primarily propose to offer is a way to select and implement the more definitive and effective psychosocial treatments that are now available. Equally important, we feel that this selection should reflect the phase of illness: acute, stabilization, recovery, and postrecovery, the last of these being often referred to as the "maintenance" phase (which we view as lifelong for all but a small minority of patients).

We begin with some requisite qualifications. First, the psychosocial treatments that we recommend often include components that *overlap*. Obviously, one should not engage in unnecessary redundancy when sequencing these interventions. Family psychoeducation treatment (FPT) and PT are good examples. Rather than a vehicle that exclusively provides information on the nature of schizophrenia and its treatment (together with some recommendations for coping), FPT as designed by Falloon et al. (1985); Leff, Kuipers, Berkowitz, Eberlein-Vries, and Sturgeon (1982); Tarrier et al. (1989); and our own group uses psychoeducation as a tool for facilitating stabilization and the day-to-day management of schizophrenia, primarily a method for implementing the *patient's* treatment plan. Following the initial strategies for *connecting with family* and the *psychoeducation workshop*, the approach thus becomes *patient* rather than *family* centered. Prior to PT, FPT was the most effective stabilization strategy available for patients compared to the prominent individual approaches of skills training and supportive psychotherapy. PT has now been shown to be more effective than the later stages of FPT for stabilizing patients and enhancing social and vocational functioning (see Chapter 2 and Hogarty, Greenwald, et al., 1997). Thus, our recommended algorithm will often shift the patient's treatment plan to PT following the initial strategies of FPT. Social skills training (SST), although it offers precise prescriptions for specific and important deficits such as medication self-monitoring, friendship formation, job interviewing, and money management, will be largely reserved to the problems suffered by patients who are characterized by more severe and enduring impairments and disabilities, as reflected in empirical studies. As described earlier in this volume, selected skills training approaches are used in PT for stabilization, but less so once patients are able to function autonomously. Newer cognitive interventions such as integrated psychological treatment (IPT) [see Brenner et al., 1992; Spaulding et al., 1999]) and the schizophrenia modifications of cognitive-behavioral therapy (CBT) directly address the issues of social problem solving and basic cognitive operations, or medication-refractory symptoms in the case of CBT (see Fowler et al., 1995; Garety et al., 2000). In our own cognitive-enhancement therapy (CET), the improvement of *social* cognitive ability is uniquely targeted (see Hogarty & Flesher, 1999a, 1999b), with encouraging early results. Unfortunately, full implementation of our suggested algorithm needs to await the preparation of the CET manual (which is in progress), training tapes, and software for distribution.

The algorithm that we suggest will initially be relatively costly, but one needs to take the long view in terms of psychosocial treatment requirements over a life time. Once a patient has "passed through" our suggested treatment algorithm, for example, it is likely that continuing medication management and supportive therapy will be the principal treatment requirements needed throughout the age of risk. For those that maintain recovery or achieve an optimal level of functioning, "booster sessions" of specific PT coping strategies or CET strategies or SST and CBT principles can be used. Any patients who relapse subsequent to formal exposure to the recommended intervention(s) can return for a brief time to an *earlier* phase of an appropriate treatment, where a review of the relevant stabilizing strategies can be made and the necessary "polishing" of previously acquired coping skills can be undertaken. Once a patient has received the initial and full exposure to an intervention, subsequent decompensations should be manageable using less intensive versions of the intervention.

The choice of specific psychosocial treatments within our algorithm will be based on levels of *functional disability,* and less so on psychiatric history or symptom presentation. We shall classify disability as mild, moderate, or severe. As described earlier, the foremost goals of psychosocial treatment are to achieve and maintain stabilization, avoid relapse, and promote greater social and vocational functioning. Achieving stabilization following an episode is primarily accomplished through pharmacotherapy and the psychosocial control of sources of stress, both external and internal. Except for the effects of CBT on refractory positive symptoms, the best evidence of psychosocial treatment symptom specificity is reserved to a resolution of residual impairments of affect and secondary negative symptoms in the later stages of treatment.

The recommended algorithm does not directly consider the number of prior episodes, contacts with police, types of commitment, treatment compliance history, or other course descriptors in our definition of the disability typologies. (Implied, of course, is that episodes, compliance problems, and other indicators of a poor history might definitely favor one of the typologies.) Some could argue for alternative definitions of disability. We provide definitions for the three levels of disability below, with the essential qualification that a given patient can (and likely will) fluctuate among these levels of disability as environments and biology change over time, including the positive influence of increasingly more effective medications. The use of any typology, of course, carries with it the risk of stereotyping. "Chronic" is one term that comes to mind that often contains the sentence of hopelessness and therapeutic neglect. Viewing levels of disability as dynamic and not static processes might therefore serve to avoid the negative implications of pejorative classification.

When the clinician is selecting one of the three treatment pathways from the algorithm, the patient's level of functional disability can be assessed using the rating system outlined in Tables 7.1 and 7.2. The operational definitions derive from our current study of CET, although health care providers or agencies could just as likely use their own method for classifying patients, especially one that has shown to be useful in extended practice. Table 7.1 offers descriptive definitions of cognitive disability that reflect the cognitive styles that have found broad validation in the phenomenological study of symptom presentation in schizophrenia, including its important associations with underlying neuropsychological and neurobiological functions (see Hogarty & Flesher, 1999b). Impoverished cognition, for example, is most often disabling for patients whose clinical state is characterized by negative symptoms in the pre- and postepisode phases. Disorganized cognition reflects both symptoms of the acute phase and the cognitive operations that are frequently prominent during stabilization and recovery. Only the rigid (reality distortion) cognitive style is relatively difficult to assess; from a symptom perspective, these patients are typically hallucinated and delusional when acutely ill, but following symptom remission this cognitive style is not easily categorized. Most patients manifest a residually rigid, suspicious, and often paranoid style. One can "lump" the ratings of each type of cognition when deciding whether a patient suffers mild, moderate, or severe disability, since individual pa-

TABLE 7.1. Global Assessment of Cognitive Disability and Handicaps

Impoverished cognition	Very mild	Mild	Moderate	Severe	Very severe
Effortful planning and/or problem solving; difficulty initiating behavior; effortful retrieval (recall) of information from memory. Language does not adequately express needs, preferences, or opinions; does not give credible account of behavior; lack of stamina, slowed down; socially withdrawn, disinterested, apathetic, inactive; amotivated; poverty of speech.	1	2	3	4	5

Disorganized cognition	Very mild	Mild	Moderate	Severe	Very severe
Chaotic or imprecise planning; difficulty selecting a preferable problem-solving alternative; difficulty staying on task; easily distracted; failures to organize memory stores or use working memory "on-line." Inappropriate responses are not self-edited or monitored; difficulty using language coherently; readily changes goals, plans, or opinions; hard to follow train of thought; loose or impoverished ideas; impulsive; emotionally labile.	1	2	3	4	5

Rigid (reality distortion) cognition	Very mild	Mild	Moderate	Severe	Very severe
Plans, goals, problem solving limited by inflexible thinking or odd ideas. Behavior restricted by obsessive preoccupation with details; tends toward stereotyped, suspicious, or irrational views of individuals, events, and relationships; single-minded pursuit of inappropriate goals, career plans.	1	2	3	4	5

Note. Scoring system: Mild impairment = score of 3–6 (no "severe" or "very severe" score); moderate impairment = score of 7–10 (no "very severe" score); severe impairment = score of 11–15.

TABLE 7.2. Global Assessment of Social–Vocational Disability

Vocational ineffectiveness	Very mild	Mild	Moderate	Severe	Very severe
Unemployed or working below potential; reduced mental or physical stamina; uncooperative; unable to establish or maintain routine; unable to use feedback from coworkers, supervisors, or authority figures; unrealistic or absent career goals relative to vocational abilities or liabilities.	1	2	3	4	5

Interpersonal ineffectiveness	Very mild	Mild	Moderate	Severe	Very severe
Lack of empathy, flexibility, or understanding; inability to negotiate conflicts, express needs, control behavior when necessary, take the view of another person, or see self as others do; failures to act wisely in relationships (poor social judgment).	1	2	3	4	5

Lack of foresight	Very mild	Mild	Moderate	Severe	Very severe
Inability to assess long-term consequences (good and bad) of behavior; difficulty forming long-range plans.	1	2	3	4	5

Social context deficits	Very mild	Mild	Moderate	Severe	Very severe
Inability to understand formal or informal rules of conduct as social contexts change; inability to get central point, norm, or "gist" in a social situation.	1	2	3	4	5

Denial of disability	Very mild	Mild	Moderate	Severe	Very severe
Inability to temporarily revise expectations; failure to understand and/or accept residual limitations imposed by illness.	1	2	3	4	5

Note. Scoring system: Mild disability = score of 5–10 (no "severe" or "very severe" scores); moderate disability = score of 11–18 (no more than one "very severe" score or one "very mild" score); severe disability = score of 19–25.

tients will often share features of more than one style. For example, it would be most unusual for a patient to score "very mild" on one type of cognitive style and "very severe" on another.

Table 7.2 provides an operational definition of social and vocational disability that we have found to be a useful way to approach the rehabilitation needs of individual patients. However, we again acknowledge that the field is awash in descriptive definitions of social and vocational dysfunctioning. Our definitions rely on concepts that we have found best describe the constraints against social and vocational adjustment. If the ratings of cognitive disability and social–vocational disability differ, we would recommend that the social–vocational criterion be used whenever it indicates disability that is greater than cognitive disability, since the rating of cognitive operations might be less familiar to the practicing clinician. We offer these guidelines not as a rigid formula for classifying patients but simply as a guide to appropriate treatment. For example, a score of 18 on the social–vocational disability criterion that represents the upper limit of "moderate disability" could, in the judgment of the clinician, indicate a need for selected CBT or SST strategies that we might consider for the seriously disabled. Similarly, a score of 10 (the upper limit of mild disability), could lead the clinician to choose the "moderate disability" guideline in the face of other evidence. Such supplemental information might include the unavailability of needed community supports, or comorbid medical and/or psychiatric disorders.

The algorithm for mild and moderate disability assumes that a patient being evaluated is acutely ill and new to the provider system. The algorithm for severe disability should be reserved for patients that are known to the system and are currently in the stabilization or recovery phases. For example, many patients in the acute phase will clearly present as being "severely disabled" prior to active treatment. Not only could prior history suggest otherwise, but the response to appropriate medication and the recommended psychosocial interventions of the acute and stabilization phases for mild or moderately disabled patients will often result in symptom remission and behavioral integration that reflects a more appropriate mild or moderate disability. Thus, the rating of severe disability should be reserved for the status that follows the receipt of first-line interventions. The principal differences in the treatment strategies among levels of disability will be in the relative length and sequencing of treatment exposure for the mildly and moderately disabled, and in the nature of treatments that are recommended for the severely disabled.

The Mildly Disabled Patient

Figure 7.1 attempts to illustrate the treatment pathways that might be
followed for differently disabled patients. The upper register describes
the mildly disabled patient. It will be highly unlikely that a mildly disabled patient will quickly recover from an acute episode of schizophrenia and resume premorbid levels of functioning with no evidence of disability. (In the rare cases of a transient psychotic episode, one should

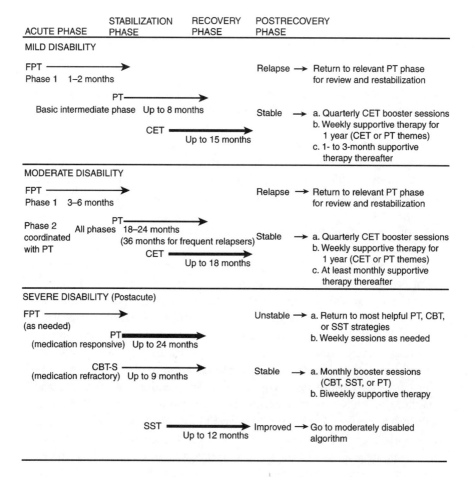

FIGURE 7.1. A psychosocial treatment algorithm for disabled patients with
schizophrenia. FPT, family psychoeducation treatment; PT, personal therapy;
CET, cognitive-enhancement therapy; CBT-S, cognitive-behavioral therapy for
schizophrenia; SST, social skills training.

look for evidence of substance abuse, extreme psychosocial stressors, or medical disorders that present with psychotic features. The last-named category may account for as many 8% of cases [Goldman, 1999], including neurological, central nervous system [CNS], autoimmune, metabolic, infectious [e.g., HIV], and endocrine disorders that evoke psychotic symptoms.)

Status as a first-episode patient should not mislead the clinician into concluding that recovery will be rapid and the subsequent course benign. (Recall the significant long-term morbidity of most first-episode patients that was cited earlier [Robinson et al., 1999].) Our experience has suggested that much in the way of patient and family psychoeducation will be needed, since denial of illness and medication noncompliance are often very high among first-episode patients. Achievement of clinical stabilization can also be extraordinarily difficult among these patients since the fullness of symptom presentation and deficit accretion are often most prominent processes in the early years of illness.

During the *acute* phase, when symptom presentation is greatest, the mildly disabled patient will likely spend but a brief period of time on an inpatient unit, one that is often measured in days or weeks. Partial hospitalization or outpatient alternatives to inpatient care will similarly require daily interventions for a period of weeks rather than months in most cases. A clue to the length of the acute phase (for all levels of disability) can often be found in the length of time that acute symptoms developed; that is, remission of symptoms will often be the "mirror image" of positive symptom onset. Active psychosocial intervention should be held to a minimum during the acute phase, since the goal is to achieve a remission of severe symptoms by establishing a therapeutic dose of an antipsychotic medication and the provision of a safe, stimuli-controlled environment. This means no exploratory group or individual psychotherapy, loud music, or forced social interactions that are often common on acute inpatient units, no matter how seemingly intelligent or verbal the patient might be. Peace, quiet, and a time to heal (asylum) are paramount. Our suggested psychosocial intervention during the acute phase represents the early (phase 1) components of family psychoeducation (i.e., connecting with the family, serving as an ombudsman, and providing a formal educational workshop, without the patient). The format for this manual-guided treatment can be found in our FPT volume (Anderson et al., 1986, pp. 28–130). Otherwise, acute phase programming should include the formation of a postacute treatment plan, an appraisal of the circumstances that might have precipitated the current episode, unsuccessful coping or problem solving regarding likely precipitants, and unmet needs and available resources. The plan to connect with the appropriate postepisode care providers should be initiated as soon as possible. For most mildly disabled patients, this process should not extend much beyond 4–6 weeks.

In the immediate postepisode, or *stabilization*, phase, the rudiments of basic and intermediate PT should begin as an alternative to the stabilizing strategies that previously were part of the FPT approach (described in Anderson et al., 1986, pp. 132–193). Most mildly disabled patients should be able to acquire the basic and intermediate PT strategies within 8 months. Once clinical stabilization is ensured, the treatment plan would then shift to CET in the *recovery* phase, an intervention that would attempt to advance social cognitive capacities beyond the selected strategies of advanced phase PT. The interactive software and social cognitive group curricula of CET will likely be completed by most mildly disabled patients within 15 months. Appropriate use of vocational and educational community services should be maintained.

If the mildly disabled patient has a subsequent relapse or otherwise becomes destabilized in the *postrecovery* phase (except for minipsychotic episodes that are readily aborted in 2–3 weeks), the patient should return to the last successfully negotiated stage of PT. Coping strategies designed to control the escalation of symptoms should be revisited and the curriculum maintained until restabilization is achieved. If the patient maintains stability and optimal social and vocational functioning, quarterly "booster" CET group sessions in the first *postrecovery* year are recommended. (Booster sessions will be defined in the forthcoming CET manual, which is being prepared for publication.) Weekly individual supportive therapy sessions in the first post-CET year that review CET or PT themes are also essential, since this is the period when most patients are likely to take on the challenges of a fuller life, yet also experience difficulty implementing CET skills. Monthly-to-trimonthly sessions geared to medication management and supportive psychotherapy (and relevant CET themes) should be routinely provided thereafter or until, in rare instances, the patient demonstrates that treatment is no longer needed. Treatment of the mildly disabled patient can be offered in the traditional outpatient clinic or the psychosocial rehabilitation center. Aside from the necessary assessments made by the primary clinician that are related to entitlement eligibility, food and clothing, housing, health care, and supported work or education, formal case management services will likely be unnecessary in most cases.

The Moderately Disabled Patient

The treatment guidelines for the moderately disabled patient will differ from those with mild disability in the length and sequencing of interventions. The moderately disabled patient will either present initially to the treatment system or enter by way of a reclassification of status from mildly or severely disabled. In the *acute* phase, programming should follow the recommendations made for mildly disabled patients, except that FPT will likely continue for a longer period of time (at least 3 months), extending into the *stabilization* phase in light of the need for families to become effective in managing this level of disability in a loved one (see Anderson et al., 1986, Ch. 4). As families become more secure and confident in the negotiated treatment plan and in their ability to cope and problem solve, treatment with PT will continue throughout the stabilization phase but formal FPT will end. Subsequent family contacts will focus on issues of support and information sharing. PT should continue until stability is ensured, a process that will likely include the social and vocational strategies of the advanced phase for patients who have experienced frequent episodes. For most patients, this treatment exposure will likely continue up to 24 months (36 months for advanced phase participants). In the *recovery* phase, CET should be considered for patients whose interests extend to a fuller social and vocational life but who continue to meet social and vocational disability criteria. An IQ of 85 or higher and symptom stability are currently the prerequisites for CET participation. Whether CET is appropriate for comorbid substance-misusing patients is untested at the moment. CET exposure up to 18 months following PT is recommended.

When moderately disabled patients experience a relapse in the *postrecovery* phase, they should also return to the PT phase that was last mastered for a review and practice of relevant coping strategies. Patients should remain in this treatment program until stability is reestablished. The booster sessions of CET described for the mildly disabled patient should also be pursued once the moderately disabled patient is stable and functional. (In a large program, these booster sessions can include mildly and moderately disabled patients.) The booster (group) sessions should be supplemented with weekly individual supportive psychotherapy sessions throughout the first postrecovery year that will include a review of status-relevant PT and/or CET principles . Again, most CET recipients will have the greatest difficulty implementing strategies in the first postrecovery year. Thereafter, at least monthly (and, for many patients, biweekly) therapy sessions are recommended throughout the age of risk. PT and CET can be provided either in the traditional outpatient clinic, the psychosocial (psychiatric) rehabilitation center, or the day treatment center, and supplemented by the vocational and educational services of community programs. Tasks related to eligible entitlements, housing, medical care, and other basic needs should be assumed by the primary clinician, supplemented by the services of an independent case manager when needed. A minority of patients will likely require the services of a the Program for Assertive Community Treatment (PACT).

The Severely Disabled Patient

Again, this determination should be reserved to the postacute phase for patients that are well known to the treatment system, although changes in status from mild and moderate disability will and do occur. In the *acute* phase, beyond the provision of early-stage FPT (which should have been provided earlier in the patient's history), we feel that the weight of treatment efficacy clearly favors a form of CBT for those with medication-refractory symptoms. Most patients in this typology will experience persistent positive symptoms. The CBT-S approach (see Garety et al., 2000) has been modified for schizophrenia patients who continue to experience a persistence of positive symptoms or otherwise remain refractory to medication. The course of treatment with CBT-S should continue up to 9 months until an optimal level of symptom stability is ensured.

Obviously, persistent and medication-refractory symptoms are neither readily nor easily defined. Recall, for example, that nearly all PT patients initially presented to the clinic with positive symptoms that had "persisted" throughout their recent inpatient stay, and throughout the postdischarge phase, albeit at a less severe level. But with appropriate medication, only 7% went on to persistent positive symptoms. The phenomenon of short-term persistent symptoms will likely become more common as inpatient lengths of stay continue to decrease. Thus, this classification requires time and a determination that medication strategies have been appropriate. Has the patient received an optimal dose of antipsychotic medication? Has this dose continued for at least 3 months? Has clozapine been introduced in the face of a suboptimal response to a first-line antipsychotic medication? Are noncompliance, substance abuse, or concurrent medical illness contributing to symptom persistence? Since all but 9 of 74 patients in our recent study responded to PT, we feel that PT also is clearly indicated for patients who are classified as being severely disabled, especially those that are able to achieve a decent remission of symptoms (i.e., who are medication responsive).

Severe social and vocational dysfunctioning (or persistent symptoms that fail CBT) can be addressed with a variety of SST modules that address specific patient needs and/or selected procedures of IPT (Liberman et al., 1999; Liberman & Eckman, 1989; Brenner et al., 1992; Spaulding et al., 1999). A 6- to 12-month exposure is recommended, depending on patient needs and responsiveness. The entire PT package might not be relevant for all patients, but the symptom-monitoring and control strategies of the basic and intermediate phases could be helpful, as would the program for prodromal management of Herz et al. (2000).

When severely disabled patients continue to do poorly at the symptom or functional levels in the *recovery* or *postrecovery* phases, the psychosocial literature provides little in the way of an alternative. At this point, one would want to look to the availability of investigational drugs (or electroconvulsive therapy) and then reevaluate the level of disability. Patients who remain severely disabled but have reached what is considered to be an optimal level of stability and community functioning should continue with relevant monthly booster sessions of PT, CBT, or SST and at least biweekly supportive psychotherapy sessions that include PT, CBT, or SST themes which were applied earlier and felt to be helpful. Patients whose level of disability improves should be returned to the guideline for moderately disabled patients. While the approach to treating severely disabled patients is capable of being implemented in the traditional outpatient clinic for some patients, most will likely be better served in the context of the psychosocial or psychiatric rehabilitation center, the day treatment center, or—depending on clinical status—the inpatient or partial hospital service. Intensive case management addressed to entitlements, housing, medical care, and other basic needs will frequently be required for a significant minority, most often provided in a comprehensive community treatment program (i.e., PACT).

In summary, we hope that PT's position in the treatment of schizophrenia and related disorders is more clear. PT can be considered a core psychosocial treatment for achieving and maintaining stabilization, as well as an important aid to the enhancement of social and vocational functioning for patients who do not qualify for CET. It should be preceded by a brief, manual-guided family intervention directed toward joining, informing, and supporting family members. For patients who subsequently have a successful exposure to at least the basic and intermediate phases of PT, a course of CET would ideally prepare them for either self-directed social and vocational initiatives or a more profitable use of vocational and educational training programs, as well as case management and PACT services. Agencies that are inclined to implement this psychosocial treatment algorithm might want to begin with patients that are new to the system. Once trained professionals and other resources are in place, these interventions can be made more broadly available to patients that are currently in the health care system. The psychosocial treatment algorithm will be relatively more costly to implement initially, but in time it will become less expensive as the reacquisition of previous coping strategies and booster sessions replace formal treatment programs. Avoiding relapse and rehospitalization, let alone enhancing personal and social adjustment, should eventually convince even the skeptic that strategic psychosocial treatments, when combined with modern psychopharmacology and the necessary service delivery systems, will constitute the most cost-effective and humane approach to managing severe mental illness in the foreseeable future.

To those who have persevered in the careful reading of this text, we express our gratitude for your interest in our work and for your dedication to the care of the severely mentally ill. We close this volume with a reminder that the PT principles and strategies discussed do not constitute an unchanging and rigid treatment formula. Rather, the process is intended to be vital and dynamic, with the various therapeutic strategies being selected according to the patient's needs and abilities. We have often indicated that the various components of PT have undergone dramatic development in the hands of behavior theorists, psychopharmacologists, stress management experts, and other schizophrenologists since PT was first designed and implemented. Undoubtedly this process will continue, particularly in response to neurobiological insights on pathoetiology, new developments in clinical psychopharmacology, as well as information related to psychosocial development, treatment mechanisms of action, and the contribution of genes and the environment to serious mental disorder. PT, as we have attempted to described it, simply provides a therapeutic scaffold from which this growing body of knowledge can be creatively shaped, molded, and tailored to the needs of the individual patient.

A Statistical Primer
for Clinicians

In this appendix, we shall take the opportunity to describe a few principles that characterize the various statistical procedures we have used in the evaluation of PT (and many of our previous interventions as well). We hope this brief review will be useful and provide confidence to readers who are perusing the clinical research literature in general. However, we shall only be discussing basic concepts, and the reader who wishes to learn more could profitably consult relevant textbooks. A valuable resource is the Dawson-Saunders and Trapp (1994) paperback entitled *Basic and Clinical Biostatistics* that provided much useful guidance. It is an excellent introductory text that is rich with many clinical examples.

BASIC STATISTICAL CONCEPTS

When researchers attempt to learn whether the clinical outcome of one treatment is better (or worse) than the outcome of another treatment, they most often use statistical tests that examine the *difference* between the *means* of an outcome measure. A mean, of course, is an average of many individual scores, and unless the scores are widely scattered, or one wishes simply to describe the scores (as we did in our description of the more individualized outcomes), the mean is preferable to other averages such as the *median* (a score at which 50% of cases are greater and 50% are less than the middle score). In clinical studies, the mean can represent the average score of some characteristic based on many ratings made on the same patient over time, or more often the average score for one or more groups of patients at one or more periods of time, especially when these groups have received different treatments. The score can represent a "subjective" judgment or rating of a patient's mood or behavior that has been made by the patient, the treating clinician, an independent observer, or a family member, for example. Or it can be a more "objective" assessment of some characteristic, such as the demographic measures of age and years of education, or a formal test that measures neuropsychological or intellectual abilities. If the rating is more subjective in nature, the clinician will want some assurance that multiple raters were "on the same page," so to speak (or a single rater agreed with an expert rater) regarding the meaning of the behavior being rated (called interrater reliability). While one might have more confidence in objective measures, nevertheless in the assessment of certain characteristics, such as measures of neuropsychological performance, the clinician will also want to be assured that the tests were administered consistently from one patient to another. These scores can be numerical measures (e.g., age), dichotomous measures (e.g., male or female), or ordinal measures (e.g., a measure that is ordered by some construct such as "severity"). The type of score often lends itself to one form of statistical testing more than another, as we shall see below. Since the question of a mean difference is so paramount in understanding clinical trials, one might ask what the statistical fuss is all about if one simply needs to determine whether the two means in a given study really differ from one another in an important and clinically meaningful way.

As it turns out, means can be misleading, or "misbehaved." This might be especially true when the scores derived from mentally ill patients are likely to be quite different in shape from the distribution of scores one would obtain in the "normal" population. Take, for example, two groups or samples of 10 people, and each sample has a mean score of 50 on a test that ranges from 0 to 100. The first group has 6 scores at 50, 2 scores at 45, and 2 scores at 55. In this sample, the mean is a decent or "reliable" average of these scores, with a symmetrical distribution of scores at or around the mean. The second sample has 4 scores at 60, 4 scores at 40, but 1 score at 0 and yet another at 100. Here the two large deviations from the mean (the scores of 1 and 100) would render this average "misbehaved" or in statistical terms "unreliable." Aside from the fact that the second sample might likely contain patients from a different population (something that we would not want to see in clinical treatment trials), these "outliers" would likely violate the assumptions that govern the use of more traditional approaches used to test the difference between the means. Therefore, before we proceed to test the difference between two means, we want to know at least three things:

1. Are the *distributions* of scores from which the means are calculated similar in shape (or symmetry) for both groups?
2. Are the sample means *reliable* or fairly true averages of the scores one would find with repeated sampling?
3. Can the difference between the means be explained away in *clinical* terms without using any tests?

Most of us can remember the familiar bell-shaped curve used to illustrate a distribution of scores that is "normal,"; that is, most scores are peaked at the top of the curve (which is typically where the mean lies), with some symmetrical distribution of scores trailing off to the left (below the mean) and to the right (above the mean) as in Figure A.1. In this normal distribution, the mean of our hypothetical outcome measure is 50, but one can also imagine curves with a mean of 40 or 60 that has individual scores that are also distributed around the mean in roughly the same proportions as those seen in Figure A.1. We would then say that the *variability* in scores and hence the shape of the score distributions around the mean of these latter two samples are *similar* and *consistent*, and we could more confidently proceed to test whether the means of 40 and 60 were in fact really different. In the real clinical world, more often the distribution of patient scores is not so symmetrically distributed, and we need a way to determine whether the means that are based on these distributions are sufficiently "well behaved" that we can legitimately test the difference. Ordinary statistical textbooks often overemphasize the importance of scores being "normally distributed," but in the case of clinical studies one would primarily want assurance that the shapes of the distributions (whether they are normal or skewed to the left or skewed to the right) are consistent between samples or across repeated attempts to collect scores from the same sample on different occasions. A way to conveniently estimate the *consistent vari-*

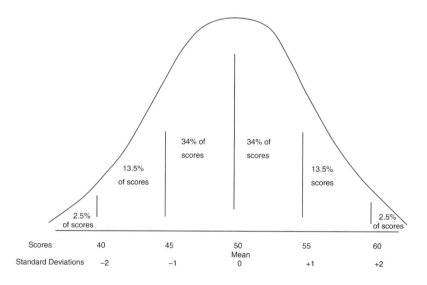

FIGURE A.1. Illustration of a normal distribution of scores with a mean of 50 and a standard deviation of 5.

ability or deviations among individual scores from the sample mean is, not surprisingly, called the *standard deviation* of the sample (written as *SD* or σ). (A "deviation" is the difference between an individual raw score and the mean of all scores in a sample.) The sample *SD* is calculated as the square root of the summed, *individual deviation raw scores* from the mean, once each of these deviations itself has been squared (i.e., multiplied by itself) and divided by the number of cases. It is written as $SD = \sqrt{\frac{\Sigma x^2}{N}}$ where Σ is the cumulative sum, x^2 is an individual deviation score squared, N the number of cases in the sample, and $\sqrt{}$ is the square root sign.

The *SD*, then, is the first clue for the clinician as to whether the distribution of scores is appropriate for testing, that is, roughly similar *SD*'s for each of the means being contrasted. Equally important, the SD provides information regarding the *spread* of individual scores around the mean. Again from Figure A.1 we can see that about 68% of all scores in the normal distribution would fall within 1 *SD* of the mean (34% below the mean and 34% above the mean). An *SD* of 2 would include about 95% of scores (almost 48% above the mean and almost 48% below), and by the time we get to 3 *SD*'s, nearly 100% of all scores would be accounted for. In the example used in Figure A.1, the mean is 50 and the *SD* is 5, such that 68% of our scores would fall between the scores of 45 and 55 and 95% of scores would fall between the scores of 40 and 60. Obviously, then, the larger the *SD*, the less accurate the sample mean will be as an indicator of the true population mean. In our earlier example, for the 10 people in the first sample (who showed a symmetrical distribution of scores), the *SD* is 3.1, thus illustrating that the mean of 50 is fairly close to all individual scores, even those that are the farthest away. In the second sample that contained the outliers, the *SD* is 24, indicating that some scores are indeed quite removed from the mean of 50. In the real world, however, as sample size increases, the scores and hence the standard deviations tend to become more normally distributed.

Having determined that there is an adequate compactness and similar shape to the scores within each of the samples we wish to compare, but before we actually apply a test of the mean difference, we need to be assured that the means themselves are *reliable,* or really good indicators of the true averages one would find in repeated sampling, by correcting for any sampling *error* that would have moved our specific sample means away from the true population mean. Two factors greatly influence the reliability of the mean: the *number* of subjects in the sample, and of course the *SD* that we just discussed. If we have a small sample, say, of 10 patients, an additional case might change the mean dramatically. On the other hand, if we had 100 patients, one additional score should have little influence on the mean. In order to account for differences that arise from different sample sizes, or sampling error, as well as the variability of scores around the means that we wish to contrast, statisticians use a measure called the *standard error of the mean,* written as *SE* or σ_m. A small *SE* indicates that the mean of our sample is likely to be very close to the mean of the entire population were we to go out, for example, and survey many samples, say of patients with the same diagnosis. This *SE* is obtained by first calculating the *SD* (the variability of the scores) in a given sample and then dividing this *SD* by the square root of the number of cases or, in small samples, the number of cases minus 1. The *SE* is thus the standard deviation of a specific *mean* from the population *mean*, according to sample size! Again, the *SE* gets smaller as the number of subjects (*N*) gets larger (or, more accurately, as the square root of *N* gets larger). In short, the *SD* represents variability in *individual scores*, whereas the *SE* represents variability in individual *means* and rises or falls depending on the number of cases. A sample of 100 patients with a mean of 50 and an *SE* of 1 indicates that the true mean likely to be found in future sampling of the population from which the sample was drawn would fall between 49 and 51. However, a contrasting sample with a larger *SE*, say, of 10 points, and a mean of 50 would leave us in the dark as to whether the mean of this sample was anywhere near the true mean of the larger population (somewhere between 40 and 60), thus making the test of a difference between two means that included this unusual mean very questionable and difficult indeed. Again, it is important to remember that the *larger* the sample the *smaller* the standard error tends to be, whereas the *SD* should be *similar* across samples and times when the sample sizes are adequate (30 or more) and representative of the larger population.

In a significant number of clinical studies of psychotherapy, the contrasting samples have often been so small and the *SE*'s of the means sufficiently large that it has been almost impossible to determine what the true means actually were that were being tested for a "significant" difference. Small samples open the door to the possibility that the scores are randomly distributed and the mean difference observed is not real, but rather is a *chance* finding. (We shall return to this problem a bit later.) The ultimate tests of mean differences that depend on clear assumptions about how the distribution of scores should be shaped or whether the scores and their means fall within acceptable "parameters" or boundaries of variability, given the number of cases involved, are appropriately called *parametric tests*. Now that we have considered the mean, its reliability, and how it is affected by the number of cases in the sample, when we discuss the more common parametric tests used in clinical studies the latter should be easier to understand.

Before turning to the actual tests themselves, we should comment on the third line of defense against the "misleading mean," the practitioner's own informed clinical judgment! In a clinical study of acute depression, for example, if the *pretreatment* means for both samples being compared were about 16, with an *SD* of 8 on the popular Hamilton Depression Scale, the clinician would be correct in thinking that a good number of these patients might only have been mildly "sad" to begin with (e.g., those with a score of 8 or less). If a form of psychotherapy applied to one sample ultimately proved to be "significantly" better than a medication given to the other sample, it would probably not be legitimate to boast that psychotherapy is "better than medication for depression" (which has some-times happened). Rather, in a sample that contained a proportion of mildly "de-pressed" individuals, one could only say that psychotherapy was effective, and lit-tle or nothing could be said about the medication. Medication would probably have been *contraindicated* in those patients who were 1 or more *SD*'s below the mean. Thus, the treatment test might not have been appropriate in the first place, since medication is not usually a treatment of choice for people who only suffer the "blues" from time to time. At least, one would want to know a great deal more about these patients, including their past history of depression, prior response to treatments, social dysfunctioning, and the like.

Recently, we had the chance to examine a report on a new cognitive rehabili-tation approach in schizophrenia that showed no apparent increase in benefit over a standard treatment. When we examined the mean scores of the pretreatment, neuropsychological subtests that likely reflected IQ, we concluded that the rela-tively low mean scores and the large *SD*'s around these means probably indicated that a substantial number of patients were being included in the study who had *mental insufficiency*. No reasonable clinician would conclude that a cognitive inter-vention should be judged to be ineffective if it failed to generate "normal" neuro-psychological functioning among the mildly retarded. Thus, the clinical "meaning of a mean," when understood in terms of its point on a scale, can often inform the practitioner whether any subsequent statistical test would be clinically warranted or informative.

Otherwise, whenever a researcher resorts to a "parametric test," namely, one that assumes a consistency in the distribution of scores when testing mean differ-ences (such as the *t* test or the analysis of variance [ANOVA] and its associated *F* test, described below), the clinician will again want to ask whether there are any *outliers*, or "oddball" cases who have extreme scores. This is a most serious concern in small samples, since a single, extreme outlier could eliminate a difference. For example, while the mean difference might appear to be large, the outlier also in-flates the error term, often rendering the difference to be nonsignificant (see the *t* test below). A clue that outliers might be present can often be found in the form of a relatively larger *SD* or *SE* for one of the means. But we have also seen in our own studies that a few outliers in a sample can influence test results even when each sample contained nearly 100 patients! (The researcher should inspect the ac-tual distribution of scores before applying a test.) When outliers are present, the researcher should have either (1) not used parametric tests or (2) if the problems were minor, then the scores should have been "normalized" by taking the log or the square root of all scores, for example. The major lesson to be learned, how-ever, is that a large mean difference in *small* samples (e.g., 10 or 15 cases) *might* mean that an atypical, randomly varying case or two has accounted for the "signif-icant" difference or lack thereof, rather than indicating an outcome that is true for the majority of cases in the sample!

PARAMETRIC TESTS

When a researcher applies a statistical test in order to determine whether the observed difference between two means is *significant*, the question or *hypothesis* is stated in such a way as to make it difficult to claim that the observed difference is really important. The beginning assumption that the observed difference is not real or not significantly different from a zero difference is called the "null" hypothesis and it will take a lot in the way of well-behaved *SD*'s and *SE*'s of the means to reject this hypothesis of "no difference" between the means. Generally, we will say that the observed difference is significant if it would occur by chance or *randomly* only 5 times in 100 independent studies. This "probability" (called alpha) of a chance finding is designated as the *p* value, and in this case the *p* would be written as $p = .05$ if it were exactly determined, or $p < .05$ if the probability of a chance finding is less than 5 out of 100 trials. (If the exact probability of being *less than* five out of 100 is known, the probability of a chance finding can be written as 1 out of 100 [$p = .01$] or 1 in 1,000 [$p = .001$].) If we tested two treatment means and had made no real assumptions before the experiment as to whether the new (experimental) treatment was better or worse than the standard treatment, we would be accounting for the variability, or distribution of scores that are both above and below each mean (e.g., the "tails" of the distribution noted as $\pm$ in Figure A.1. We would indicate that our *p* value in this instance is from a "two-tailed test." If an efficacious treatment, such as family psychoeducation, had already shown positive results in a number of prior studies that sought to lower relapse, we could in our next study of this approach legitimately use a "one-tailed test" of relapse on the assumption that our patients' relapse rate would not likely be greater with family treatment and in fact would likely be skewed in the direction of surviving without relapse. In general, the *p* value for a one-tailed test is *twice as great* as that for a two-tailed test, for example, a *p* of .05 two-tailed is about .025 in a one-tailed test (a 2.5% probability of a chance finding in every 100 trials), and similarly a *p* of .10 two-tailed (a 10% "trend" that does not represent an acceptable level of significance) could be deemed acceptable in a one-tailed test, where *p* would then equal .05. In the clinical literature, the reader should know that most editors and peer reviewers tend to frown on the use of one-tailed testing. However, because of increased costs associated with clinical trials, the noted statistician H. C. Kraemer (1991) suggests that one-sided tests might be used when differences in only one direction have regulatory significance.

The *t* Test

The *t* test between two samples is one of the most frequent parametric tests that a clinician will encounter when reading the results of clinical trials. Most often a clinical study will be comparing two or more treatments, and the *t* test provides a simple estimate of whether the observed difference between two means of interest is important or statistically significant. It is calculated by simply taking the observed *mean difference* (the numerator) and dividing this difference by the *SE* of the two means (the denominator). (Note in this example involving two treatment groups that the *SE* of the difference between the two treatment means would be calculated using the *pooled SD*'s of the two means being contrasted and the respective sample sizes.) The mean difference has thus been *standardized* once it is divided by the SE of the mean (i.e., converted to *SD* units), and one can look up the standardized difference on a table of *t* that is contained in most statistical textbooks to determine whether the difference is significant at the 1%, 2%, or 5% levels. We provide an abbreviated example of the *t* table in Table A.1. The statistical significance of a given *t* value will absolutely depend on the size of the sample, which is expressed as "degrees of freedom" (*df*), that is, the number of cases minus 1. For example, Table A.1 illustrates that a total sample with 10 *df* would require a *t* of 2.23 in order to be significant at the $p = .05$ level, but a sample with 100 *df* would only require a *t* of 1.98.

The clinician will recall that the majority of studies that have contrasted two forms of psychotherapy (typically without a control condition) have often failed to demonstrate that the outcome means were different. More often than not, this lack of difference can again be traced to the fact that the samples were simply too small (or that one mean *might* have differed from the control group mean had a control condition been included in the study; see Persons & Silberschatz, 1998). As mentioned above, an inadequate number of patients in a sample will frequently result in more variable scores and thus a larger *SD* and larger *SE* (a large denominator) as well as fewer degrees of freedom and therefore the need for a "really big" difference between the two means in order to be significant. Studies that lack the sample sizes needed for appropriate testing (or that suffer problems in sampling) are often referred to as being "underpowered," or unable to detect a true difference. They are subject to what is called type II error, that is, detecting no differ-

TABLE A.1. Examples from the Table of *t*

Degrees of freedom (*df*)	Probability (*p*) value			
	.10	.05	.02	.01
10	*t* = 1.81	2.23	2.76	3.17
20	*t* = 1.72	2.03	2.53	2.84
30	*t* = 1.70	2.04	2.46	2.75
50	*t* = 1.68	2.01	2.40	2.68
100	*t* = 1.66	1.98	2.36	2.63
200	*t* = 1.65	1.97	2.35	2.60
Infinity	*t* = 1.65	1.96	2.33	2.58

ence when in fact a larger or more appropriate sample would likely have found a difference. (Type I error, on the other hand, follows upon misbehaved means, differently shaped distributions, or outliers, and hence random variation that leads the researcher to claim that the treatments are really different when in fact they are not. In such a case, the study might indeed be one of the "5 in 100" experiments where the mean difference is, in fact, a chance finding. Type I error is considered to be the larger problem.) Often the difference between the two means can be "eye-balled" for significance—for example, by graphically drawing the two distributions and their *SD*'s (like the bell-shaped curve) and inspecting the amount of *overlap* between the curves to see if the overlap is small and thus significantly different, or large and not different. Larger overlapping curves remind us that when we accept the null hypothesis of "no difference," we do not necessarily imply that the two means are identical. Rather, we acknowledge that there is a relatively small range of scores within which the two means might fall but that such minor mean differences would not be significantly different statistically.

When the samples being contrasted share characteristics (such as carefully matched cases with the same diagnosis that were randomly assigned to two different treatments), or when the same patients were assessed (sampled) at two different times (e.g., at pre- and posttreatment), then the clinician will want to be assured that the "paired *t* test" was used. The advantage here is that the *SE* of the mean difference (the denominator) can be made smaller by literally subtracting from the error term the *correlation* that exists between the scores in each sample. Decreasing the denominator, obviously, provides for a more sensitive test of the mean difference.

Simple though the formula might be, a failure to appreciate the meaning of a *t* value (or any other statistic) and the *confidence* that we can place in its value might often serve as an obstacle to understanding study results. Although some might cringe at the following explanation, think of the *t* value as an *SD of the difference between the means of interest and how far this SD is from zero*. Again, a *t* is essentially the mean difference score that has been standardized (i.e., converted to a score that has a mean of zero and an *SD* of 1). Now, from our earlier discussion, remember that the *SD* gives us a clue as to where scores (or in this case the *mean differences*) would fall if normally distributed after many experiments: about 68% of the standardized difference scores would fall within ± 1 *SD* of zero, 95% of the difference scores would fall within ± 2 *SD*'s, and 99% of the difference scores would be within ± 3 *SD*'s from zero. If, in a sample of 200 patients randomly assigned to treatment A and B, a *t* of 1.97 (or nearly a 2 *SD* difference from zero) would allow us to conclude that the probability of observing this difference by chance would be only 5 out of 100 trials (i.e., *p* = .05). We would have 95% confidence that this was a real difference. As confident as we might be, we would still be close to saying that no difference exists, since the .05 level places us closer to a zero difference than an .01 or .001 level of significance. The *confidence interval,* the range of difference scores within which the mean difference is likely to be found based on the *SD* of a specific mean difference, or *t*, is often used in place of the *t* value, but it essentially provides us with the same information as the *t* value itself. In essence, what we need to remember when interpreting *t* values is that the observed mean difference will be significant or not depending on its difference from zero when converted to a standard deviation unit. The closer our *observed* raw score difference and its standardized *range* gets to 0, the less assured are we that the difference is real.

Figure A.2 attempts to graphically illustrate what the *t* value for a .05-level test would be like in order to say whether a mean difference *is* significantly different from zero (reject the null hypothesis of no difference) or whether it is *not* significantly different from zero (accept the null hypothesis) using a two-tailed test. Figure A.2 again reminds us that every parametric statistic (or value) that we calculate has its own *distribution*. In the case of the *t* statistic (again, a measure of the mean difference expressed essentially in the form of a standard deviation), we are simply indicating that the value is significantly greatly than zero, given the *SD* and the number of subjects. For a *one-tailed test* of $p = .05$ (or $p = .10$ two tailed), the standard deviation *t* value needed would only be about 1.65 instead of 1.96 (as can be seen from Table A.1), that is, a *t* greater than +1.65 would represent a significant difference. We would in this case ignore the other "tail" (−1.65). However 1.65 is a bit closer to zero than 1.96.

When calculating *t* tests on many measures that are characteristic of the two samples, we need to guard against the "error" or mistake that often comes from

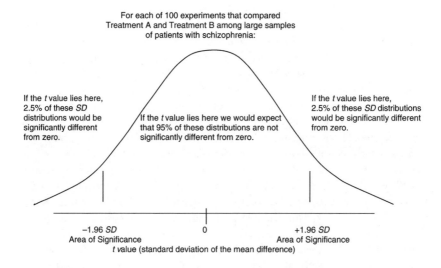

FIGURE A.2. Illustration of a *t* test at the $p = .05$ level of significance using a two-tailed test.

multiple testing. Think of this as a case where a whole construct (comprising, e.g., numerous symptoms of schizophrenia) should first be shown to be significantly different between the two groups before examining each of the symptoms one by one. (In the major results of PT [Chapter 2], all of our *t* tests were protected by an overall, larger multivariate test, such as the initial tests of the multivariable composite measures in our multivariate regression analysis.)

When performing individual univariate tests, if we did one 5% test on a specific psychotic symptom (e.g., hallucinations) to see if it were different between the groups, there would be a 1 in 20 chance of obtaining an erroneous finding. If we then did another 5% test on another specific symptom (e.g., delusions), our potential error (called the experiment-wise error rate) could rise to 2 in 20, or 10% (i.e., the chance that only one of the two tests is significant). With six specific tests of six symptoms (.05 × 6) our error rate could conceivably rise to almost 30% (actually 27% using a more exact formula). This type of error calculation is useful with a small number of tests, since theoretically it is impossible to have a 100% chance of error. In the example of two tests, we could limit the chance for increased error that follows multiple univariate testing by requiring a more stringent *p* value in the first place (e.g., *p* = .025 rather than .05), or by making an adjustment to our *p* value (such as the Bonferroni adjustment) that takes the 5% error rate and divides it by the number of tests being made in order to derive a more stringent *p* value. (We tend not to use this type of adjustment in our own work for reasons that go beyond this discourse.) In our description of the predictors of PT outcome (Chapter 2), we were using univariate tests not as tests of specific hypotheses but rather as suggestions of possible associations between treatment, outcomes, and individual patient characteristics (i.e., posthoc exploratory analyses). There are, however, a number of ways to test multiple hypotheses at the same time without encountering this type of error (e.g., comparing three different treatment groups) such as using the ANOVA approach described below. Or one could also test an overall hypothesis using many characteristics of the samples at the same time by way of a test called the discriminant function analysis, which is powerful in detecting complex patterns.

Effect Size

Much attention in the clinical literature these days has been drawn to a statistic known as the effect size (*ES*), which is an extension of the *t* value. The *ES*, even though it can be described at a statistically significant level, attempts to convey the clinical *magnitude* of a treatment effect. The *ES* can be for a correlation, or a proportion, or—in the case of the PT studies a mean difference. Here the meaning of the effect size bears a very close relationship to the *t* test itself. Whereas the *t* value represents a conversion of the absolute mean difference to a standard deviation of the difference from a mean of zero, the ES returns to the absolute mean difference and expresses this difference in standard deviation units around the actual observed means. The t value and the ES can be directly derived from one another. From Table A.1, for example, a t value of 2.0 with approximately 50 patients in the study ($p = .05$), would convert to an ES of 0.28. Similarly a t of 2.8 derived from a sample of about 20 patients ($p = .01$) would have an ES of 0.63. Most often, it is authors of a meta-analysis (see below) that will use the t (or the F statistic) from many studies and convert these values to an ES. Just as in the case of t or F, however, the ES needed to be judged statistically significant in a meta-analysis will decrease as the different sample sizes increase. From a clinical point of view, we would say that a mean difference between two groups that is one-third of an SD different ($ES = 0.33$) would be very suggestive of a clinically important dif ference; an ES of one-half and SD (0.50) would absolutely be clinically meaningful, and an ES greater than 0.75 or even 1.0 could likely provide the basis for a clinical mandate if independently validated.

The F Test and the Analysis of Variance

The analysis of variance (ANOVA) is a way to test multiple hypotheses at one time. The principle used in calculating an SD provides a good transition to the principle used in calculating the F ratio. Recall that the SD takes the square root of the sum of the squared deviations of individual scores from the sample mean, divided by N. Now the F test sums the *variance* in these scores (which is essentially the SD of a given mean that has been squared) and compares these variances around *different* means as a ratio (called the F ratio). The sums of the squared scores are additive, so they can be divided into component parts. The F test is most often used in clinical research when three or more groups are being compared. If we have three groups—A, B, and C—we have three possible tests: A versus B, A versus C, and B versus C. (If we add a fourth group D, then six tests are possible.) ANOVA gives us a way to "protect" the 5% chance level by treating all the subsample comparisons as one experiment, but the overall difference would have to be greater than a simple t test. ANOVA begins by summing the squared deviation of each patient's score from the *grand mean* of the entire population of patients being studied (i.e., the total sum of the squares). ANOVA simply takes this total amount of variance and divides it up into the summed squared deviations (variances) of individual patient scores *within* their own *group mean* and the sum squared deviations (variances) *among* the group means themselves, calculated in terms of the individual group mean deviations from the grand mean. The F test comes into play as a ratio between these different "sums of squares." If the variance among the individual group means is much larger than the variance of scores around the grand mean, this ratio will be expressed as a significant F statistic for a group difference. If the ratio is not significant, the test tells us that the variance among patients within each of the groups is about the same as the variance among the groups themselves. Thus the ANOVA, while relying on the variance around the different group means, is really a test that determines whether the group means are truly equal or not. The F ratio for a group difference is the sum of the squared deviations from the grand mean for all the group means being tested (three or more), called the *among group mean squares*, which is then divided by the variance within the groups called the *mean square error* term. Unfortunately, and this is most important, when the ANOVA yields a significant F ratio, it only indicates that the groups being compared are different *overall*. It does not tell us which specific groups are different from each other!

Here one needs to return to the t test in order to determine which pairs of means are significantly different from each other. The clinician might ask, "Why not just do the various t tests without the hassle of computing an ANOVA?" The reason once again is that we need to protect our univariate t testing (i.e., reduce the probability of a chance finding that follows multiple testing) with a multivariate, significant F ratio. The various post hoc comparisons between the means of interest (such as the A vs. B, A vs. C, and B vs. C contrasts noted above) can be made in a more stringent or conservative manner than the simple t test. When there is a significant F test from the ANOVA, most ad hoc tests of the individual mean differences assume that there is a common error term for the various tests and that the group sizes do not differ randomly. With these restrictions, various procedures try to hold the number of tests (and the need for correction) to a minimum. One that is often used when testing independent pairs of means following ANOVA is the *Tukey test*, a procedure that makes corrections similar to the Bonferroni approach by adjusting for the number of independent groups or levels in the ANOVA. The *Sheffé procedure* is a more conservative approach (e.g., a special case that will accommodate any number of tests or combination of means), but it requires a larger value for the t test. The *Student's range test* is a t test of the largest differences among many comparisons, while the *Newman–Keuls test* is a form of multiple t testing when the comparisons involve ranks rather than raw means.

The process described above, a test of multiple group means, is called a "one-way" ANOVA; that is, we are simply testing three groups at one point in time on a single factor, in this case different forms of treatment. In clinical trials research, however, we often want to describe our various groups in terms of one or more additional variables called "factors" that might affect outcome. When we add another factor, such as sex, we now have a "two-way" analysis of variance and thus more groups for our numerator; that is, we are able to test both the effects of the different treatments among our groups and the treatment effects on the two sex groups. In our example, we would have three treatment groups × two sex groups in our design, or six cells available for possible tests or hypotheses that we could approach in a single analysis. (If we tested this sample at another time(s), we would also have another group term called "periods.") We can determine the main effect of treatment by calculating the F ratio as described above, that is, the among group mean squares (or sums of squares) for the groups divided by the mean square error (or the within treatment groups sums of squares). And we can determine the main effect of sex independent of the treatment received (the sums of squares for the two sex groups divided by the within sex group error) and, perhaps more important, we can also test the *interaction* between treatment and sex (e.g., whether a treatment has a positive effect among females vs. a negative effect among males).

Sometimes, we might not be interested in an interaction at all if, using our example, females had traditionally been shown to do better than males on all previous tests of these treatments. But we still might want to remove the variance associated with sex from the error term (making the denominator smaller) when testing the treatment group effect, thus producing a larger F ratio. The error variance within the six treatment by sex groups would be less than the error variance within the three treatment groups themselves. While this seems counterintuitive (since six means are twice the number of the three treatment means), remember that the six individual subsamples would be smaller, their means might likely better fit or represent the scores within each group, the deviations from each subsample mean would accordingly be smaller, and hence their "squares" or variances would be less. While this might sound a bit confusing, this is precisely how researchers remove (or "control for") the effect of an independent variable when calculating an F test on treatment outcome. Otherwise, we might want some reassurance that the females in our new experiment continued to show a superiority over males, as they had in past studies. If, using this example, there is not a sex effect in our new study, we would need a good explanation for its absence. Were these females really representative of the larger female population of patients? Or does one of the treatment groups have considerably more females than another treatment group so that treatment and sex are *confounded* in such a way that we do not know which factor is causing the effect?

Finally, when we have two or more assessment periods on the same treatment groups, we could conduct what is called a *repeated measures* ANOVA. Here we are calculating a new "group" measure or numerator, namely, a *change* score between pre- and posttreatment that accounts for the fact that the two sets of scores are derived from the same patients. Again, the change score can be adjusted in terms of the independent variable(s) of interest. The F test on the amount of change in a two-group repeated measures ANOVA essentially resolves to a t test that has been squared. For the most part, however, we tend to avoid formal applications of the repeated measures ANOVA in our studies because of technical problems that might arise when scores on an individual patient are missing at a rating period and when an initial level difference exists in spite of random assignment. Rather, we often prefer a careful analysis of covariance (ANCOVA) as our test of treatment effects at each assessment period.

ANCOVA is a version of ANOVA that allows us to "covary" or correct the posttreatment means in terms of many important independent variables such as the patient's sex, age, race, and particularly the baseline rating of the dependent variable itself (i.e., the initial level). The effect is to take the variance attributed to the independent variable and remove it from the error term (the denominator), thus yielding a more robust *F* test. Adjusting posttreatment means in terms of initial-level or other variables is quite legitimate when the minor group differences at baseline have occurred by chance, as is true in the random assignment design. But when random assignment has not been used, it is questionable whether ANCOVA results should be showcased since the initial differences might be real and not chance and thus reflect a systematic bias in sampling or even confounding that one would not want to conceal statistically.

Interpreting the *F* ratio at different levels of probability and with different sample sizes is much the same as interpreting the *t* value. (As indicated above, if we had conducted an ANOVA using just two groups, the F value would be identical to the *t* value squared.) The principal difference in interpreting a table of *F* and a table of *t* is how the degrees of freedom are calculated. Whether an *F* value is significant at a given *p* value depends on the degrees of freedom (*df*) for both the denominator and the numerator—not exclusively for the denominator as in the *t* test. The *df* for the numerator is the number of groups being compared minus 1. In our example of three treatment groups, the *df* for the numerator would be 3 minus 1, or 2. If we had 50 patients in each of the three groups, the *df* for the denominator would be 150 minus the 2 *df* for the groups (or 148) minus 1 (a correction for our *N*), resulting in 147 *df* for the denominator. From a table of *F* we could determine that with 2 *df* and 147 *df* we would need an *F* of 3.00 for an .05 level test of significance, and an *F* of 4.61 for an .01 level of significance.

In summary, the ANOVA simply takes the total sum of all squared deviations from the grand mean, then divides this total variance into its component parts: the variance attributed to groups, the variance associated with any interaction, and the variance within each group being contrasted.

The Correlation

Nothing is more common (but often misinterpreted) than the simple Pearson linear correlation that is expressed as *r*. (There are other forms of correlation that we shall only describe briefly.) Much like the mean and *SD*, the Pearson correlation also has a special relationship with the normal distribution if the measures of the two variables being compared are continuous and normally distributed. Unfortunately, this is often not the case and a very high or very low correlation might indicate a problem with sampling. For example, if we wanted a measure of association (or correlation) between height and weight but only sampled people who were between 6'1" and 6'2", our correlation would erroneously be very low because the measure of height was not widely distributed and thus had very little variance to account for. The mental health literature too often contains studies of sorts that are essentially one-time, "single-shot," cross-sectional associations of variables within a sample. The correlations that are presented are sometimes explicitly or implicitly inferred as being "causal," or predictive of future status, when they are not (see Kraemer, Yesavage, Taylor, & Kupfer, 2000). As an extreme example, if we correlated the number of taxi cabs with the number of chronic schizophrenia patients in an urban sector, we could hardly conclude that the taxi cabs caused schizophrenia. Most often these correlations are examples of antecedents and consequences (like the night following the day), rather than cause and effect.

The correlation is often a clinical research concern when it is used as an estimate of the agreement between the raters of treatment outcome, an estimate that is called *interrater reliability*. Essentially, this form of reliability has two dimensions: whether the scores of the raters are parallel (i.e., in a similar direction) and whether the actual levels are similar (i.e., the number of identical ratings made, subject by subject). The researcher can satisfy one direction but not the other and still have relatively poor agreement although the *r* might appear to be high. Say, for example, that an expert had determined that the total symptom scores of five criterion patients were all 30. Now rater A rated the five patients 25, 26, 27, 28, and 29, and rater B rated the patients 31, 32, 33, 34, and 35, respectively. The correlation *r* would be high since the scores are parallel and in a similar direction that corresponds to the criterion. But we could not necessarily conclude that there was agreement between the raters regarding level. In fact, a *t* test of the mean differences between raters A and B would likely show them to be significantly different. Conversely, levels could appear to be similar although the scoring is not parallel. Say, both raters classified five patients as mildly ill and five as moderately ill, but rater A's mildly ill patients were rater B's moderately ill patients and vice versa. Sometimes, a researcher will report a form of rater agreement called the *intraclass correlation coefficient* that accommodates both the direction and the level (but not very well, in our opinion). We tend to inspect each dimension of rater reliability separately, for example, by using the simple Pearson *r* for direction, and applying a paired *t* test to see if the raters are different. For categorical (but not continuous variables) we will sometimes construct 2×2 tables and estimate the identical matches that occur beyond chance (or guessing) using a summary measure called the *kappa coefficient*.

If the truth be known, attempting to maintain interrater reliability for many years over the course of a clinical trial has often been as difficult as catching flies in the dark. Critics can be overly harsh, discounting studies that have not reported high rater agreement on all measures used in the study. While we look for assurances that our raters are using the same criteria when we introduce a new rating scale, rarely is it possible to achieve near-identical ratings on the same criterion subjects when numerous rating scales are used on many occasions. (Some investigators appear to harass clinical staff for variations in the "reliability" of their ratings, and in other instances have been moved to actually fire otherwise good clinicians.) When patients in our studies have been randomly assigned to a treatment and essentially to different clinician-raters, and the same clinicians rater with his or her individual tendencies continues to evaluate the same assigned patients throughout the clinical trial, then the variance attributed to raters is likely to have been distributed equally across the treatment conditions and can be accounted for in the error term when testing treatment differences. A far greater source of error comes from replacing clinician-raters during a study, something to which funding agencies and journal editors need to give more attention. In these instances, when a clinician-rater is replaced midway in a study, the variance between the two different raters of a given patient will often be greater than the variance attributed to treatment. (Of 151 patients in the PT studies, only four PT patients, three family psychoeducation treatment patients, and four control patients had a different rater over the 3 years of treatment.) Our relative interest has more often been in the *validity* of treatment differences, rather than in the scoring tendencies of our raters. Reliability does not at all ensure validity (that the treatment difference is real), but demonstrable validity can build a very strong case for the underlying reliability of the measures.

There are clear exceptions to this maxim. In comparative treatment studies, when the therapist-raters of treatment A are different individuals than the therapist-raters of treatment B, the clinical "horse race" that inevitably develops regarding therapy allegiance can often (but not always) bias results in the absence of interrater reliability. We have suspected that the absence of robust adjustment differences in our previous study of family psychoeducation and social skills training (and the studies of others) might have, in part, followed upon this phenomenon. Unfortunately, the options for correcting the problem are few, and also problematic. If one uses many rating scales that contain literally hundreds of items, as we do in our studies, it is nearly impossible to ensure interrater reliability for each and every item across many clinician raters and many rating periods. As is typically the case in studies of clinical depression, researchers will often turn to a *single* criterion rating scale, such as the Hamilton Depression Scale, which is administered by a highly reliable and *independent* assessor. The problem here is that a narrow focus on one scale can seriously curtail the amount of important information needed to comprehensively account for treatment effects. Of greater importance, such independent raters consistently learn less about the patient in a brief (often 20-minute) interview than the treating clinician who has had an ongoing experience with the patient over the course of an episode and recovery. Knowledge of the patient offers the best assurance of valid observations, in our experience. Still other investigators will resort to having the treating clinician use "structured" interviews (as we did in the PT studies with the Social Adjustment Scale II), but the context becomes somewhat artificial—formally inquiring about the behavior and adjustment of a patient that the clinician might have been seeing weekly for many months or years. In other instances, (again, as we did in the PT studies), one can seek the opinion of different *observers*, such as the patient and a family member as well as the therapist, and look for a consistency in reported effects, especially when the various rating scales are moderately intercorrelated. Thus, there is no ideal solution to the problem of interrater reliability when raters as well as patients have not been randomized.

    Correlations are expressed anywhere from a perfect positive correlation of
1.0 to a perfect negative correlation of –1.0. (The statistical significance of a specific *r* will also depend on the sample size, as was the case with the *t* test, although
a relatively small *r* could be judged to be statistically significant in a very large sample, as is often true in epidemiology studies.) The overall magnitude of an *r* should
guide our judgment of clinical importance: An *r* of .25 or less in clinical studies
such as ours typically indicates a low correlation; one between .25 and .50 suggests a relationship that might indeed be important; between .50 and .75 there is a
demonstrably good relationship (such as one will often find between pre- and
posttreatment ratings); and above .75 a very strong relationship exists, such as one
that we would want between raters. (But once again we would need to be cautious
as to whether these very high or very low correlations are spurious, i.e., artifacts of
our sampling.) However, the *r* should ultimately be interpreted in the context of
the actual study. For example, an *r* of .40 between a treatment and relapse could
be an indicator of a very large correlation. However, a very small *r* in an epidemiology study of mortality risk following exposure to a toxin could also be important, but here the sample size might be 100 times larger to detect an *r* that is only
about one-tenth of that found in a smaller clinical trial (e.g., an *r* of .40 in a clinical
trial of 30 subjects might compare to a sample of 3,000 for a significant *r* of .04).
Sometimes we can actually "eyeball" an estimated correlation by simply plotting
our *X* and *Y* scores on a scatter plot. Figure A.3 is an illustration of three different

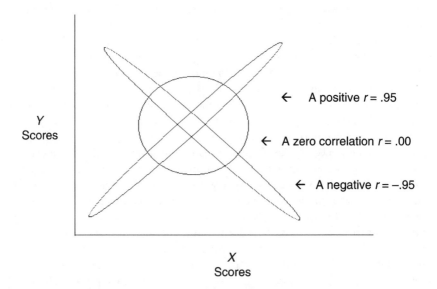

FIGURE A.3. Illustrations of correlation.

correlations from a scatter plot: a very positive correlation, a zero correlation when scores are within a "circle," and a very negative correlation. Differently shaped scores skewed to the right (positive) or the left (negative) can thus give is a quick estimate of the degree of correlation that lies between −1.0 and +1.0.

The linear (or straight-line) Pearson "product–moment" correlation is essentially a ratio that signifies the amount of change in one variable (X) that is systematically associated with the amount of change in another variable (Y). It is thus the "product" or sum of the individual score deviations from the X mean (divided by the *SD* of the X mean), *multiplied* by the sum of the deviations from the Y mean (divided by the *SD* of the Y mean), all of which are then further divided by the number of scores. In this particular formula we are *standardizing* (or putting on the same scale) the X and Y deviations by dividing each set by its respective *SD*. We do this because the two variables being associated are often expressed in different units of measurement (e.g., height and weight, or milligrams of drug and psychopathology scores).

Other names exist for the Pearson correlation. When both variables are dichotomous measures (such as sex and "ever married") the correlation calculated is referred to as a *phi coefficient*. When one variable is a continuous measure (such as age) and the other is dichotomous, the correlation can be designated a *point biserial correlation*. The *Spearman rho* is a "nonparametric" correlation (see below) that ignores the original distribution and calculates the association between *ranks* instead of the association between the original scores (e.g., the lowest score is placed in category 1, the next lowest score is placed in category 2, and so on), and ties are given separate ranks, which can become something of a problem. The ranks are then averaged and compared. Its value lies in minimizing the influence of outliers in the original distribution of scores. The *Kendall tau* is similarly used when the original distribution of scores is skewed or contained outliers (that would have precluded an ANOVA) and scores have been transformed, for example, by taking the log or the square root of the original scores. Compared to the Spearman rho, it gives less weight to extreme discrepancies between ranks and more weight to slight discrepancies. There are also refined versions of *r* such as the *partial correlation* between the X and Y scores, controlling for another variable (Z), or the combined, *multiple correlation* of the X and Y (or other) variables when one is assessing this association with Z. (The multiple correlation is equivalent to a Pearson *r* that is calculated between a criterion [outcome] variable and the best possible equation using multiple independent variables.) Sometimes the multiple correlation itself is squared (R^2) as an indicator of the amount of variance in the outcome measure that is accounted for by the independent variables. Partialing out the variance of X and Y while controlling for Z is similar in many ways to the goals of the ANOVA that were described above. The combined association of X and Y when correlated with (or predicting) Z is often the task of yet another somewhat complex statistical method called *regression* (see below). Sometimes the relationship between variables is not linear. These curvilinear relationships can be calculated with more complex statistical approaches that are beyond the scope of this brief description. More often we will simply transform the scores, thus allowing more linear approaches to be used.

Finally, when faced with many behavioral measures contained in a single rating scale that has been applied to a large number of patients, rather than analyze each item or total scale score when analyzing data, the researcher can look for dimensions or factors that represent sets of highly intercorrelated items within the scale. *Factor analysis* variably combines these intercorrelated items in a series of discrete linear analyses such that the first factor (set of items) explains most of the variance among the group of correlated items, the second set of items explains the next largest amount of variance after controlling for the factor set, etc. Once the factors are extracted they are "rotated," that is, statistically manipulated in a search for the combination of items that make the most clinical sense. As we saw in Chapter 2, factor analysis was an important correlational approach used in the PT studies in order to derive somewhat intracorrelated yet reasonably independent dimensions of personal and social adjustment. In order to create valid factors, the number of patient ratings in the analysis should be at least 10 times greater than the number of items being factored.

Regression

While the simple linear correlation estimates the association between two sets of scores, say X and Y, regression attempts to *predict* the y scores from the x scores (i.e., called "regressing" y scores on x scores), or vice versa. To make this prediction, the mathematical equation that needs to be calculated uses much of the same information regarding the characteristics of these scores that we described earlier in the calculation of t, F, and r. This information includes the deviation of individual scores from their respective means, the *SD* of each mean, an estimate of the measurement error, and—not surprisingly—the correlation between the scores in each sample. The equation generated will essentially tell us that for each change in x scores, y scores will also change by a fixed amount that falls within a range. (The range here is once again determined by the error in measurement, in this case called the *standard estimate of the error*.) Obviously, predicting an *individual y* score from an individual x score will be far less accurate (a much greater chance of error) than predicting how a *group* of Y scores will change as the group of X scores change. (As in calculating the t test, the error term or denominator will decrease as the N increases.) It was a version of this type of linear regression that characterized our analysis of adjustment in the PT studies (Chapter 2).

In our discussion of linear correlation, Figure A.3 illustrated the shapes of scores for a positive or negative correlation. In regression analysis, a line is typically drawn through these shapes in a way that best reflects or "fits" the distribution of scores. How a line slants (left to right or right to left), is called its *slope*, designated by the letter b. Where the line crosses the y axis (the vertical set of scores) is called the *intercept* and is designated as *a*. If *x* increases and *y* also increases, the slope is considered to be positive. If *y* decreases when *x* increases, the slope is considered to be negative. Thus the *regression equation* designed to "predict" a *y* score (say, a person's weight) from knowledge of one *x* score (say, a person's height) becomes $y = a + bx$, where *x* is the amount of known change (say, an inch increase), *a* is the intercept, and *b* is the *beta coefficient*, or slope. In this case we can calculate *b* by simply taking the *correlation coefficient* (*r*) and multiplying it by the *SD* of the Y scores divided by the *SD* of the X scores. We calculate *a* by taking the mean of the Y scores, minus *b* times the mean of the X scores, or $a = Y - bX$. The test on the slope of the regression line (the beta coefficient) and the Pearson *r* (the correlation) between *x* and *y* will be equivalent.

In the PT studies, our approach was to calculate the slope or beta coefficient of the change scores between the baseline assessment and one of the outcome periods for the PT and the no-PT treatment conditions. Our statistical analyses of treatment *differences* ultimately resolved to a *t* test of the difference between the two beta coefficients or slopes being compared! We used what is called multiple regression since the change scores (our *x* scores) had been adjusted for random initial level differences (our *y* scores) as well as the effects of other categorical (independent) variables of interest such as age, sex, and chronicity. Like other tests, regression also assumes that the distribution of scores for X and Y are similarly shaped, that the means are reliable, and that the correlation is not spurious, assumptions that are sometimes not met in published studies.

NONPARAMETRIC TESTS

We conclude our review of statistical testing with a brief comment on tests that are often used when the assumptions for a normal distribution of scores are not met, that is, when the distributions are described apart from such parametric characteristics as means, *SD*'s and their error terms. Applications can also arise when distributions are differently skewed and the researcher is less concerned that there might be valuable evidence represented by the extreme scores or is hesitant about transforming scores by taking the square root or log of the scores. Nonparametric tests typically rely on a contingency table that includes categorical variables such as race or sex, different treatment groups, or some other continuous outcome measure experienced, for example, as ranks.

The Ranks Test

A frequently used nonparametric approach is called the *Wilcoxon ranks test*, where the two sets of scores (e.g., X and Y) are grouped into numerical ranks (e.g., from the highest to the lowest group of scores) and the difference between the two sets of ranks then become tested much like a *t* test. But rather than using the *raw* means and *SD*'s as in the *t* test, the means and *SD*'s used are those of the two sets of *ranks* being compared. The rank difference between the two groups is the numerator, and the *SE* of the ranks for both groups becomes the denominator.

The (Contingency Table) Chi-Square

In clinical research, the most common nonparametric test encountered is the chi-square (χ^2), a way to test differences in proportions or percentage between two or more independent samples. The question being answered with the chi-square in clinical trials is whether the difference in proportions or percentage is independent of treatment or due to the treatment, by calculating whether the treatment differences are greater or less than one might have simply expected by chance. Chi-square is thus a way to estimate whether the observed frequencies or proportions are significantly different from the frequencies or proportions that one would expect by chance. It is calculated by taking the observed frequency minus the expected frequency (squared) for each of the cells being compared and then dividing this difference by the expected frequency for each cell. These values are then summed, cell by cell, to get the chi-square.

Table A.2, which we shall use to illustrate the chi-square, is a 2×2 contingency table: two treatment groups (drug and placebo) by two outcomes (relapse and no relapse). The table reflects the relapse experience of patients treated in one of our earlier studies Hogarty et al., 1974). The point that needs to be emphasized when calculating chi-square tests of contingency tables is that the subjects in each cell should be independent of subjects in other cells (i.e., each person should be counted only once). Further, if we were comparing symptom frequencies in two treatment groups, it would be appropriate to construct a contingency table that distinguished between patients with "no symptoms" and those with "some symptoms," but it would be less appropriate to compare people with 0, 1, 2, 3, 4, or more symptoms since these continuous distributions are more suited to parametric testing.

TABLE A.2. Observed Frequencies of Patients with Schizophrenia Relapsing or Surviving after 1 Year of Drug or Placebo Treatment ($N = 200$)

	Drug	Placebo	Marginal row totals
Relapse	40 (cell A)	80 (cell B)	120
No relapse	60 (cell C)	20 (cell D)	80
Marginal column totals	100	100	200

The clinician might best grasp the concept of chi-square by walking through Table A.2 that describes the *observed* frequency of relapse on drug and placebo. We begin by computing the *expected* frequency in each of the cells that have been identified as A, B, C, and D. The cell A expected frequency (i.e., the proportion relapsing on drug) is the relapse *row* marginal total (120) multiplied by the corresponding marginal *column* total for drug (100), which is then divided by the grand total of all our patients (200). The result is 120×100, or $12{,}000 \div 200 = 60$. The difference between the observed frequency of relapse in cell A (40) and that to be expected by chance (60) is thus 20. When this difference is squared (20^2) the result is 400, which in turn is divided by the expected frequency for that cell ($400 \div 60 = 6.67$). Cell A's contribution to the final chi-square is thus 6.67. Using the same formula for placebo relapse (cell B) yields the same value, such that cell B's contribution to the chi-square is also 6.67. One can continue the process by calculating the contributions from cells C and D which in this case are both 10. The final chi-square value then becomes $6.67 + 6.67 + 10 + 10 = 33.34$. Clearly one can see that the ultimate chi-square value depends on the addition of all the difference calculations between expected and observed frequencies in each of the cells. With 1 *df* (see below), a chi-square of 33.34 is significant well beyond the .001 level. (In fact, all we would have needed for a .05 level difference was a chi-square of 3.84.) We would conclude from our example that relapse is not independent of treatment and thus reject the null hypothesis. *Degrees of freedom* in the chi-square test depend upon the number of *rows* minus 1, *times* the number of *columns* minus 1. (In our example, 2 relapse rows minus 1 row equals 1, and 2 treatment columns minus 1 column equals 1. Thus the product 1×1 equals 1 *df*.) If we had used three different drug treatment columns—say, high dose, low dose, and placebo—our degrees of freedom would have been 2: ($3 - 1$ columns $= 2)(2 - 1$ rows $= 1$), thus $2 \times 1 = 2 \, df$. Similarly, if we had these three drug levels and three relapse rows (e.g., a psychotic relapse, an affective relapse, and no relapse) our degrees of freedom would have been 4: ($3 - 1$ rows $= 2)(3 - 1$ columns $= 2$), thus $2 \times 2 = 4$ *df*. As can be seen from any table of chi-square, the size of the value needed for significance increases as the degrees of freedom increase (i.e., as more cells are added).

The same data in Table A.2 can serve to illustrate two additional simple but popular statistics, the *relative risk ratio* and the *odds ratio*. While the latter is often recommended for epidemiology studies and the former for longitudinal clinical trials, we prefer the odds ratio in clinical trials as well because it gives more consistent estimates in spite of different base rates. For example, the relative risk of relapse in patients exposed to placebo (the risk factor) compared to those not exposed (i.e., those maintained on drug) is 2, or twice the risk on placebo compared to drug (e.g., $80 \div 100$ patients relapsed on placebo and $40 \div 100$ relapsed on drug, such that $.80 \div .40 = 2$). However, the odds ratio gives a much more meaningful and accurate estimate of the odds of relapsing in one treatment group compared to the other. In the placebo group, the odds are 80 to 20 (or 4 to 1) for relapse but only 40 to 60 on drug, or 2 to 3; 4 divided by ⅔ gives an odds ratio of 6, such that the odds of relapsing are six times greater for placebo than for drug in this example. The relative risk measure tends to underestimate risk when the percent differences are larger (e.g., 80% relapse vs. 20% survival). It has more utility when these percent differences or fractions are smaller, and it has less utility as the fractions become larger (e.g., a 5-point relapse difference of 5% vs. 10% means something more than a 5-point relapse difference of 94% vs. 99%).

One can also compare proportions or ranks between two groups using ANOVA or the *t* test with results that are very similar to the chi-square or other nonparametric tests. The approaches differ slightly in that the error term used in the parametric tests reflect the corrected number of subjects (i.e., the degrees of freedom) whereas the chi-square does not use the *N* for scores or subjects as an error term; rather, degrees of freedom are based on the rows and columns of the contingency table used to divide the various proportions as described above. Recall that for a $p = .05$ test using the *F* or *t* ratio, we would consider that 5% of the scores lie beyond ± 1.96 *SD*'s, characteristic of the normal distribution. But in the 1 *df* chi-square test, the 5% of scores needed for significance lie beyond 3.84 *SD*'s, as can be seen in any chi-square table found in statistical textbooks.

Survivorship Analyses

Again, using the example in Table A.2, let us say that we had studied these 200 patients assigned to drug or placebo for *10* years rather than 1 year and found that, given sufficient time, all 200 patients eventually had a relapse! Does it mean that the drug is no better than placebo regarding relapse? Clearly the answer is no, since we had earlier observed that the vast majority of assignees to placebo had already relapsed at the end of a single year while less than half the patients had experienced a relapse on medication. Frequently the superiority of a treatment lies in its ability to forestall or to *delay* relapse (or some other poor outcome) rather than prevent it. This is a common prophylactic effect not only of medication but of psychosocial treatment as well, as described in Chapter 1. Thus the *speed* of relapse, or average time to relapse, is also an important criterion that tells us whether our treatments differ significantly in their effects over time. In these cases we use *survivorship* or *life table* analyses that essentially compare the proportions of patients surviving or relapsing at various times, in a nonparametric manner. While these tests were originally used in health fields other than psychiatry, survivorship without relapse is typically used in the mental health field; mortality or organ failure are often the relevant outcomes in general medicine. To our knowledge, we were the first to apply survivorship analysis to schizophrenia treatment studies (Hogarty & Ulrich, 1977). We have also used other outcomes in these life table analyses, such as "mini" psychotic episodes, and even episodes of "affective disorder," as in the PT studies.

Essentially, survivorship analysis is an extension of the chi-square statistic described above: the observed versus the expected rates of surviving (without relapse in our case) over a determined period of time. In the PT studies, the period for which relapse or survivorship was calculated was 3 years, divided into monthly time intervals. The underlying principle is that, all things being equal, the expected incidence of relapse for each treatment group being compared should be equal at each successive period of time. (We do, however, acknowledge that the risk or probability of relapse at later periods of times is likely to decrease the longer a sample is followed after the index psychotic episode [Hogarty & Ulrich, 1977].) If the observed number of relapse events differs (in the same direction) at various time intervals, the treatments could be shown to be significantly different in their ability to delay relapse. In the PT studies we could, of course, have calculated the time intervals of study at every 3 months or 6 months, for example, over the 3 years of treatment. We chose to use monthly intervals because survivorship analysis assumes that a relapse (or a dropout) occurs at the midpoint of the time interval, a rather risky assumption if our time intervals had been in 6-month blocks.

Life table analysis will generate a survivorship curve for each treatment condition being compared, based on the relapse or withdrawal experiences at each time interval (i.e., month by month in the PT studies). Different statistics can be applied to test whether the curves are significantly different, the most popular in the psychiatry literature being the *Mantel–Haenszel test*. Nearly identical to the 1 *df* chi-square test, the Mantel–Haenszel approach uses a series of 2×2 contingency tables in order to assess the proportions of patients relapsing and surviving at each time interval. (In the PT studies these contingency tables typically represented the two treatment conditions of either PT or no PT according to the two outcomes, relapse or survival.) At each time interval the expected and observed relapses are determined and summed across the proportions (cells) and across the time periods in order to generate the Mantel–Haenszel statistical value.

In our analysis of relapse rates in the PT studies, we compared the survivorship curves for those patients in the PT and the various no-PT conditions using a nonparametric test called the *Gehan statistic*, a test which is a variation of the Wilcoxon rank test described earlier. The Gehan statistic essentially ranks the number of patients in a treatment who are surviving each time a patient relapses, and the ranks between treatments are then tested. Since the Gehan statistic differentially weights the sheer number of patients surviving at the beginning of a time interval, it will of necessity place more emphasis on the larger number of patients available in the early months of observation compared to the fewer number of patients available in later months. The Mantel–Haenszel procedure, on the other hand, weights each time interval equally, relatively speaking.

There are a few other characteristics of survivorship analysis that might help the clinician to understand how these proportions are assessed. Once one accounts for the number of relapses and withdrawals within a time interval (say, month 1) and proceeds to calculate the proportion of patients surviving without relapse (called the "censored" cases) in the next interval (month 2), the survivorship analysis assumes that the probability of surviving in month 2 was in fact a *condition* of having survived month 1. This "conditional probability" is often referred to as the *hazard rate* and is the basis for calculating the cumulative probability of surviving without relapse month by month throughout the period of study. By way of example, let us say that 10 of our 100 placebo-treated patients described in Table A.2 relapsed within month 1 (and there were no dropouts), such that the probability of surviving at the end of month 1 was 90%. Now in month 2 another 10 of these 90 surviving patients also had a relapse, such that the probability of surviving month 2 is 89%. In the life table method, the cumulative probability of having *continuously* survived without relapse for the *entire* 2 months is only 80% (.90 × .89 = .80). The survivorship curve graphically describes (sometimes in logarithmic units) these cumulative probabilities month by month over the 1, 2, 3, or more years of study. As the number of patients surviving at the beginning of a month declines over time, obviously the cumulative probability of surviving will also decline month by month. It is these monthly proportions of expected and observed survivorship that are summed and tested either at a given point of time during the study (e.g., at 6 months) or across the whole period of study itself (e.g., 3 years in the PT studies).

Finally, researchers will often make reference to another nonparametric test of survivorship called the *Cox proportional hazard method*. Now that we have dealt with testing proportions and calculating the conditional probability of surviving (the "hazard"), this approach should not be too intimidating. The Cox approach is a form of multiple regression analysis used to evaluate the influence of other proportions of risk factors on survivorship or relapse, such as the dichotomous measures of age, sex, or good and poor premorbid status. In essence, the Cox method estimates the effects of these independent variables (having accounted for their intercorrelations) on the probability of surviving each time interval.

Meta-Analysis

Following this brief overview of statistics, we hope the clinician's appreciation of the conditions that can adversely affect the mean, its difference from another mean, and the subsequent test of significance has increased. But now let us consider the problem for clinicians when some well-intended "reviewers" of the clinical literature combine the statistical results of *all* studies on a given treatment in a search for its "real" effect, a modern example of sound-bite science, called *meta-analysis*. (The approach allegedly saves clinicians from reading the literature, synthesizing the results, and getting the "big picture" on their own.) Entered into the meta-analysis are the *pooled* statistical effects from different studies: those that have small samples and those with large samples; studies with asymmetrical distributions of scores and those that have symmetrical distributions; studies with misbehaved means and those that have reliable means, those with spurious correlations and those without—and studies with unrecognized type I or type II errors along with those whose results are more valid! Some meta-analyses list requirements for the studies to be selected, such as that the patients had to be randomized to treatment or that the diagnostic criteria needed to be similar. But even these standards rarely offer protection from the "garbage in–garbage out" phenomenon attributed to the data. Kraemer (2000) has gone so far as to challenge the pooling of studies that might have used different sampling methods, different treatment delivery systems, or different outcome measures. Even in the case of "replication" studies that do not agree, "someone," she claims, "is doing bad science" (p. 328). For one thing, meta-analysis does not explain why the studies differed in their effects in the first place.

In recent years, meta-analyses have even grown to include the pooled tests of all, and often markedly different, "psychosocial" treatments for schizophrenia, independent of the patients' course of illness, characteristics, therapist skill, or the likely difference in mechanisms of action among treatments (e.g., Mojtabai, Nicholson, & Carpenter, 1998). In a nutshell, the overall effect of meta-analysis (even if it is supportive of a decent treatment) is to give greater weight to the poor and often smaller studies, and to dilute the effects of the appropriately conducted and more often larger studies! In the last analysis, there is rarely a need for a meta-analysis at all, in our admittedly minority opinion. A colleague once wrote that there are so few scientifically sound studies of a specific treatment with a specific population available that the reviewer would serve the clinical audience best by simply describing the results of those few good studies (Kazdin, 1983). A much heralded meta-analysis on the effects of social work intervention among the seriously mentally ill can serve as a good example of just about everything that can go wrong with meta-analysis when it is applied to treatment studies (see Videka-Sherman, 1988, and the subsequent critique by Hogarty, 1989). This particular meta-analysis led to the seriously flawed conclusions (1) that antipsychotic medication was ineffective and (2) that very brief treatment was better than continued treatment for psychotic patients! The present author's most unhappy occasion in a long science career has been to observe the immolation of otherwise well-designed and efficacious studies on the altar of meta-analysis. In short, one needs to be very cautious when basing treatment decisions on the results of a meta-analysis; it is *far better to read the few good studies oneself*. The only arguments that have impressed us regarding the justification of meta-analysis are the rare instances when there is a large number of really well-conducted studies on a specific treatment that do not agree and the reviewer wants to increase the sample size (or power) that supports an overall effect size, or wants to correct for a number of possible "file drawer" studies with negative effects that were never published. (Again, the test will not tell you why these studies disagreed.) The approach might have its greatest utility as a form of "mega-analysis" where the results of multiple centers or studies are combined for thousands of patients as a way to increase the power needed to detect rare outcomes.

With this brief review of statistical theory and methods, we hope the design and analysis of the PT studies will not only be more understandable but will provide a more acceptable basis for clinical practice as well.

APPENDIX B

The Process Rating Scale

Instructions: Please circle the category for each question that best describes the patient's status over the past month.

Basic Phase Status	Almost never/ No	Sometimes/To a small extent	Often/Quite a bit	Usually/To a large extent	Almost always/ Definitely yes	Unknown or N/A
1. Patient's dose of medication is stable	1	2	3	4	5	9
2. Serious medication side effects are absent	1	2	3	4	5	9
3. Patient sees need for medication	1	2	3	4	5	9
4. Patient is aware of and reports side effects if present	1	2	3	4	5	9
5. Patient takes medication as prescribed	1	2	3	4	5	9
6. Any physical illness is under reasonable medical control	1	2	3	4	5	9
7. Patient attends clinic regularly (75% of appointments)	1	2	3	4	5	9
8. Patient gives evidence of understanding schizophrenia as a psychosociobiological illness that requires treatment	1	2	3	4	5	9
9. Patient knows one or more of his or her individual prodromal signs of psychotic relapse	1	2	3	4	5	9
10. Patient calls possible prodromal signs to the attention of the therapist	1	2	3	4	5	9

	Almost never/ No	Sometimes/To a small extent	Often/Quite a bit	Usually/To a large extent	Almost always/ Definitely yes	Unknown or N/A
11. Patient can define what stress means to him or her	1	2	3	4	5	9
12. Patient views therapist as a competent person who can be trusted	1	2	3	4	5	9
13. Patient calls upon therapist in times of crises	1	2	3	4	5	9
14. Family is a source of emotional and/or material support	1	2	3	4	5	9
15. Housing is secure and stable	1	2	3	4	5	9
16. Entitlements and basic needs have been secured	1	2	3	4	5	9
17. Patient can restructure role if needed (e.g., limit hours on job or socializing)	1	2	3	4	5	9
18. Patient can identify and appropriately apply an autoprotection strategy	1	2	3	4	5	9
19. Patient can maintain attention during a session for at least half an hour	1	2	3	4	5	9
20. Patient expresses positive statements/ feelings (compliments or appreciation) when indicated	1	2	3	4	5	9
21. Patient avoids or extricates self from conflict situations when indicated	1	2	3	4	5	9
22. Patient performs self-care activities (diet, hygiene, dress, transportation, etc.) without prompting	1	2	3	4	5	9
23. Patient performs basic household tasks as expected	1	2	3	4	5	9
24. Patient manifests appropriate eye contact, speech latency, and voice tone and/or quality	1	2	3	4	5	9

Intermediate Phase Status

	Almost never/ No	Sometimes/To a small extent	Often/Quite a bit	Usually/To a large extent	Almost always/ Definitely yes	Unknown or N/A
1. Patient maintains stability achieved in basic phase	1	2	3	4	5	9
2. Patient acknowledges one or more potential disabilities of schizophrenia	1	2	3	4	5	9

3. Patient has some appreciation of symptom progression (from cues to minor symptoms to an episode)   1   2   3   4   5   9

4. Patient appropriately expresses personal preferences and opinions (e.g., "I would rather" [positive assertion])   1   2   3   4   5   9

5. Patient appropriately expresses dislikes (e.g., "I don't like it when" [negative assertion])   1   2   3   4   5   9

6. Patient manifests internal coping skills in simulated (office) interpersonally stressful circumstances   1   2   3   4   5   9

7. Patient seems able to apply relaxation techniques when aroused or upset outside of office   1   2   3   4   5   9

8. Patient is able to achieve a level of relaxation below baseline arousal using deep breathing (in or out of office)   1   2   3   4   5   9

9. Patient listens well (appropriate eye contact, nodding, questions, commenting)   1   2   3   4   5   9

10. Patient accurately evaluates other person's feelings in a potentially conflicted situation   1   2   3   4   5   9

11. Patient accurately evaluates the volatility of a potential conflict situation (e.g., knows other is getting angry)   1   2   3   4   5   9

12. Patient responds appropriately in a potential conflict situation   1   2   3   4   5   9

13. Patient correctly describes what might cause a new episode (stress, loss, conflict, alcohol and drugs, etc.)   1   2   3   4   5   9

14. Patient uses a physical, affective, cognitive, or behavioral cue to identify a stress signal   1   2   3   4   5   9

15. Patient can identify one or more circumstances that might lead to his or her affective dysregulation   1   2   3   4   5   9

16. Patient seems more able to prevent or minimize stressful encounters outside the office   1   2   3   4   5   9

17. Patient gives evidence of not appearing unduly anxious, angry, or depressed when stressed   1   2   3   4   5   9

Advanced Phase Status	Almost never/ No	Sometimes/To a small extent	Often/Quite a bit	Usually/To a large extent	Almost always/ Definitely yes	Unknown or N/A
1. Patient maintains stability from the basic and intermediate phases	1	2	3	4	5	9
2. Patient takes initiative to improve an existing relationship	1	2	3	4	5	9
3. Patient takes initiative to form a new relationship or reestablish an old relationship	1	2	3	4	5	9
4. Patient takes initiative to return to work or school	1	2	3	4	5	9
5. Patient performs expected household tasks that involve cooperation with others	1	2	3	4	5	9
6. Patient applies learned coping strategies with friends or family	1	2	3	4	5	9
7. Patient is able to negotiate pressure to drink or use drugs	1	2	3	4	5	9
8. Patient can distinguish between just and unjust criticism	1	2	3	4	5	9
9. Patient responds well to valid criticism by apologizing, explaining circumstances, offering a solution	1	2	3	4	5	9
10. Patient responds well to invalid criticism (e.g., redefines criticism, stands up for self)	1	2	3	4	5	9
11. Patient appears to use internal controls in the face of criticism (e.g., reframing, denial, deep breathing, relaxation responses)	1	2	3	4	5	9
12. Patient gives evidence of using reciprocity in relationships	1	2	3	4	5	9
13. Patient is aware how his or her mood and behavior affect others	1	2	3	4	5	9
14. Patient plans vocational objectives that are appropriate to skills, education, and disabilities	1	2	3	4	5	9
15. Patient relaxes (below baseline) using progressive muscle relaxation or "letting go" relaxation	1	2	3	4	5	9
16. Patient relaxes (below baseline) using guided imagery	1	2	3	4	5	9

17. Patient is aware of personal   1   2   3   4   5   9
    vulnerabilities that can be exploited by
    relationships or the workplace

18. Patient is aware of instrumental role   1   2   3   4   5   9
    limitations

19. Patient manifests interpersonal coping   1   2   3   4   5   9
    skills in simulated (office) vocationally
    stressful circumstances

20. Patient is aware of prevocational or   1   2   3   4   5   9
    vocational circumstances in which affect
    becomes dysregulated

21. Patient applies learned coping strategies   1   2   3   4   5   9
    in a vocational or prevocational setting

References

Acosta, F. Z., Yamamoto, J., & Wilcox, S. A. (1978). Application of electromyographic biofeedback to the relaxation training of schizophrenic, neurotic, and tension headache patients. *Journal of Consulting and Clinical Psychology*, *46*(2), 383–384.

Albrecht, K. (1979). *Stress and the manager*. Englewood Cliffs, NJ: Prentice-Hall.

American Psychiatric Association. (1987). *Diagnostic and statistical manual of mental disorders* (3rd ed., rev.). Washington, DC: Author.

American Psychiatric Association. (1994). *Diagnostic and statistical manual of mental disorders* (4th ed.). Washington, DC: Author.

American Psychiatric Association. (1997). Practice guidelines for the treatment of patients with schizophrenia. *American Journal of Psychiatry*, *54*(Suppl.), 1–63.

Anderson, C. M., Hogarty, G. E., & Reiss, D. J. (1980). Family treatment of adult schizophrenic patients: A research based psycho-educational approach. *Schizophrenia Bulletin*, *6*, 490–505.

Anderson, C. M., Reiss, D. J., & Hogarty, G. E. (1986). *Schizophrenia and the family: A practitioner's guide to psychoeducation and management*. New York: Guilford Press.

Andrews, G. (1993). The essential psychotherapies. *British Journal of Psychiatry*, *162*, 447–451.

Arieti, S. (1974). *Interpretation of schizophrenia*. New York: Basic Books.

Ball, R. A., Moore, E., & Kuipers, L. (1992). Expressed emotion in community care staff. *Social Psychiatry and Psychiatric Epidemiology*, *27*, 35–39.

Bandura, A. (1969). *Principles of behavior modification*. New York: Holt, Rinehart & Winston.

Barlow, D. H., Chorpita, B. F., & Turovsky, J. (1996). Fear, panic, anxiety and disorders of emotion. In D. A. Hope (Ed.), *Nebraska symposium on motivation: Perspectives on anxiety, panic and fear* (pp. 251–328). Lincoln: University of Nebraska Press.

Baronet, A. M., & Gerber, G. J. (1998). Psychiatric rehabilitation: Efficacy of four models. *Clinical Psychology Review, 18*, 189–228.

Bellack, A. S., & DiClemente, C. C. (1999). Treating substance abuse among patients with schizophrenia. *Psychiatric Services, 50*, 75–80.

Bellack, A. S., & Mueser, K. T. (1993). Psychosocial treatment for schizophrenia. *Schizophrenia Bulletin, 19*, 317–336.

Benson, H. (1975). *The relaxation response*. New York: Avon Books.

Benson, H. (1996). *Timeless healing*. New York: Scribner.

Bentley, K. J., & Walsh, J. (2000). *The social worker and psychotropic medication* (2nd ed.). Pacific Grove, CA: Brooks/Cole.

Bernstein, D. A., & Borkovec, T. D. (1973). *Progressive relaxation training*. Champaign, IL: Research Press.

Blanchard, J. J., Brown, S. A., Horan, W. P., & Sherwood, A. R. (2000). Substance use disorders in schizophrenia: Review, integration and a proposed model. *Clinical Psychology Review, 20*, 207–234.

Braden, W. (1984). Vulnerability and schizoaffective psychoses: A two-factor model. *Schizophrenia Bulletin, 10*, 71–86.

Breggin, P. R. (1997). *Brain disabling treatments in psychiatry: Drugs, electroshock and the role of the FDA*. New York: Springer.

Breier, A., & Strauss, J. S. (1983). Self-control in psychotic disorders. *Archives of General Psychiatry, 40*, 1141–1145.

Breier, A., Wolkowitz, O. M., Doran, A. R., Roy, A., Boronow, J., Hommer, D. W., & Pickar, D. (1987). Neuroleptic responsivity of negative and positive symptoms in schizophrenia. *American Journal of Psychiatry, 144*, 1549–1553.

Brenner, H. D., Boker, W., & Muller, J. (1987). On autoprotective efforts of schizophrenics, neurotics and controls. *Acta Psychiatrica Scandinavica, 75*, 405–414.

Brenner, H. D., Hodel, B., Roder, V., & Corrigan, P. (1992). Treatment of cognitive dysfunctions and behavioral deficits in schizophrenia. *Schizophrenia Bulletin, 18*, 21–26.

Brown, R. (1996). Politeness in schizophrenia. In S. Matthyese, D. L. Levy, J. Kagan, & F. M. Benes (Eds.), *Psychopathology: The evolving science of mental disorder* (pp. 336–350). New York: Cambridge University Press.

Buckly, P. F., & Lys, C. (1996). Psychotherapy and schizophrenia. *Journal of Psychotherapy Practice and Research, 5*, 185–201.

Budzynski, T. H. (1974). *Relaxation training program* [Audiotape]. New York: Guilford Publications.

Burns, D. D. (1980). *Feeling good: The new mood therapy*. New York: Morrow.

Bustillo, J., Buchanan, R. W., & Carpenter, W. T. (1995). Prodromal symptoms vs. early warning signs and clinical action in schizophrenia. *Schizophrenia Bulletin*, *21*, 553–561.

Caldwell, C. B., & Gottesman, I. H. (1990). Schizophrenics kill themselves too: A review of risk factors for suicide. *Schizophrenia Bulletin*, *16*, 571–589.

Cameron, N., & Margaret, H. (1951). Desocialization. In N. Cameron & H. Margaret (Eds.), *Behavior pathology* (pp. 478–503). New York: Houghton Mifflin.

Carlson, G. A., & Goodwin, F. K. (1973). The stages of mania: A longitudinal analysis of the manic episode. *Archives of General Psychiatry*, *28*, 221–228.

Carpenter, W. T., Buchanan, R. W., Kirkpatrick, B., & Breier, A. F. (1999). Diazepam treatment of early signs of exacerbation in schizophrenia. *American Journal of Psychiatry*, *156*, 299–303.

Carpenter, W. T., Heinricks, D. W., & Wagman, A. M. I. (1988). Deficit and non-deficit forms of schizophrenia: The concept. *American Journal of Psychiatry*, *145*, 578–583.

Carpenter, W. T., Schooler, N. R., & Kane, J. M. (1997). The rationale and ethics of medication-free research in schizophrenia. *Archives of General Psychiatry*, *54*, 401–407.

Carr, V. J. (1983). Recovery from schizophrenia: A review of patterns of psychosis. *Schizophrenia Bulletin*, *9*, 95–121.

Carr, V. J. (1988). Patients' techniques for coping with schizophrenia: An exploratory study. *British Journal of Medical Psychology*, *61*, 339–352.

Carter, C. S., & Barch, D. M. (2000). Attention, memory and language disturbances in schizophrenia: Characteristics and implications. In C. Andrade (Ed.), *Advances in psychiatry* (pp. 45–72). London and New Delhi: Oxford University Press.

Charlesworth, E. A., & Nathan, R. G. (1984). *Stress management: A comprehensive guide to wellness*. New York: Atheneum.

Cloward, R. A. (1998). Letter: The decline of education for professional practice. *Social Work*, *43*, 584–586.

Cohen, C. I., & Berk, L. A. (1985). Personal coping styles of schizophrenic outpatients. *Hospital and Community Psychiatry*, *36*, 407–411

Conley, R. R., & Buchanan, R. W. (1997). Evaluation of treatment-resistant schizophrenia. *Schizophrenia Bulletin*, *23*, 663–674.

Conley, R. R., & Mahmoud, R. (2001). A randomized double-blind study of risperidone and olanzapine in the treatment of schizophrenia or schizoaffective disorder. *American Journal of Psychiatry*, *158*, 765–774.

Corrigan, P. W. (1991). Social skills training in adult psychotic populations: A meta-analysis. *Behavioral Therapeutics and Experimental Psychology*, *22*, 203–210.

Coryell, W., Grove, W., vanEerdwigh, M., Keller, M., & Endicott, J. (1987).

Outcome in RDC schizo-affective depression: The importance of diagnostic subtyping. *Journal of Affective Disorders, 12*, 47–55.

Coursey, R. D. (1989). Psychotherapy with persons suffering from schizophrenia. *Schizophrenia Bulletin, 15*, 349–353.

Coursey, R. D., Keller, A. B., & Farrell, E. W. (1995). Individual psychotherapy and persons with serious mental illness: The client's perspective. *Schizophrenia Bulletin, 21*, 283–301.

Davidson, L., Stayner, D., & Haglund, K. E. (1998). Phenomenological perspectives on the social functioning of people with schizophrenia. In K. Mueser & N. Tarrier (Eds.), *Handbook of social functioning in schizophrenia* (pp. 97–120). Boston: Allyn & Bacon.

Dawson-Saunders, B., & Trapp, R. G. (1994). *Basic and clinical biostatistics.* Norwalk, CT: Appleton & Large.

DeLoach, C., & Greer, B. G. (1981). *Adjustment to severe physical disability: A metamorphosis.* New York: McGraw-Hill.

Devlin, M. J., Yanovski, S. Z., & Wilson, G. T. (2000). Obesity: What mental health professionals need to know. *American Journal of Psychiatry, 157*, 854–866.

Dittman, J., & Schuttler, R. (1990). Disease consciousness and coping strategies of patients with schizophrenic psychosis. *Acta Psychiatrica Scandinavica, 82*, 318–322.

Dixon, L., Adams, C., & Lucksted, A. (2000). Update on family psychoeducation for schizophrenia. *Schizophrenia Bulletin, 26*, 5–20.

Dixon, L., & Lehman, A. F. (1995). Family interventions for schizophrenia. *Schizophrenia Bulletin, 21*, 631–643.

Dixon, L., Lyles, A., Scott, J., Lehman, A. F., Postrado, L., Goldman, H., & McGlynn, E. (1999). Services to families of adults with schizophrenia: From treatment recommendations to dissemination. *Psychiatric Services, 50*, 233–238.

Doherty, N. M. (1996). Affective reactivity of symptoms as a process discriminator in schizophrenia. *Journal of Nervous and Mental Disease, 184*, 535–541.

Donenberg, G. R. (1999). Reconsidering "between-group psychotherapy outcome research and basic science": Applications to child and adolescent psychotherapy outcome research [comment]. *Journal of Clinical Psychology, 55*, 181–190, discussion, 191–200.

Donlon, P. T., & Blocker, K. H. (1973). Stages of schizophrenics' decompensation and integration. *Journal of Nervous and Mental Disease, 157*, 200–209.

Drake, R. E., & Brunette, M. F. (1998). Complications of severe mental illness related to alcohol and other drug use disorders. In M. Galanter (Ed.), *Recent developments in alcoholism: Vol. 14. Consequences of alcoholism* (pp. 285–299). New York: Plenum Press.

Drake, R. E., Mercer-McFadden, C., Mueser, K. T., McHugo, G. J., & Bond, G. R. (1998). A review of integrated mental health and substance abuse treatment for patients with dual disorders. *Schizophrenia Bulletin*, *24*, 589–608.

Drake, R. E., & Mueser, K. T. (2000). Psychosocial approaches to dual diagnosis. *Schizophrenia Bulletin*, *26*, 105–118.

Drake, R. E., & Sederer, L. I. (1986). The adverse effects of intensive treatment of chronic schizophrenia. *Comprehensive Psychiatry*, *27*, 313–326.

Drake, R. E., Yie, H., McHugo, G. J., & Green, A. I. (2000). The effects of clozapine on alcohol and drug use disorders among patients with schizophrenia. *Schizophrenia Bulletin*, *26*, 441–449.

Eaton, M. (1996). The psychotherapy of schizophrenia. In W. R. Breakey (Ed.), *Integrated mental health services: Modern community psychiatry* (pp. 206–221). New York: Oxford University Press.

Egan, M. F., Apud, J., & Wyatt, R. J. (1997). Treatment of tardive dyskinesia. *Schizophrenia Bulletin*, *23*, 583–609.

Eisenberg, L. (1995). The social construction of the human brain. *American Journal of Psychiatry*, *152*, 1563–1575.

Ellenbroek, B. A., & Cools, A. R. (2000). The long-term effects of maternal deprivation depend on the genetic background. *Neuropsychopharmacology*, *23*, 99–106.

Falloon, I. R. H., Boyd, J. L., McGill, C. W., Williamson, W., Razoni, J., Moss, H. B., Gilderman, A. M., & Simpson, G. M. (1985). Family management in the prevention of morbidity of schizophrenia. *Archives of General Psychiatry*, *42*, 887–896.

Falloon, I. R. H., Lindley, P., McDonald, R., & Marks, I. M. (1977). Social skills training of out-patient groups: a controlled study of rehearsal and homework. *British Journal of Psychiatry*, *131*, 599–609.

Falloon, I. R. H., & Talbot, R. E. (1980). Persistent auditory hallucinations: Coping mechanisms and implications for management. *Psychological Medicine*, *11*, 329–339.

Fenton, W. S. (2000). Evolving perspectives on individual psychotherapy for schizophrenia. *Schizophrenia Bulletin*, *26*, 47–72.

Fenton, W. S., Blyler, C. R., & Heinssen, R. K. (1997). Determinants of medication compliance in schizophrenia: Empirical and clinical findings. *Schizophrenia Bulletin*, *23*, 637–651.

Fenton, W. S., & Cole, S. A. (1995). Psychosocial therapies of schizophrenia: individual, group and family. In G. O. Gabbard (Ed.), *Treatment of psychiatric disorders* (pp. 987–1018). Washington, DC: American Psychiatric Press.

Fenton, W. S., & McGlashan, T. H. (1999). Schizophrenia: Individual psychotherapy. In B. J. Sadock & V. Sadock (Eds.), *Kaplan and Sadock's comprehensive textbook of psychiatry* (pp. 1217–1231). Philadelphia: Lippincott Williams & Wilkins.

Forrest, D. V. (1994). Psychotherapy of patients with neuropsychiatric disorders. In S. Yudofsky & R. Hales (Eds.), *Synopsis of neuropsychiatry* (pp. 533–558). Washington, DC: American Psychiatric Press.

Fowler, D., Garety, P., & Kuipers, E. (1995). *Cognitive behavior therapy for psychosis*. Chichester, UK: Wiley.

Frank, A. F., & Gunderson, J. G. (1990). The role of the therapeutic alliance in the treatment of schizophrenia. *Archives of General Psychiatry, 47*, 228–236.

Frank, E., Kupfer, D. J., Perel, J. H., Cornes, C., Jarrett, D. B., Mallinger, A. G., Thase, M. E., McEachran, A. B., & Grochocisnki, V. J. (1990). Three-year outcomes for maintenance therapies in recurrent depression. *Archives of General Psychiatry, 47*, 1093–1099.

Gabbard, G. O. (1992). Psychodynamic psychiatry in the "decade of the brain." *American Journal of Psychiatry, 149*, 991–998.

Garety, P. A., Fowler, D., & Kuipers, E. (2000). Cognitive-behavioral therapy for medication-resistant symptoms. *Schizophrenia Bulletin, 26*, 73–86.

Garrett, H. E., & Woodworth, R. S. (1953). *Statistics in psychology and education* (p. ii). New York: Longmans, Green.

Gilbert, P., Harris, M., McAdams, L., & Jeste, D. (1995). Neuroleptic withdrawal in schizophrenic patients: A review of the literature. *Archives of General Psychiatry, 52*, 173–188.

Glass, L. L., Katz, H. M., Schnitzer, R. D., Knapp, P. H., Frank, A. F., & Gunderson, J. G. (1989). Psychotherapy of schizophrenia: An empirical investigation of the relationship of process to outcome. *American Journal of Psychiatry, 146*, 603–680.

Goldberg, S. C., Schooler, N. R., Hogarty, G. E., & Roper, M. (1977). Prediction of relapse in schizophrenic outpatients treated by drugs and social therapy. *Archives of General Psychiatry, 34*, 171–184.

Goldfried, M. R., & Davison, G. C. (1976). *Clinical behavior therapy*. New York: Holt, Rinehart & Winston.

Goldman, L. S. (1999). Medical illness in patients with schizophrenia. *Journal of Clinical Psychiatry, 60*(Suppl. 21), 5–10.

Gomes-Schwartz, B. (1984). Individual psychotherapy of schizophrenia. In A. Bellack (Ed.), *Schizophrenia: Treatment, management, and rehabilitation* (pp. 307–335). Orlando, FL: Grune & Stratton.

Greenough, W. T., & Black, J. E. (1992). Induction of brain structure by experience: Substrates for cognitive development. In M. R. Grunnar & C. A. Nelson (Eds.), *Developmental behavioral neuroscience* (pp. 155–200). Hillsdale, NJ: Erlbaum.

Grinspoon, L., Ewalt, J. R., & Shader, R. I. (1968). Psychotherapy and pharmacotherapy in chronic schizophrenia. *American Journal of Psychiatry, 124*, 1645–1652.

Grinspoon, L., Ewalt, J. R., & Shader, R. I. (1972). *Schizophrenia: Pharmacotherapy and psychotherapy*. Baltimore: Williams & Wilkins.

Gunderson, J. G., Frank, A. F., Katz, H. M., Vannicelli, M. L., Frisch, J. P., & Knapp, P. H. (1984). Effects of psychotherapy in schizophrenia: II. Comparative outcome of two forms of treatment. *Schizophrenia Bulletin*, *10*, 564–598.

Guy, W., Gross, M., & Hogarty, G. E. (1969). A controlled evaluation of day hospital effectiveness. *Archives of General Psychiatry*, *20*, 329–338.

Hafner, H., an der Heiden, W., Behrens, S., Gattaz, W. F., Hambrect, M., Loffler, W., Maurer, K., Munk-Jorgensen, P., Nowotny, B., Riecher-Rossler, A., & Stein, A. (1998). Causes and consequences of the gender difference in age at onset of schizophrenia. *Schizophrenia Bulletin*, *24*, 99–113.

Hansen, T. E., Casey, D. E., & Hoffman, W. F. (1997). Neuroleptic intolerance. *Schizophrenia Bulletin*, *23*, 567–582.

Hartwell, C. E. (1996). The schizophrenogenic mother concept in American psychiatry. *Psychiatry*, *59*, 274–297.

Hatfield, A. G. (1989). Patients' accounts of stress and coping in schizophrenia. *Hospital and Community Psychiatry*, *40*, 1141–1145.

Havassy, B. E., Shopshire, M. S., & Quigley, L. A. (2000). Effects of substance dependence on outcomes of patients in a randomized trial of two case management models. *Psychiatric Services*, *51*, 639–644.

Hawkins, R. C., Doell, S. R., Lindseth, P., Jeffers, V., & Skaggs, S. (1980). Anxiety reduction in hospitalized schizophrenics through thermal biofeedback and relaxation training. *Perceptual and Motor Skills*, *51*, 475–482.

Heinssen, R. K., Liberman, R. P., & Kopelowicz, A. (2000). Psychosocial skills training for schizophrenia: Lessons from the laboratory. *Schizophrenia Bulletin*, *26*, 21–46.

Henderson, D. C., Cagliero, E., Gray, C., Nasrallah, R. A., Hyden, D. L., Shoenfeld, D. A., & Goff, D. C. (2000). Clozapine, diabetes mellitus, weight gain, and lipid abnormalities: A five-year naturalistic study. *American Journal of Psychiatry*, *15*, 975–981.

Herz, M. I. (1985). Prodromal symptoms and prevention of relapse in schizophrenia. *Journal of Clinical Psychiatry*, *46*(Suppl.), 22–25.

Herz, M. I., Glazer, W., Mirza, M., Mostert, M., & Hafez, H. (1989). Treating prodromal episodes to prevent relapse in schizophrenia. *British Journal of Psychiatry*, *155*, 123–127.

Herz, M. I., Lamberti, J. S., Munetz, J., Scott, R., O'Dell, S. P., McCartan, L., & Nix, G. (2000). A program for relapse prevention in schizophrenia. *Archives of General Psychiatry*, *57*, 277–283.

Herz, M. I., & Melville, C. (1980). Relapse in schizophrenia. *American Journal of Psychiatry*, *137*, 801–805.

Hirsch, S. R., & Leff, J. P. (1975). *Abnormalities in the parents of schizophrenics*. London: Oxford University Press.

Hodel, B., & Brenner, H. D. (1994). Cognitive therapy with schizophrenic patients. *Acta Psychiatrica Scandinavica*, *90*, 108–115.

Hoffart, M. B., & Keene, E. P. (1998). The benefits of visualization. *American Journal of Nursing, 98,* 44–47.

Hogarty, G. E. (1984). Depot neuroleptics: The relevance of psychosocial factors. *Journal of Clinical Psychiatry, 45*(Sec. 2), 36–42.

Hogarty, G. E. (1985). Expressed emotion and schizophrenic relapse: Implications from the Pittsburgh study. In M. Alpert (Ed.), *Controversies in schizophrenia* (pp. 354–365). New York: Guilford Press.

Hogarty, G. E. (1989). Meta-analysis of the effects of practice with the chronically mentally ill: A critique and reappraisal of the literature. *Social Work, 43*(4), 363–373.

Hogarty, G. E. (1998). Efficacy vs. effectiveness in psychiatric research: Reply to Summerfelt and Meltzer. *Psychiatric Services, 49,* 834–835.

Hogarty, G. E., Anderson, C. M., Reiss, D. J., Kornblith, S. J., Greenwald, D. P., Javna, C. D., & Madonia, M. J. (1986). Family psychoeducation, social skills training, and maintenance chemotherapy in the aftercare treatment of schizophrenia: I. One-year effects of a controlled study on relapse and expressed emotion. *Archives of General Psychiatry, 43,* 633–642.

Hogarty, G. E., Anderson, C. M., Reiss, D. J., Kornblith, S. J., Greenwald, D. P., Ulrich, R. F., & Carter, M. (1991). Family psychoeducation, social skills training, and maintenance chemotherapy in the aftercare treatment of schizophrenia: II. Two-year effects of a controlled study on relapse and adjustment. *Archives of General Psychiatry, 48,* 340–347.

Hogarty, G. E., & Flesher, S. (1999a). Developmental theory for a cognitive enhancement therapy of schizophrenia. *Schizophrenia Bulletin, 25,* 677–692.

Hogarty, G. E., & Flesher, S. (1999b). Practice principles of cognitive enhancement therapy for schizophrenia. *Schizophrenia Bulletin, 25,* 693–708.

Hogarty, G. E., & Goldberg, S. C. (1973). Drug and sociotherapy in the aftercare of schizophrenic patients: One-year relapse rates. *Archives of General Psychiatry, 28,* 54–64.

Hogarty, G. E., Goldberg, S. C., & Schooler, N. R. (1974). Drug and sociotherapy in the aftercare of schizophrenic patients: III. Adjustment of nonrelapsed patients. *Archives of General Psychiatry, 31,* 797–805.

Hogarty, G. E., Goldberg, S. C., Schooler, N. R., & Ulrich, R. F. (1974). Drug and sociotherapy in the aftercare of schizophrenic patients: II. Two-year relapse rates. *Archives of General Psychiatry, 31,* 609–618.

Hogarty, G. E., Greenwald, D., Ulrich, R. F., Kornblith, S. J., DiBarry, A. L., Cooley, S., Carter, M., & Flesher, S. (1997). Three-year trials of personal therapy among schizophrenic patients living with or independent of family: II. Effects on adjustment of patients. *American Journal of Psychiatry, 154*(11), 1514–1524.

Hogarty, G. E., Kornblith, S. J., Greenwald, D., DiBarry, A. L., Cooley, S., Ulrich, R., Carter, M., & Flesher, S. (1997). Three-year trials of personal therapy among schizophrenic patients living with or independent of family:

I. Description of study and effects on relapse rates. *American Journal of Psychiatry*, *154*(11), 1504–1513.

Hogarty, G. E., Kornblith, S. F., Greenwald, D., DiBarry, A. L., Cooley, S., Flesher, S., Reiss, D., Carter, M., & Ulrich, R. (1995). Personal therapy: A disorder-relevant psychotherapy for schizophrenia. *Schizophrenia Bulletin*, *21*, 379–393.

Hogarty, G. E., McEvoy, J. P., Munetz, M., DiBarry, A. L., Bartone, P., Cather, R., Cooley, S. J., Ulrich, R. F., Carter, M., & Madonia, M. J. (1988). Dose of fluphenazine, familial expressed emotion, and outcome in schizophrenia: Results of a two-year controlled study. *Archives of General Psychiatry*, *45*, 797–805.

Hogarty, G. E., McEvoy, J. P., Ulrich, R. F., DiBarry, A. L., Bartone, P., Cooley, S. J., Hammill, K., Carter, M., Munetz, M. R., & Perel, J. (1995). Pharmacotherapy of impaired affect in recovering schizophrenia. *Archives of General Psychiatry*, *52*, 29–41.

Hogarty, G. E., Schooler, N. R., & Baker, R. W. (1997). Efficacy vs. effectiveness. *Psychiatric Services*, *48*, 1107.

Hogarty, G. E., Schooler, N. R., Ulrich, R. F., Mussare, F., Herron, E., & Ferro, P. (1979). Fluphenazine and social therapy in the aftercare of schizophrenic patients: Relapse analyses of a two-year controlled study of fluphenazine decanoate and fluphenazine hydrochloride. *Archives of General Psychiatry*, *36*, 1283–1294.

Hogarty, G. E., & Ulrich, R. F. (1977). Temporal effects of drug and placebo in delaying relapse in schizophrenic outpatients. *Archives of General Psychiatry*, *34*, 297–301.

Hogarty, G. E., & Ulrich, R. (1998). The limitations of antipsychotic medication on schizophrenia relapse and adjustment and the contributions of psychosocial treatment. *Journal of Psychiatric Research*, *32*, 243–250.

Hollis, F. (1964). *Casework: A psychosocial therapy*. New York: Random House.

Huskamp, H. A. (1998). How a managed behavioral health care carve-out plan affected spending for episodes of treatment. *Psychiatric Services*, *49*, 1559–1562.

Hyman, R. B., Feldman, H. R., Harris, R. F., Levin, R. F., & Malloy, G. B. (1989). The effects of relaxation training in clinical symptoms: A meta-analysis. *Nursing Research*, *38*, 216–220.

Johnson, D. A. W. (1981). Studies of depressive symptoms in schizophrenia: IV. A double-blind trial of nortriptyline for depression in chronic schizophrenia. *British Journal of Psychiatry*, *139*, 97–101.

Kabat-Zinn, J. (1990). *Full catastrophe living* (pp. 47–58). New York: Dell.

Kanas, N. (1986). Group therapy with schizophrenics. *International Journal of Group Psychotherapy*, *36*, 339–351.

Kane, J. M. (1996). Schizophrenia (drug therapy). *New England Journal of Medicine*, *333*, 34–41.

Kanter, J. (1989). Clinical case management: Definition, principles, components. *Hospital and Community Psychiatry*, *40*, 361–368.

Kapur, S., & Seeman, P. (2001). Does fast dissociation from the dopamine D$_2$ receptor explain the action of atypical antipsychotics?: A new hypothesis. *American Journal of Psychiatry*, *158*, 360–369.

Karon, B. P., & VandenBos, G. R. (1972). The consequence of psychotherapy for schizophrenic patients. *Psychotherapy: Theory, Research and Practice*, *9*, 111–119.

Kates, J., & Rockland, L. H. (1994). Supportive psychotherapy of the schizophrenic patient. *American Journal of Psychotherapy*, *48*, 543–561.

Katz, H. M., Frank, A., Gunderson, J. C., & Hamm, D. (1984). Psychotherapy of schizophrenia: What happens to treatment dropouts. *Journal of Nervous and Mental Disease*, *172*, 326–331.

Katz, M. M., & Warren, W. L. (1999). *Katz Adjustment Scales: Relative report form (KAS-R)*. Los Angeles: Western Psychological Services.

Kavanagh, D. J. (1992). Recent developments in expressed emotion and schizophrenia. *British Journal of Psychiatry*, *160*, 601–620.

Kazdin, A. E. (1983). Meta-analyses of psychotherapy: Criteria for selecting investigations. *Behavioral and Brain Sciences*, *6*, 296.

Keshavan, M. S., & Hogarty, G. E. (1999). Brain maturational processes and delayed onset in schizophrenia. *Development and Psychopathology*, *11*, 525–543.

Keshavan, M. S., & Murray, R. M. (Eds.). (1997). *Neurodevelopment and adult psychopathology*. Cambridge, UK: Cambridge University Press.

Knights, A., & Hirsch, S. R. (1981). "Revealed" depression and drug treatment for schizophrenia. *Archives of General Psychiatry*, *38*, 806–811.

Kraemer, H. C. (1991). To increase power in randomized clinical trials without increasing sample size. *Psychopharmacology Bulletin*, *27*, 217–225.

Kraemer, H. C. (2000). Statistical analyses to settle ethical issues? *Archives of General Psychiatry*, *57*, 327–328.

Kraemer, H. C., Yesavage, J. A., Taylor, J. L., & Kupfer, D. (2000). How can we learn about developmental processes from cross-sectional studies, or can we? *American Journal of Psychiatry*, *157*, 163–171.

Kramer, M. S., Vogel, W. H., DiJohnson, C., Dewer, D. A., Sheves, P., Cavicchia, S., Little, P., Schmidt, R., & Kimes, I. (1989). Antidepressants in "depressed" schizophrenic inpatients. *Archives of General Psychiatry*, *46*, 922–928.

Leff, J. P. (1981). The interaction of social and pharmacological treatments. In J. K. Wing, P. Kielholz, & W. M. Zinn (Eds.), *Rehabilitation of patients with schizophrenia and with depression* (pp. 137–148). Bern, Switzerland: Hans Huber.

Leff, J. P. (2001). Cultural influences in schizophrenia. In J. A. Lieberman & R. M. Murray (Eds.), *Comprehensive care of schizophrenia* (pp. 303–314). London: Dunitz.

Leff, J. P., Kuipers, L., Berkowitz, R., Eberlein-Vries, R., & Sturgeon, D. (1982). A controlled trial of social intervention in the families of schizophrenic patients. *British Journal of Psychiatry*, *141*, 121–134.

Leff, J. P., Kuipers, L., Berkowitz, R., & Sturgeon, D. (1985). A controlled trial of social intervention in the families of schizophrenic patients: Two-year follow-up. *British Journal of Psychiatry*, *146*, 594–600.

Leff, J. P., & Vaughn, C. E. (1985). *Expressed emotion in families*. New York: Guilford Press.

Lehman, A. F. (1995). Vocational rehabilitation in schizophrenia. *Schizophrenia Bulletin*, *21*, 645–656.

Lehman, A. F., Carpenter, W. T., Goldman, H., & Steinwachs, D. M. (1995). Treatment outcomes in schizophrenia: Implications for practice, policy and research. *Schizophrenia Bulletin*, *21*, 669–675.

Lehman, A. F., & Steinwachs, D. M. (1998). Patterns of usual care for schizophrenia: Initial results from the schizophrenia patient outcomes research team (PORT) client survey. *Schizophrenia Bulletin*, *24*, 11–20.

Leslie, D. L., & Rosenheck, R. (1999). Shifting to outpatient care?: Mental health care use and cost under private insurance. *American Journal of Psychiatry*, *156*, 1250–1257.

Liberman, R. P., DeRisi, W. J., & Mueser, K. T. (1989). *Social skills training for psychiatric patients*. New York: Pergamon Press.

Liberman, R. P., & Eckman, T. A. (1989). Dissemination of skills training modules to psychiatric facilities. *British Journal of Psychiatry*, *155*(Suppl. 5), 117–122..

Liberman, R. P., Wallace, C. J., Blackwell, G., Kopelowicz, A., Vaccaro, J. V., & Mintz, J. (1998). Skills training versus psychosocial occupational therapy for persons with persistent schizophrenia. *American Journal of Psychiatry*, *155*, 1087–1091.

Lieberman, J. A., Sheitman, B. B., & Kinon, B. J. (1997). Neurochemical sensitization in the pathophysiology of schizophrenia: Deficits and dysfunction in neuronal regulation and plasticity. *Neuropsychopharmacology*, *17*, 205–229.

Linn, M. W., Caffey, E. M., Klett, C. J., & Hogarty, G. E. (1977). Hospital vs community (foster) care for psychiatric patients: A Veterans Administration cooperative study. *Archives of General Psychiatry*, *34*, 78–83.

Linn, M. W., Caffey, E. M., Klett, C. J., Hogarty, G. E., & Lamb, R. (1979). Day treatment and psychotropic drugs in the aftercare of schizophrenic patients. *Archives of General Psychiatry*, *36*, 1055–1066.

Linn, M. W., Klett, C. J., & Caffey, E. M. (1980). Foster home characteristics and psychiatric patient outcome. *Archives of General Psychiatry*, *37*, 129–132.

Luborsky, L. (1996). Onset conditions for psychological and psychosomatic symptoms during psychotherapy: A new theory based on a unique data set. *American Journal of Psychiatry*, *153*(Suppl.), 11–23.

Mace, C., & Margison, F. (2000). Psychotherapy for psychosis. In H. Maxwell

(Ed.), *Clinical psychotherapy for health professionals* (pp. 114–123). London: Whurr.

Malm, U. (1982). The influence of group therapy on schizophrenia. *Acta Psychiatrica Scandinavica, 65*(Suppl. 297), 1–65.

Marder, S. R., Wirshing, W. C., Van Putten, T., Mintz, J., McKenzie, J., Johnston-Cronk, K., Lebell, M., & Liberman, R. P. (1994). Fluphenazine vs. placebo supplementation for prodromal signs of relapse in schizophrenia. *Archives of General Psychiatry, 51*, 280–287.

May, P. R. A. (1968). *Treatment of schizophrenia: A comparative study of five treatment methods.* New York: Science House.

May, P. R. A. (1975). Schizophrenia: evaluation of treatment methods. In A. M. Freedman, H. I. Kaplan, & B. J. Sadock (Eds.), *Comprehensive textbook of psychiatry* (pp. 955–981). Baltimore: Williams & Wilkins.

May, P. R. A., & Tuma, A. H. (1970). Methodologic problems in psychotherapy research. *British Journal of Psychiatry, 117*, 569–570.

McEvoy, J. P., & Freter, S. (1989). The dose–response relationship for memory impairment by anticholinergic drugs. *Comprehensive Psychiatry, 30*, 135–138.

McEvoy, J. P., Hogarty, G. E., & Steingard, S. (1991). Optimal dose of neuroleptic in acute schizophrenia: A controlled study of the neuroleptic threshold and higher haloperidol dose. *Archives of General Psychiatry, 48*, 739–745.

McEvoy, J. P., Howe, A., & Hogarty, G. E. (1984). Differences in the nature of relapse and subsequent inpatient course between medication-compliant and -noncompliant schizophrenic patients. *Journal of Nervous and Mental Disease, 172*, 412–416.

McEvoy, J. P., Scheifler, P. L., & Frances, A. (1999). The Expert Consensus Guideline Series: Treatment of schizophrenia. *Journal of Clinical Psychiatry, 60*(Suppl. 11), 1–80.

McEwen, B. S. (2000). Effects of adverse experiences for brain structure and function. *Biological Psychiatry, 48*, 721–731.

McGlashan, T. H. (1983). Intensive individual psychotherapy of schizophrenia. *Archives of General Psychiatry, 40*, 909–920.

McGlashan, T. H. (1984). The Chestnut Lodge follow-up study: II. Long-term outcome of schizophrenia and the affective disorders. *Archives of General Psychiatry, 41*, 486–601.

McGlashan, T. H. (1994). What has become of the psychotherapy of schizophrenia? *Acta Psychiatrica Scandinavica, 90*(Suppl. 384), 147–152.

McKay, M., Davis, M., & Fanney, P. (1981). *Thoughts and feelings: The art of cognitive stress intervention.* Richmond, CA: New Harbinger.

Meehl, P. E. (1973). Why I do not attend case conferences. In P. E. Meehl (Ed.), *Psychodiagnosis: Selected papers* (pp. 225–302). Minneapolis: University of Minnesota Press.

Meichenbaum, D., & Cameron, R. (1973). Training schizophrenics to talk to themselves: A means of developing attentional controls. *Behavior Therapy, 4*, 515–534.

Meichenbaum, D., & Cameron, R. (1974). The clinical potential of modifying what clients say to themselves. *Psychotherapy: Theory, Research and Practice, 11*, 103–117.

Meichenbaum, D., & Novaco, R. (1985). Stress inoculation: A preventative approach. *Issues in Mental Health Nursing, 7*, 419–435.

Miller, W. P., & Rollnick, S. (2002). *Motivational interviewing* (2nd ed.). New York: Guilford Press.

Miyashita, Y. (1995). How the brain creates imagery: Projection to primary visual cortex. *Science, 268*, 1719–1720.

Mojtabai, R., Nicholson, R. A., & Carpenter, B. N. (1998). Role of psychosocial treatments in management of schizophrenia: A meta-analytic review of controlled outcome studies. *Schizophrenia Bulletin, 24*, 569–587.

Morley, J. A. (1998). People matter: Client-reported interpersonal interaction and its impact on symptoms of schizophrenia. *Social Work, 43*, 437–444.

Morrison, E. (1992). *The city on the hill: A history of the Harrisburg State Hospital*. Harrisburg, PA: Triangle Press.

Mortimer, A., & McKenna, P. J. (1994). Levels of explanation: Symptoms, neuropsychological deficit and morphological abnormalities in schizophrenia. *Psychological Medicine, 24*, 541–555.

Mosher, L. R., & Menn, A. Z. (1978). Community residential treatment for schizophrenia: Two year follow-up. *Hospital and Community Psychiatry, 29*, 715–723.

Mueser, K. T., & Berenbaum, H. (1990). Psychodynamic treatment of schizophrenia: Is there a future? *Psychological Medicine, 20*, 253–262.

Mueser, K. T., Bond, G. R., Drake, R. E., & Resnick, S. G. (1998). Models of community care for severe mental illness: A review of research on case management. *Schizophrenia Bulletin, 24*, 37–74.

Mueser, K. T., Drake, R. E., & Noordsy, D. L. (1998). Integrated mental health and substance abuse treatment for serious psychiatric disorders. *Journal of Practical Psychiatry and Behavioral Health, 4*, 129–139.

Mueser, K. T., Yarnold, P. P., Rosenberg, S. D., Swelt, C., Miles, K. M., & Hill, D. (2000). Substance use disorder in hospitalized severely mentally ill psychotic patients. *Schizophrenia Bulletin, 26*, 179–192.

Naparstek, B. (1993). *General wellness*. New York: Time Warner Audio Books.

Narrow, W. E., Regier, D. A., Rae, D. S., Mandersheid, R. W., & Locke, B. Z. (1993). Use of services by persons with mental and addictive disorders. *Archives of General Psychiatry, 50*, 95–107.

Nemiah, J. (1984). Psychoanalysis and individual psychotherapy. In T. B. Karasu (Ed.), *The psychiatric therapies* (pp. 321–346). Washington, DC: American Psychiatric Association.

NIMH Consortium of Editors. (1999). Editorial statement. *Psychiatry*, *62*, 287–288.

Novacek, J., & Raskin, R. (1998). Recognition of warning signs: A consideration for cost-effective treatment of severe mental illness. *Psychiatric Services*, *49*, 376–378.

Novaco, R. W. (1976). The functions and regulation of the arousal of anger. *American Journal of Psychiatry*, *33*, 1124–1128.

Nuechterlein, K. H., & Dawson, M. E. (1984). A heuristic vulnerability/stress model of schizophrenic episodes. *Schizophrenia Bulletin*, *10*, 300–312.

Paul, G. L., Tobias, L. L., & Holly, B. L. (1972). Maintenance psychotropic drugs in the presence of active treatment programs. *Archives of General Psychiatry*, *27*, 106–115.

Pearsall, R., Glick, I. D., Pickar, D., Sujapes, T., Tausher, J., & Jobson, K. O. (1998). A new algorithm for treating schizophrenia. *Psychopharmacology Bulletin*, *34*, 349–354.

Persons, J. B., & Silberschatz, G. (1998). Are the results of randomized clinical trials useful to psychotherapists? *Journal of Consulting and Clinical Psychology*, *66*, 126–135.

Pies, R. W. (1998). *Handbook of essential psychopharmacology*. Washington, DC: American Psychiatric Press.

Pitschel-Walz, G., Leucht, S., Bauml, J., Kissling, W., & Engel, R. R. (2001). The effect of family intervention on relapse and rehospitalization in schizophrenia: A meta-analysis. *Schizophrenia Bulletin*, *27*, 73–92.

Richmond, M. E. (1917). *Social diagnosis*. New York: Russell Sage.

Rickard, H. C., Collier, J. B., McCoy, A. D., & Christ, D. A. (1993). Relaxation training for psychiatric inpatients. *Psychology Reports*, *72*, 1267–1274.

Robinson, D., Woerner, M. G., Alvin, J. M. J., Bilder, R., Goldman, R., Geesler, S., Koreen, A., Sheitman, B., Chakos, M., Mayerhoff, D., & Lieberman, J. A. (1999). Predictors of relapse following response from a first episode of schizophrenia or schizoaffective disorders. *Archives of General Psychiatry*, *56*, 241–247.

Rosenfarb, I. S., Nuechterlein, K. H., Goldstein, M. J., & Subotnik, K. L. (2000). Neurocognitive vulnerability, interpersonal criticism, and the emergence of unusual thinking by schizophrenic patients during family transactions. *Archives of General Psychiatry*, *57*, 1174–1179.

Rosenheck, R. A., Dausey, D. J., Frisman, L., & Kasprow, W. (2000). Outcomes after initial receipt of social security benefits among homeless veterans with mental illness. *Psychiatric Services*, *51*, 1549–1554.

Rosenheck, R., Tehell, J., Peters, J., Cramer, J., Fontana, A., Yu, W., Thomas, J., Henderson, W., & Charney, D. (1998). Does participation in psychosocial treatment augment the benefit of clozapine. *Archives of General Psychiatry*, *55*, 618–625.

Rubin, A., Cardenas, J., Warren, K., Pike, C. K., & Wambach, K. (1998). Outdated practitioner views about family culpability and severe mental disorder. *Social Work*, *43*, 412–422.

Sanger, T. M., Lieberman, J. A., Token, M., Grundy, S., Beasley, C., & Tollefson, G. D. (1999). Olanzapine versus haloperidol treatment of first-episode psychosis. *American Journal of Psychiatry*, *156*, 79–87.

Sarti, P., & Cournos, F. (1990). Medication and psychotherapy in the treatment of chronic schizophrenia. *Psychiatric Clinics of North America*, *13*, 215–228.

Schachter, S., & Singer, J. E. (1962). Cognitive, social and physiological determinants of emotional state. *Psychological Review*, *69*, 379–399.

Schafer, W. (1983). *Wellness through stress management*. Davis, CA: International Dialogue Press.

Schatzberg, A. F., Cole, J. O., & DeBallista, C. (1997). *Manual of clinical psychopharmacology* (3rd ed.). Washington, DC: American Psychiatric Press.

Schooler, N. R., & Hogarty, G. E. (1987). Medication and psychosocial strategies in the treatment of schizophrenia. In H. Y. Meltzer (Ed.), *Psychopharmacology: The third generation of progress* (pp. 1111–1119). New York: Raven Press.

Schooler, N. R., & Keith, S. J. (1993). The clinical research base for the treatment of schizophrenia. In *Health care reform for Americans with severe mental illness: Report of the National Advisory Mental Health Council* (pp. 2–30). Washington, DC: U.S. Government Printing Office.

Schooler, N. R., Keith, S. J., Severe, J. B., Matthews, S. M., Bellack, A. S., Glick, I. S., Hargreaves, W. A., Kane, J. M., Ninan, P. T., Frances, A., Jacobs, M., Lieberman, J. A., Mance, R., Simpson, G. M., & Woerner, M. G. (1997). Relapse and rehospitalization during maintenance treatment of schizophrenia: The effects of dose reduction and family treatment. *Archives of General Psychiatry*, *54*, 453–463.

Schooler, N. R., Levine, J., Severe, J. B., Brauzer, B., DiMascio, A., Klerman, G. L., & Tuason, V. B. (1980). Prevention of relapse in schizophrenia: An evaluation of fluphenazine decanoate. *Archives of General Psychiatry*, *37*, 16–24.

Scott, J. E., & Dixon, L. B. (1995). Psychological interventions for schizophrenia. *Schizophrenia Bulletin*, *21*, 621–630.

Searles, H. F. (1965). *Collected papers on schizophrenia and related subjects.* New York: International Universities Press.

Selye, H. (1974). *Stress without distress*. Philadelphia: Lippincott.

Selye, H. (1976). *The stress of life*. New York: McGraw-Hill.

Sharma, V., Whitney, D., Kazarian, S. S., & Manchanda, R. (2000). Preferred terms for users of mental health services among service providers and recipients. *Psychiatric Services*, *51*, 203–209.

Shatz, C. J. (1992, September). The developing brain. *Scientific American*, *267*, 60–67.

Simpson, G. M., Shih, J. C., Chen, K., Flowers, G., Kumazawa, T., & Spring, B. (1999). Schizophrenia, monoamine oxidase activity, and cigarette smoking. *Neuropsychopharmacology, 20,* 392–394.

Sippel, M. O., Tubesing, D., & Halpern (1982). *Relax—let go—relax.* Duluth, MN: Whole Person Associates.

Siris, S. G. (2000). Depression in schizophrenia: Perspective in the era of "atypical" antipsychotic agents. *American Journal of Psychiatry, 157,* 1379–1389.

Siris, S. G., Bermanzohn, P. C., Mason, S. E., & Shuwall, M. A. (1994). Maintenance imipramine therapy for secondary depression in schizophrenia: A controlled trial. *Archives of General Psychiatry, 51,* 109–115.

Spaulding, W. P., Reed, D., Sullivan, M., Richardson, C., & Weiler, M. (1999). Effects of cognitive treatment in psychiatric rehabilitation. *Schizophrenia Bulletin, 25,* 657–676.

Stellar, J. R., & Stellar, E. (1985). *The neurobiology of motivation and reward.* New York: Springer-Verlag.

Stone, M. H. (1986). Exploratory psychotherapy in schizophrenia-spectrum patients. *Bulletin of the Menninger Clinic, 50,* 287–306.

Strauss, J. S. (1989). Mediating processes in schizophrenia. *British Journal of Psychiatry, 155*(Suppl. 5), 22–28.

Stuart, H. L., & Arboleda-Florez, J. E. (2001). A public health perspective on violent offenses among persons with mental illness. *Psychiatric Services, 52,* 654–659.

Sullivan, E. V., Deshmukh, A., Desmond, J. E., Mathalon, D. H., Rosenbloom, M. J., Lim, K. O., & Pfferbaum, A. (2000). Contributions of alcohol abuse to cerebellar volume deficits in men with schizophrenia. *Archives of General Psychiatry, 57,* 894–902.

Sullivan, G., Wells, I. B., & Leake, B. (1992). Clinical factors associated with better quality of life in a seriously mentally ill population. *Hospital and Community Psychiatry, 43,* 794–798.

Sullwold, L., & Herrlich, J. (1992). Providing schizophrenic patients with a concept of illness: An essential element of therapy. *British Journal of Psychiatry, 161*(Suppl. 18), 129–132.

Suomi, S. J. (1997). Long-term effects of different early rearing experiences on social, emotional, and physiologic development in non-human primates. In M. S. Keshavan & R. M. Murry (Eds.), *Neurodevelopment and adult psychopathology* (pp. 104–116). Cambridge, UK: Cambridge University Press.

Takai, A., Ulmatsu, M., Kaiza, H., Inoue, M., & Ueki, H. (1990). Coping styles to basic disorders among schizophrenics. *Acta Psychiatrica Scandinavica, 82,* 289–294.

Tarrier, N., Barrowclough, C., Vaughn, C., Bamrak, J. S., Porceddu, K., Watts, S., & Freeman, H. (1989). Community management of schizophrenia: A two-year follow-up of a behavioural intervention with families. *British Journal of Psychiatry, 154,* 625–628.

Taubes, T. (1998). "Healthy avenues of the mind": Psychological theory building and the influence of religion during the era of moral treatment. *American Journal of Psychiatry, 155*, 1001–1008.

Taylor, E. H., & Cadet, J. L. (1989). Social intelligence: A neurological system? *Psychological Reports, 64*, 423–444.

Tessler, R. C., Bernstein, A. G., Rosen, B. M., & Goldman, H. H. (1982). The chronic mentally ill in community support systems. *Hospital and Community Psychiatry, 33*, 208–211.

van der Kolk, B. A., Pelcovitz, D., Roth, S., & Mandel, F. S. (1996). Dissociation, somatization and affect dysregulation: The complexity of adaptation to trauma. *American Journal of Psychiatry, 153*(Suppl.), 83–93.

Van Hassel, H. H., Bloom, J. J., & Gonzalez, A. M. (1982). Anxiety management with schizophrenic outpatients. *Journal of Clinical Psychology, 38*, 282–285.

Van Putten, T., & May, P. R. A. (1976). Milieu therapy of the schizophrenias. In L. J. West & D. E. Flinn (Eds.), *Treatment of schizophrenia: Progress and prospects* (pp. 217–243). New York: Grune & Stratton.

Vaughn, C. E., & Leff, J. P. (1976). The influence of family and social factors on the course of psychiatric illness. *British Journal of Psychiatry, 129*, 125–137.

Velligan, D. I., Bow-Thomas, L. C., Huntzinger, C., Ritch, J., Ledbetter, N., Prihoda, T. J., & Miller, A. L. (2000). Randomized controlled trial of the use of compensating strategies to enhance adaptive functioning in outpatients with schizophrenia. *American Journal of Psychiatry, 157*, 1317–1323.

Videka-Sherman, L. (1988). Meta-analysis of research on social work practice in mental health. *Social Work, 33*, 325–338.

Walsh, R. G., & Kelley, F. E. (1963). Short-term psychotherapy with schizophrenic patients evaluated over a 3–year follow-up period. *Journal of Nervous and Mental Disease, 137*, 349–352.

Warner, R. (1983). Recovery from schizophrenia in the Third World. *Psychiatry, 46*, 197–212.

Wasylenki, D. A. (1992). Psychotherapy of schizophrenia revisited. *Hospital and Community Psychiatry, 43*, 123–127.

Weiden, P., & Havens, L. (1994). Psychotherapeutic management techniques in the treatment of outpatients with schizophrenia. *Hospital and Community Psychiatry, 45*, 549–555.

Weinberger, D. R. (1987). Implications of normal brain development for the pathogenesis of schizophrenia. *Archives of General Psychiatry, 44*, 660–667.

Wing, J. K., & Brown, G. W. (1970). *Institutionalism and schizophrenia*. London: Cambridge University Press.

Winnicott, D. (1965). *The motivational process and the facilitating environment*. New York: International Universities Press.

Winston, A., Pinsker, H., & McCullough, L. (1986). A review of supportive psychotherapy. *Hospital and Community Psychiatry, 37*, 1105–114.

Witkin, S. L. (1998). The right to effective treatment and the effective treatment of rights: Rhetorical empiricism and the politics of research. *Social Work, 43,* 75–80.

Wyatt, R. J., & Henter, I. D. (1998). The effects of early and sustained intervention on the long-term morbidity of schizophrenia. *Journal of Psychiatric Research, 32,* 169–177.

Wykes, T. (2000). The rehabilitation of cognitive deficits. *Psychiatric Rehabilitation Skills, 4,* 234–248.

Young, A. S., Sullivan, G., Burnam, M. A., & Brock, R. H. (1998). Measuring quality of outpatient treatment for schizophrenia. *Archives of General Psychiatry, 55,* 611–617.

Zahourek, R. P. (1988). *Relaxation and imagery: Tools for therapeutic communication and intervention.* Philadelphia: Saunders.

Ziedonis, D. M., & Trudeau, K. (1997). Motivation to quit using substances among individuals with schizophrenia: Implications for a motivation-based treatment model. *Schizophrenia Bulletin, 23,* 227–238.

Zubin, J., & Spring, B. (1977). Vulnerability: A new view of schizophrenia. *Journal of Abnormal Psychology, 86,* 103–126.

Index